The Macrophage in Neoplasia

Edited by

MARY A. FINK

Division of Cancer Research Resources and Centers
National Cancer Institute

1976

ACADEMIC PRESS, INC. *New York San Francisco London*

A Subsidiary of Harcourt Brace Jovanovich, Publishers

ACADEMIC PRESS, INC.
111 Fifth Avenue, New York, New York 10003

United Kingdom Edition published by
ACADEMIC PRESS, INC. (LONDON) LTD.
24/28 Oval Road, London NW1

LIBRARY OF CONGRESS CATALOG CARD NUMBER: 76–44557

ISBN 0–12–256950–4

PRINTED IN THE UNITED STATES OF AMERICA

Contents

List of Participants

Dolph O. Adams, Department of Pathology, Duke University Medical Center, Durham, North Carolina 27710

D. Bernard Amos, Duke University Medical Center, Box 3010, Durham, North Carolina 27710

Rolf F. Barth, Department of Pathology and Oncology, University of Kansas Medical Center, Kansas City, Kansas 66103

Frances Cohen, Division of Cancer Research Resources and Centers, National Cancer Institute, National Institutes of Health, Westwood Building, Room 848, Bethesda, Maryland 20014

Stanley Cohen, Department of Pathology and Medicine, University of Connecticut Health Center, School of Medicine, 1280 Asylum Avenue, Farmington, Connecticut 06032

John R. David, Department of Medicine, Harvard Medical School, Boston, Massachusetts 02120

N. R. DiLuzio, Department of Physiology, Tulane University School of Medicine, New Orleans, Louisiana 70112

Harold F. Dvorak, Department of Pathology, Harvard Medical School, Massachusetts General Hospital, 32 Fruit Street, Boston, Massachusetts 02114

Robert Evans, Chester Beatty Research Institute, Belmont, Sutton, Surrey, England

I. J. Fidler, Basic Research Program, Frederick Cancer Research Center, Box B, Frederick, Maryland 20710

Mary A. Fink, Division of Cancer Research Resources and Centers, National Cancer Institute, National Institutes of Health, Westwood Building, Room 848, Bethesda, Maryland 20014

Richard K. Gershon, Department of Pathology, Yale University School of Medicine, 333 Cedar Street, New Haven, Connecticut 06510

David W. Golde, Division of Hematology and Oncology, Department of Medicine, U.C.L.A. Center for Health Sciences, Los Angeles, California 90024

M.G. Hanna, Jr., Basic Research Program, Frederick Cancer Research Center, P.O. Box B, Frederick, Maryland 21701

John B. Hibbs, Jr., Department of Medicine, Veterans Administration Hospital, Salt Lake City, Utah 84113

Ole A. Holtermann, Department of Dermatology, Roswell Park Memorial Institute, 666 Elm Street, Buffalo, New York 14205

Alan M. Kaplan, Department of Surgery, Medical College of Virginia, P.O. Box 756, Richmond, Virginia 23298

LIST OF PARTICIPANTS

R. Keller, Immunological Research Group, University Zurich, Schonleinstrasse 22, CH-8032, Zurich, Switzerland*

G. B. Mackaness, Trudeau Institute, Box 59, Saranac Lake, New York 12983

Peter W.A. Mansell, Department of Surgery, Royal Victoria Hospital, 687 Pine Avenue, Montreal 112, Canada

Keith L. McIvor, Department of Bacteriology, Washington State University, Pullman, Washington 99163

Monte S. Meltzer, Biology Branch, National Cancer Institute, National Institutes of Health, Building 37, Room 2C26, Bethesda, Maryland 20014

Luka Milas, Central Institute for Tumors, 41000 Zagreb, Yugoslavia

Malcolm S. Mitchell, Department of Internal Medicine, Section of Medical Oncology, Yale University School of Medicine, 333 Cedar Street, New Haven, Connecticut 06510

Carl F. Nathan, Immunology Branch, Division of Cancer Biology and Diagnosis, National Cancer Institute, National Institutes of Health, Building 10, Room 4B08, Bethesda, Maryland 20014

Benjamin W. Papermaster, Department of Biochemistry, University of Texas Medical Branch, 181 Shriners Burns Institute, Galveston, Texas 77550

William Regelson, Division of Medical Oncology, Medical College of Virginia/VCU, Box 273, Richmond, Virginia 23298

Stephen W. Russell, Department of Immunobiology, Scripps Clinic and Research Center, 476 Prospect Street, La Jolla, California 92037

Ralph Snyderman, Duke University Medical Center, Box 3892, Durham, North Carolina 27710

Osias Stutman, Sloan-Kettering Institute for Cancer Research, New York, New York 10021

Bruce S. Zwilling, Department of Microbiology, Ohio State University, Columbus, Ohio 43210

*R. Keller was invited to the workshop but was unable to attend. His paper was not presented at the workshop but has been included in this volume.

Preface

The macrophage has for years been in and out of vogue as a major participant in the host's immunity to malignant tumors. In recent years, the excitement attendant to evaluation of knowledge of T and B lymphocytes has tended to obscure the macrophage. For various reasons, many revealed in this volume, the macrophage has refused to be "put down." Several of the many faceted activities of this elegant cell are detailed on the following pages.

The need for this workshop was conceived at the time of a large national meeting when it became evident that macrophage workers had no forum for discussion of their current concepts. With the knowledgeable and enthusiastic collaboration of Dr. I. Fidler and Dr. N. DiLuzio a workshop was planned and held at the Marine Biological Laboratory, Woods Hole, Massachusetts October 8-11, 1975. This volume represents the written results of that effort.

The interest and advice of Dr. Thomas King, Director, Division of Cancer Research Resources and Centers, National Cancer Institute, the helpful editorial assistance of Ms. Frances Cohen, and the expert secretarial backup of Ms. Barbara Huffman are much appreciated.

Mary A. Fink

SESSION I

Role of Tumor Macrophages In Vivo

Chairman: William Regelson

ROLE OF MACROPHAGES IN HOST DEFENSE MECHANISMS

G. B. Mackaness

Instead of dealing with the role of macrophages in resistance to tumors, the theme here will be based upon some new findings in Dr. R. J. North's laboratory. This paper will begin by reconsidering the analogy between resistance to infectious disease and resistance to tumors; for it now seems that the parallel is even closer than envisaged in previous reviews (1,2,3), and fundamental to any concept of the host-tumor relationship.

INNATE RESISTANCE

Let us begin by noting that mononuclear phagocytes, in the apparent absence of aid from any acquired immunological mechanism, have four important qualities which equip them to serve as the effectors of a native form of immunity which is often called "innate resistance": they possess a primitive mechanism for distinguishing foreigness; are actively phagocytic; can destroy ingested material by a remarkable sequence of endocytic events (4); and may even to able to perform aggressive acts exocytically (5). The discriminatory capacity of macrophages is obviously not very highly developed; if it were, phagocytes would have little use for the antibodies which we know to be important in facilitating their capacity to distinguish between self and non-self. It seems to be sufficient, however, to allow at least the activated macrophage to recognize a difference between the surfaces of normal and transformed cells (6).

We must also note that there are at least two separate components to the monocyte-macrophage system of phagocytic cells: the fixed phagocytes, such as Kupffer cells and alveolar macrophages; and a mobile pool of monocytes which originate from rapidly replicationg precursors in bone marrow. Evans, Bowman and Winternitz (7) made the first attempt to determine the relative importance of these fixed and free phagocytes in resistance to infection. They hoped to measure the contributions made by monocytes and Kupffer cells to the formation of tubercles in the livers of tuberculous rabbits; but they could not settle the question with the simple labeling techniques available to them. However, with modern methods North (8) was able to show that the monocyte is by far the more important cell in expressing resistance to infection with *L. monocytogenes*. It seems, in fact, that the Kupffer cell functions mainly to scavenge the blood of parasites or other particulate material. Its very immobility precludes it from taking a more active part in any defensive operation. By contrast, circulating monocytes can be called to service in practically unlimited numbers and at virtually any location. Indeed, the concept of "cellular immunity" has to do, among other things, with the processes whereby monocytes are brought into effective contact with an immunological target.

As a rule, pathogenic organisms do not invade by routes that bring them into immediate contact with fixed phagocytes. But whether they do or not, they must be able to survive their first encounter with host phagocytes. This is well illustrated by an experimental infection of the lung (9). Here it is immediately apparent that only those organisms which escape a fatal interaction with resident alveolar macrophages have any chance of ever becoming established in the lung. It is almost certain, however, that microorganisms entering by other routes must also endure an early encounter with phagocytic cells. Even the least irritant of parasites, those which do not provoke the least semblance of an acute inflammatory response, are probably met at the portal of entry by immigrant monocytes. Even substances as bland as purified egg albumin cause these cells to accumulate at the site of inoculation (10).

It was apparent to Metchinkoff that phagocytic cells, even in the absence of specific immunity, have powerful antimicrobial properties. But his faith in cells was unbounded, for he also believed that acquired resistance was due to "the perfecting of the phagocytic and digestive properties of phagocytic cells". It is true that very few microorganisms can survive ingestion, either by polymorphonuclear leucocytes or mononuclear phagocytes. The post-phagocytic half-life of most pathogenic microorganisms can usually be reckoned in minutes. The role of phagocytic cells in innate resistance to infection thus depends upon three variables: rate of delivery of phagocytic cells to an infectious focus; rate of phagocytosis relative to the rate of parasite replication; and capacity of phagocytes to kill ingested organisms. So important is the distinction between parasites which can survive ingestion and those which cannot that Suter (11) divided infectious agents into three classes: obligate extracellular parasites, and facultative or obligate intracellular parasites. The latter can subsist only in an intracellular habitat. But even for them there is usually a strong statistical probability that they will not survive their first encounter with the host's native defenses. Just as it takes a certain threshold dose of tumor cells for successful transplantation, so too does it require at least one minimal infective dose to start an experimental infection. Even highly macrophage-adapted strains of *L. monocytogenes* (12) or *S. typhimurium* (13) lose more than half their numbers to the fixed phagocytes of the reticuloendothelial system within the first few hours of intravenous inoculation.

It now seems certain that tumor cells are subject to the same hazard. North's unpublished observations suggest (14,15,16) that the mouse possesses an innate defense mechanism which operates against both allogeneic and syngeneic tumor cells in the apparent absence of any known immunological mechanism. They also show that this mechanism of resistance is counteracted by the tumor itself, thus providing a means of escape from the body's innate defenses. This aggressive quality in tumor cells is analogous to the anti-phagocytic properties or the capacity to survive ingestion that characterize many infectious agents.

While studying the phenomenon of concomitant immunity North and his colleagues discovered that all of five unselected syngeneic tumors of mice caused a profound depression of natural resistance to infection (14). Within 12 hours of implanting 10^5 or 10^6 tumor cells subcutaneously in the foot, host resistance to intravenous challenge with a sublethal dose of *L. monocytogenes* was abolished. This organism, after an initial kill which eliminates a majority of the organisms implanted in spleen and liver, replicates in these organs until acquired immunity develops and the rate of destruction exceeds their rate of growth. In tumor bearing animals, the initial kill does not occur and acquired resistance does not develop. Even more extraordinary was the finding that animals which have recently recovered from a Listeria infection, and are already equipped with highly activated macrophages and everything else required to deal with this organism, lose most of their capacity to resist a challenge with the same organism if tumor cells are implanted in the foot at the time of reinfection.

This impairment of native and acquired resistance to an infectious agent was attributed to a factor which could be detected in serum within 12 hours of implanting tumor cells in the foot. As little as 0.03 ml of tumor bearing serum (drawn 24 hours after tumor implantation) caused the Listeria populations of the liver to rise tenfold higher in treated mice during the first 24 hours of infection. An infection with *Yerisinia enterocolitica* was similarly affected.

The inhibitor of host resistance is of low molecular weight. It is heat labile, but otherwise stable on storage. It is too potent in its effects to be a corticosteroid, and does not cause lymphoid atrophy as cortisone does in the doses needed to abolish antimicrobial resistance. It must act through its ability to interfere with the activities of mononuclear phagocytes, and circulating monocytes in particular, because these are the only cells that are directly involved in resistance to *L. monocytogenes*. Some indication of its mode of action was obtained by studying the mobilization of leucocytes into a peritoneal exudate. The presence of a tumor in the foot, or an injection of serum from a tumor bearing animal, caused a sharp reduction (as much as 80%) in the number of cells entering a casein-induced exudate. The inhibitory mechanism and the cell type most affected have not yet been determined; but in light of the information reported in papers by Snyderman and Meltzer in this volume, it seems certain that monocytes will be found to be the cells most affected.

However, inhibition may not be confined to monocytes, for it was found by Bernstein *et al.* (17) that migration of both monocytes and granulocytes into the peritoneal cavity was depressed despite increased production of both cell types in tumor bearing guinea pigs. Fauve *et al.* (18) have also reported that cultured tumor cells produce a low molecular weight factor which severely restricts the entry of polymorphonuclear leucocytes into an inflammatory exudate in rodents.

A factor which could interfere with the mobilization of blood-borne cells at the site of a tumor implant would conceivably bestow on tumor cells a period of grace which would allow them time to get established in an innately hostile environment. A tumor-promoting effect has in fact been demonstrated by North. A second tumor, implanted 3 days after the first, was found to grow at an accelerated pace. In keeping with its non-specific effect on antimicrobial resistance, the promoting factor was found to enhance the growth of tumor cells of a different antigenic specificity. Moreover, irradiated tumor cells had the same pro-infective and tumor-promoting effects, thus helping to explain the Révész (19) effect in which the admixing of irradiated cells reduces the threshold dose of tumor cells needed for a successful take.

It is highly significant that despite elaboration of a factor which interferes with resistance to infection, facilitates growth of a tumor and blocks the entry of cells into a peritoneal exudate, the tumor bearing host soon shows a reversal of these defects. They disappear with the advent of concomitant immunity which, once established, prevents further implantations of tumor cells even though the factor with tumor-promoting and pro-infective properties persists in the serum in almost undiminished concentrations. This seems to imply that specific, tumor-directed immunity may be powerful enough to overcome the tumor's inhibitory influence in innate resistance at a new implantation site, but not be strong enough to contend with excessive concentrations of an inhibitor within the primary tumor. The ability to express resistance in one location but not in another is also seen in infectious diseases. The phenomenon of infection-immunity or premunition is quite commonly encountered. Animals which can eradicate thousands of lethal doses of genetically marked bacteria may nonetheless succumb to their primary infections (13).

These findings are highly pertinent to the topic of the workshop because they suggest that there exists an innate mechanism of resistance to neoplasia which makes use of the same cell types that operate against microorganisms. They show, too, that if this non-immunological defense is once broached, only an *acquired* mechanism of resistance (specific immunity) can weight the balance in favor of the host. But unfortunately, even this may not be enough to deal definitively with a well established tumor, for even a thread of cotton may fail to provoke an inflammatory response within a tumor mass (20).

IMMUNOLOGICAL SURVEILLANCE

Immunological surveillance, as first expressed by Thomas (21) and elaborated by Burnet (22), is assumed to depend upon an immune response to specific antigens in the newly transformed cells. For such a mechanism to operate effectively, it would be necessary for tumor cells to appear rapidly and in sufficient numbers to produce a fully immunogenic stimulus. Anything less would result in an immune response too small to ensure an effective attack on the emerging tumor. Even in the case of microorganisms, which tend to be highly antigenic, it takes a relatively substantial antigenic stimulus to produce a measurable effect. In brucellosis, for example, the infection waxes and wanes (undulant fever) because the immunological stimulus from a declining bacterial population allows resistance to abate and permits the parasite to grow again until the antigenic stimulus is high enough to reactivate the host's defenses (23). If defense against an infectious agent demands such a strong antigenic stimulus, it seems unlikely that a transformed cell or two would provoke a protective immune response.

The existence of an innate defense against colonization of the tissues by neoplastic cells suggests a more plausible basis for the concept of immunological surveillance. As North suggests, it is easier to imagine a mechanism based on the ability of mononuclear phagocytes to discriminate between self and non-self (15). We already have simple reasons for believing that macrophages can recognize differences between normal and neoplastic cells (6). The fact that effete red blood cells are selectively removed from circulation also attests to the existence of phagocytic cells which can recognize topographical features on cell surfaces. Such differences may well be conspicuous enough to allow macrophages to discriminate between young and old, normal and neoplastic. One can imagine that if surface changes were expressed early enough in neoplastic transformation, they could be detected without any need to provoke a full-fledged immune response. If so, the elaboration of a factor which interferes with innate defenses would enable precancerous cells to go undetected until it was too late even for the onslaught of specific immunity to unseat them.

SPECIFIC IMMUNITY

Specific immunity, whether cell- or antibody-mediated, frequently functions through preexisting mechanisms. In fact, acquired immunity is often no more than an amplification of innate resistance. It is necessary, therefore, to describe how antibodies and activated T cells can enhance the functional performance of mononuclear phagocytes in defense against infectious agents as well as tumor cells.

About five ways can be visualized in which specific immunity can enhance the performance of mononuclear phagocytes: antibodies can improve the efficiency of interaction between target and phagocytic cells. This is true of both infectious agents and tumor cells. Monolayers of macrophages from immune animals can destroy allogeneic tumor cells *in vitro* (24,25). The reaction and its specificity appear to depend on cytophilic antibody (26,27). The phenomenon of antibody-mediated destruction of tumor cells by macrophages appears also to have been demonstrated *in vivo* (28,29). The alternative notion of a specific macrophage-arming factor (SMAF) of T cell origin has been proposed (30), but the interpretation of experiments purporting to show that macrophages can be rendered cytotoxic in this way is complicated by equally convincing evidence that macrophages activated by immunologically non-specific reactions can also kill tumor cells (31), and by the extreme difficulty of excluding specific antibodies from *in vitro* systems.

Apart from the capacity of antibodies to promote interaction between target cells and phagocytic cells, there are well known indications that activated T cells can influence the behavior of mononuclear phagocytes in even more helpful ways. In both viral (32) and bacterial infections (12) the attraction of mononuclear phagocytes to infectious centers is undoubtedly under the control of specifically reactive T cells. In both cases, mononuclear phagocytes are marshaled into the area of a target under the guidance of the lymphocytes which mediate delayed-type hypersensitivity (DTH) (33). The specific mediators of DTH are particularly well equipped to perform this function because they have a very pronounced tendency to enter inflamed tissues. But they can do so only while in the S phase of their mitotic cycle (34). This exudate-seeking quality befits the cell for its role in dictating the cellular composition of an inflammatory exudate. The presence of reactive T cells at any site containing specific antigen would be expected to result in the local release of lymphokines which can attract monocytes to the area and alter them in other functionally important ways.

This effect of specifically activated T cells on circulating monocytes is easy to demonstrate and quantify. Blood monocytes can be labeled with tritiated thymidine because their precursors in bone marrow are constantly dividing. The movement of labeled monocytes can thus be traced by radiometric and autoradiographic techniques. If animals with prelabeled monocytes are presented with a specific target (*L. monocytogenes*, for example), the difference in rate of accumulation of radioactive monocytes can be compared in the livers of normal and adoptively immunized subjects. In one study (35), more than five times as many radioactively labeled cells accumulated in the livers of adoptively sensitized mice. They could be found histologically as labeled cells located within the lesions of the adoptively sensitized mice. If monocytes could recognize abnormal features on neoplastic cells, and a mechanism as strong as this were available for assembling large numbers of them in a tumor bed, we would have the basic components for an effective defense against neoplasia. The phenomenon of concomitant immunity implies, however, that there are forces (presumably generated by the tumor) which militate against the successful operation of such a simple mechanism within the primary tumor. It is the aim of immunotherapy to overcome this impediment; but whether this can be done by creating bigger and better immune responses to tumor-specific antigens remains to be seen.

Promoting an influx of mononuclear phagocytes into a tumor is not the only contribution that cell-mediated immunity is capable of making to host defenses. Specifically sensitized T cells have also been credited with being able to activate macrophages. This is an important event in resistance to infection because many parasites can survive and multiply in normal, but not in activated, macrophages. Obviously, if an activated macrophage is also more efficient in its capacity to detect and destroy a transformed cell, the process of activation might be equally important in antitumor immunity. Other studies that will also be presented make it likely that immunologically activated macrophages do, in fact, display an augmented capacity to destroy tumor cells. If so, there is yet another parallel between anti-tumor and anti-microbial immunity.

There is another respect in which specific cell-mediated immunity can improve the functional capacity of the host's mononuclear phagocyte population. Infectious diseases which provoke a cellular defense mechanism cause a marked increase in the output of mononuclear phagocytes. Not only are the numbers of fixed phagocytes increased by vigorous division (36,37), but the supply of circulating monocytes is also enlarged during infection (38). Circulating monocyte levels are an unreliable index of their availability because the transit time may be much reduced in the presence of a strong demand for monocytes. However, a kinetic study by Bernstein *et al.* (17) has shown that in tumor bearing guinea pigs the rate of monocyte production is also increased.

In the course of many infections, and as a result of injecting immunopotentiating agents such as Freund's complete adjuvant, there is a substantial increase in the turnover of monocyte precursors in bone marrow. An increased output of monocytes would make them more abundantly available for a variety of purposes. This could explain, in part, the increased resistance to transplantable tumors that comes from non-specific stimulation of the reticuloendothelial system by agents such as BCG (39) or *C. parvum* (40). There are strong indications, however, that a non-specific antitumor effect also develops as a consequence of the *specific* immune response to the tumor. As in the case of infectious agents which activate the monocyte-macrophage system through immunological pathways (41), a measure of non-specific resistance also develops in tumor bearing mice. This could not be more clearly demonstrated than in North's studies which show that once the phase of negative resistance has passed (in 3–4 days), the tumor bearing mouse enters a phase of strongly increased resistance to a Listeria infection (15). The onset of increased antimicrobial resistance coincides with the appearance of concomitant, antitumor immunity.

Kearney and Nelson (42) have also detected a non-specific feature in concomitant immunity to syngeneic, carcinogen-induced tumors. At an early phase of the host's response (day 4), resistance was found to be specific and was vested in a cell with the characteristics of a T cell. But it was shown in an extension of these studies that this cell could not kill tumor cells *in vitro* without resistance from cells with the characteristics of macrophages (43). An amplifying effect of macrophages on resistance to tumors could also be detected by cell transfer studies *in vivo* (44). At a later stage of the response to these methylcholanthrene-induced tumors, when the non-specific component had become manifest, resistance was mediated in quite a different way. Though it was capable of expression against an unrelated tumor, the *development* of this form of resistance was also T-cell-dependent. Even so an enriched population of T cells was not cytotoxic, even in the presence of macrophages. The T cell dependence of this non-specific phase of antitumor immunity is reminiscent of the non-specific, macrophage-mediated resistance developed against microorganisms (41). Although the cell types involved in the non-specific resistance generated by a syngeneic tumor are still obscure, it is significant that the resistance generated against a tumor can be expressed against an infectious agent (15). This obviously tends to implicate the monocyte-macrophage system in antitumor immunity.

The experiments of Tevethia and Zarling (45) also provide inferential evidence for the direct involvement of macrophages in antitumor immunity. These authors showed that irradiated subjects cannot be immunized adoptively against SV40-transformed cells. However, the deficit could be rectified by bone marrow cells from a normal donor. In addition, protection was poor in adoptively immunized recipients which had been treated with silica, a specific macrophage toxin. These findings strike a close parallel with resistance to infection. In the case of anti-Listeria immunity specific T-cell-mediated resistance depends for its expression on macrophages. Here, too, irradiation of recipients interferes with adoptive immunization, and again the defect can be rectified by a graft of normal marrow (46). The same is true of delayed-type hypersensitivity (DTH). Irradiated animals can be adoptively sensitized with immune lymphoid cells only if they are given a bone marrow graft (47), or if peritoneal macrophages from normal donors are introduced directly into the test site (48).

It seems from this brief review that there is an almost perfect parallel between cell-mediated antimicrobial immunity and resistance to neoplasia. Since no one doubts the role of macrophages in antimicrobial immunity, why should we still be questioning their involvement in resistance to tumors. There are several reasons: phagocytosis, which is an essential step in antimicrobial immunity, is usually not a conspicuous feature of resistance to tumors; macrophages have an undoubted scavenging role, so that their presence in regressing tumors does not imply that they are playing an active part in the process; other cell types have been shown *in vitro* to be capable of killing tumor cells, so that an absolute requirement for macrophages would be difficult to prove. One might reasonably conclude, however, that the macrophage is well equipped to play an accessory role. Having regard to its more professional approach, its ability to distinguish self from non-self, its physiological make-up, its capacity to enlarge its numbers and undergo marked changes in form and function, it would be odd if the macrophage were not cast for a major role in resistance to neoplasia.

REFERENCES

1. Mackaness, G. B. and R. V. Blanden (1967). Cellular immunity. *Progr. Allergy 11*:89-140.

2. Nelson, D. S. (1972). Macrophages as effectors of cell-mediated immunity. *CRC Crit. Rev. Microbiol. 1*:353-384.

3. Nelson, D. S. (1974). Immunity to infection, allograft immunity and tumour immunity: Parallels and contrasts. *Transplant. Rev. 19*:226-254.

4. Cohn, Z. A. (1975). Macrophage physiology. *Fed. Proc. 34*:1725-1729.

5. Hibbs, J. B., Jr. (1974). Heterocytolysis by macrophages activated by bacillus Calmette-Guérin: Lysosome exocytosis into tumor cells. *Science 184*:468-471.

6. Hibbs, J. B., Jr. (1973). Macrophage nonimmunologic recognition: Target cell factors related to contact inhibition. *Science 180*:868-870.

7. Evans, H. M., F. B. Bowman and M. C. Winternitz (1914). An experimental study of the histogenesis of the miliary tubercle in vitally stained rabbits. *J. Exp. Med. 19*:283-302.

8. North, R. J. (1970). The relative importance of blood monocytes and fixed macrophages to the expression of cell-mediated immunity to infection. *J. Exp. Med. 132*:521-534.

9. Truitt, G. L. and G. B. Mackaness (1971). Cell-mediated resistance to aerogenic infection of the lung. *Am. Rev. Resp. Dis. 104*:829-843.

10. Goldman, A. S. and B. E. Walker (1962). The origin of the cells found in the infiltrates at the sites of foreign protein injection. *Lab. Invest. 11*:808-813.

11. Suter, E. (1956). Interaction between phagocytes and pathogenic microorganisms. *Bact. Rev. 20*:94-132.

12. North, R. J. (1974a). T cell dependence of macrophage activation and mobilization during infection with *Mycobacterium tuberculosis. Infect. Immun. 10*:66-71.

13. Mackaness, G. B., R. V. Blanden and F. M. Collins (1966). Host-parasite relations in mouse typhoid. *J. Exp. Med. 124*:573-583.

14. North, R. J., D. P. Kirstein and R. L. Tuttle. Subversion of host defenses by murine tumors. I. A. circulating factor that suppresses macrophage-mediated resistance to infection. In preparation.

15. North, R. J., D. P. Kirstein and R. L. Tuttle. Subversion of host defenses by murine tumors. II. The counter influence of concomitant immunity. In preparation.

16. North, R. J., D. P. Kirstein and R. L. Tuttle. Subversion of host defenses by murine tumors. III. A circulating factor that interferes withh movement of cells into inflammatory exudates. In preparation.

17. Bernstein, I. D., B. Zbar and J. J. Rapp (1972). Impaired inflammatory response in tumor-bearing guinea pigs. *J. Nat. Cancer Inst. 49*:1641-1647.

18. Fauve, R. M., B. Hevin, H. Jacob, J. A. Gaillard and F. Jacob (1974). Antiinflammatory effects of murine tumors. *Proc. Nat. Acad. Sci. 71*:4052-4056.

19. Révész, L. (1958). Effect of lethally damaged tumor cells upon the development of admixed viable cells. *J. Nat. Cancer Inst. 20*:1157-1186.

20. Mahoney, M. J. and J. Leighton (1962). The inflammatory response to a foreign body within transplantable tumors. *Cancer Res. 22:334-338.*

21. Thomas, L. (1959). *Cellular and Humoral Aspects of the Hypersensitive State.* H. S. Lawrence, Ed. Hoeber-Harper, New York.

22. Burnet, F. M. (1970). *Immunological Surveillance*. Pergamon, Sydney.

23. Mackaness, G. B. (1969). The influence of immunologically committed lymphocytes on macrophage activity *in vivo. J. Exp. Med. 129*:973-992.

24. Granger, G. A. and R. S. Weiser (1964). Homograft target cells: Specific destruction *in vitro* by contact interaction with immune macrophages. *Science 145*:1427-1429.

25. Lohmann-Matthes, M. L., H. Schipper and H. Fisher (1972). Macrophage-mediated cytotoxicity against allogeneic target cells *in vitro. Europ. J. Immol. 2*:45-49.

26. Granger, G. A., J. Rudin and R. S. Weiser (1966). The role of cytophilic antibody in immune macrophage-target cell interaction. *J. Reticulo. Soc. 3*:354.

27. Hoy, W. E. and D. S. Nelson (1969). Studies on cytophilic antibodies. V. Alloantibodies cytophilic for mouse macrophages. *Aust. J. Exp. Biol. Med. Sci. 47*:525-539.

28. Tsoi, M. S. and R. S. Weiser (1968). Mechanisms of immunity to sarcoma I allografts in the C_{57}B1/Ks mouse. III. The additive and synergistic actions of macrophages and immune serum. *J. Nat. Cancer Inst. 40*:23-30.

29. Shin, H. S., N. Kaliss, D. Borenstein and M. K. Gately (1972). Antibody mediated suppression of grafted lymphoma cells: II. Participation of macrophages. *J. Exp. Med. 136*:375-380.

30. Evans, R., C. K. Grant, H. Cox, K. Steele and P. Alexander (1972). Thymus-derived lymphocytes produce an immunologically specific macrophage-arming factor. *J. Exp. Med. 136*:1318-1322.

31. Hibbs, J. B., Jr., L. H. Lambert and J. S. Remington (1972). Possible roles of macrophage mediated nonspecific cytotoxicity in tumor resistance. *Nature (New Biol.) 235*:48-50.

32. Blanden, R. V. (1974). T cell response to viral and bacterial infection. *Transplant. Rev. 19*:56-88.

33. Mackaness, G. B. (1971). Delayed hypersensitivity and the mechanism of cellular resistance to infection. *Progress in Immol. 1*:413-424.

34. Hahn, H., T. E. Miller and G. B. Mackaness (1975). In preparation.

35. Mackaness, G. B. (1971). Cell-mediated immunity. *Cellular Interactions in the Immune Response*. S. Cohen, G. Cudkowicz and R. T. McCluskey, Eds. Karger, Basil.

36. North, R. J. (1969). The mitotic potential of fixed phagocytes in the liver as revealed during the development of cellular immunity. *J. Exp. Med. 130*:315-326.

37. North, R. J. and G. B. Mackaness (1973). Immunological control of macrophage proliferation *in vivo*. *Infect. Immun. 8*:68-73.

38. Volkman, A. and F. M. Collins (1974). The cytokinetics of monocytosis in acute salmonella infection in the rat. *J. Exp. Med. 139*:264-277.

39. Old, L. J., B. Benacerraf, D. A. Clarke, E. A. Carswell and E. Stockert (1961). The role of the reticuloendothelial system in the host response to neoplasia. *Cancer Res. 21*:1281-1300.

40. Scott, M. T. (1974). *Corynebacterium parvum* as an immunotherapeutic anticancer agent. *Sem. Oncol. 1*:367-378.

41. Mackaness, G. B. (1964). The immunological basis of acquired cellular resistance. *J. Exp. Med. 120*:105-120.

42. Kearney, R. and D. S. Nelson (1973). Concomitant immunity to syngeneic methylcholanthrene-induced tumours in mice. Occurrence and specificity of concomitant immunity. *Aust. J. Exp. Biol. Med. Sci. 51*:723-735.

43. Kearney, R., A. Basten and D. S. Nelson (1975). Cellular basis for the immune response to methylcholanthrene-induced tumor in mice. Heterogeneity of effector cells. *Int. J. Cancer 15*:438-450.

44. Simes, R. J., R. Kearney and D. S. Nelson (1975). Role of a noncommitted accessory cell in the *in vivo* suppression of a syngeneic tumour by immune lymphocytes. *Immunology 29*:343-351.

45. Tevethia, S. S. and J. M. Zarling (1972). Participation of macrophages in tumor immunity. *Nat. Cancer Inst. Monogr. 35*:279-282.

46. Hahn, H. (1975). Requirement for a bone marrow-derived component in the expression of cell-mediated antibacterial immunity. *J. Inf. Immun. 11*:949-954.

47. Lubaroff, D. M. and B. H. Waksman (1967). Delayed hypersensitivity bone marrow as the sources of cells in delayed skin reactions. *Science 157*:322-323.

48. Volkman, A. and F. M. Collins (1971). The restorative effect of peritoneal macrophages on delayed hypersensitivity following ionizing radiation. *Cell. Immol. 2*:552-566.

STUDIES ON THE HEMATOGENOUS DISSEMINATION OF TECHNETIUM–99m LABELED MALIGNANT CELLS[1]

Rolf F. Barth, M. D. and Om Singla

Department of Pathology and Oncology
University of Kansas Medical Center
College of Health Sciences and Hospital
Kansas City, Kansas 66103

Chromium-51 (1-4), ^{3}H-thymidine (5), ^{3}H-cytidine (6), I-125 iododeoxyuridine (4,7-9) and gallium-67 (10) have been employed as radioisotopic labels to study the hematogenous dissemination of malignant cells. Each of these radionuclides has disadvantages which limit its usefulness in experimental animals and none are ideally suited for clinical scintigraphic studies of tumor cell dissemination. ^{51}Cr (2,4), ^{3}H-TdR (11) and ^{67}Ga (10,12) elute from viable cells and are extensively reutilized. ^{125}I-IUDR, ^{3}H-TdR, and ^{3}H-CdR require DNA synthesis for incorporation thereby limiting their applicability to relatively rapidly dividing cells. The clinical usefulness of ^{51}Cr and ^{125}I-IUDR as cellular labels are further limited by their long half-life and low photon flux. Although ^{67}Ga has been employed clinically to demonstrate primary and metastatic tumors (13,14), its high rate of elution and rapid re-incorporation by non-malignant cells are serious limitations.

Technetium-99m (^{99m}Tc), a high specific activity metastable radioisotope, emitting a gamma photon with an energy of 140 keV, has rapidly become the most widely used radionuclide for diagnostic gamma imaging. Its short half-life, ($T_{1/2}$ = 6 hrs), high photon flux, favorable chemical properties and rapid excretion are significant advantages which have contributed to its usefulness as a scanning agent. We have developed a method for labeling nucleated cells with ^{99m}Tc (15,16) and have employed this radioisotope to

[1] Supported by grants CA 13190 and CA 16503, National Cancer Institute, National Institutes of Health.

study the distribution patterns of lymphoid cells in normal (17,18) and immunosuppressed mice (19) and in animals carrying skin allografts (20). The present report describes the applicability of ^{99m}Tc as a label to study the hematogenous dissemination of malignant cells and defines the advantages and limitations of this radioisotope for such studies.

MATERIALS AND METHODS

Tumors. The lymphocytic leukemia L1210 and the myeloid leukemia C1498 were propagated in ascitic form by serial passage in BDF_1 and C57BL/6 mice respectively. Sarcoma I and B16 melanoma were maintained *in vitro* in Nutrient Mixture F12 supplemented with 10% fetal calf serum, penicillin (100 μ/ml) and streptomycin (100 μg/ml), and periodically were passaged as subcutaneous tumors in A/J and C57BL/6 mice respectively. Tissue culture cells were disaggregated by treatment with 0.25% trypsin for 10 min at 37°C.

Labeling of tumor cells with ^{99m}Tc. Tumor cells were washed three times in Hanks Balanced Salt Solution (HBSS) and their concentration adjusted to 10^7 to 2×10^7/ml. Sodium pertechnetate ($Na^{99m}TcO_4$) was eluted from a molybdenum-technetium generator with 0.9% NaCl. Five millicuries of ^{99m}Tc were added to the cell suspension in 2 ml of HBSS and incubated for 10-15 min at 37°C. Following this the cells were sedimented by centrifugation at $400 \times g$ for 15 min and the unbound radioisotope was removed by washing them three times in HBSS. The labeled cells, having a viability of 88-98% as determined by trypan blue exclusion, were adjusted to a final concentration of 4×10^6/ml unless indicated otherwise. Previous studies had indicated that post reduction with stannous chloride in the presence of sodium chromate produced cell surface changes which resulted in a significant degree of pulmonary entrapment (18,19). For this reason, reduction with $SnCl_2$ was omitted in most of the experiments described herein. More recent data indicate that reduction in the absence of carrier Na_2CrO_4 does not significantly alter the distribution patterns of radiolabeled cells but does increase labeling efficiency ten-fold (16). In some experiments, therefore, the valence of ^{99m}Tc was reduced by the dropwise addition of 0.3 ml of a freshly prepared 0.2% solution of $SnCl_2$ dissolved in acid citrate dextrose (16). After an additional 15 min incubation at 37°C, the cells were sedimented, washed three times in HBSS and adjusted to their final concentration. In light of our most recent experience, it is recommended that post reduction with $SnCl_2$ be included in the labeling procedure.

Organ distribution experiments. Groups of 4 mice were injected via the lateral tail vein with 10^6 labeled cells suspended in 0.25 ml of HBSS, unless indicated otherwise. Animals were bled via the retro-orbital sinus immediately prior to killing by cervical dislocation, and thymus, brain, lymph nodes, heart, spleen, stomach, intestines, kidneys, liver, lungs, skin (1 cm in diameter), muscle ($\sim$ 0.5 gm), and 0.1 ml of blood were removed for gamma counting.

Gamma scintillation counting and decay corrections. ^{99m}Tc samples were counted in a Searle Analytic model 1185 gamma scintillation counter for 0.4 min. Decay follows the first order equation $A = A_o\, e^{-.693\frac{t}{T_{1/2}}}$ where A = the amount of radioactivity at time t, A_o = the amount at time t_o and $T_{1/2}$ = the half life of ^{99m}Tc (6 hrs). Accordingly, 11% of the total radioactivity would have decayed after 1 hour, 20% after 2 hours and 30% after 3 hours. Correction for decay was important in those experiments where results were expressed in terms of percent injected dose of radioactivity or where CPM were directly related to an equivalent number of cells. A computer program for this correction is available upon request. Decay could be remarkably compensated for by expressing the data as percent recoverable radioactivity. This was calculated by dividing the mean CPM of each organ by the total recoverable CPM and multiplying the quotient by 100.

RESULTS

Organ distribution of $Na^{99m}TcO_4$. In order to define the distribution of the free radionuclide, groups of four BALB/c mice were injected i.v. with 1 mCi of ^{99m}Tc-labeled sodium pertechnetate and killed after 10 min, 1, 4 and 24 hours. Urine and feces were collected whenever possible. Technetium-99m localized primarily in the stomach, intestines, blood and liver (Table 1). These organs accounted for 53% of the injected dose at 10 minutes, decreasing to 7% at 24 hrs. Urinary excretion of ^{99m}Tc increased from 12% of the injected dose at 1 hr to 66% at 24 hrs. The feces accounted for 3% of the injected dose at 4 hrs and 33% at 24 hrs. In contrast to the distribution of radiolabeled cells, the lungs had only 1% of the injected dose at 10 min and 0.03% at 24 hrs.

Organ distribution of ^{99m}Tc labeled leukemic cells. Groups of four BDF_1 mice were injected i.v. with 10^6 ^{99m}Tc labeled L1210 cells and killed after 10 min, 1, 4 and 24 hrs. Labeled cells were distributed primarily to the liver, lungs, stomach, intestines, kidneys and blood (Table 2). Except for the gastrointestinal tract, there was a gradual decline in the amount of radioactivity detected in each of these compartments as a function of time. The total percent recoverable radioactivity decreased from 74% of the injected dose at 10 min to 21% at 24 hrs. This decline may have been due to cell death and subsequent cytolysis and/or the elution of ^{99m}Tc from viable cells. Either of these events would result in an increased amount of radioactivity localized in the gastrointestinal tract since this is a major route by which ^{99m}Tc is excreted. The distribution pattern of intraperitoneally administered

TABLE 1.
Organ Distribution of ^{99m}Tc Labeled Sodium Pertechnetate

Organ[a]	Percent Injected Dose of Radioactivity			
	10 min	1 hour	4 hours	24 hours
Thymus	.22 ± .02	.13 ± .02	.04 ± .00	.00 ± .00
Muscle	1.45 ± .10	1.10 ± .09	.52 ± .04	.02 ± .00
Brain	.15 ± .00	.11 ± .00	.04 ± .00	.00 ± .00
Skin	.21 ± .03	.17 ± .05	.03 ± .00	.01 ± .00
Lymph nodes	.81 ± .05	1.59 ± .19	.39 ± .06	.04 ± .00
Heart	.63 ± .04	.31 ± .04	.09 ± .01	.01 ± .00
Spleen	.30 ± .05	.24 ± .03	.06 ± .00	.00 ± .00
Stomach	21.96 ± 2.97	31.70 ± 2.14	12.57 ± .32	2.59 ± .37
Intestine	7.29 ± .80	14.83 ± 2.16	25.28 ± 3.42	2.84 ± .72
Kidney	1.29 ± .08	.99 ± .09	.45 ± .02	.17 ± .01
Total blood	13.86 ± .73	10.17 ± 1.12	2.60 ± .34	.41 ± .05
Liver	10.21 ± .80	8.69 ± .40	4.19 ± .50	1.24 ± .03
Lung	1.40 ± .11	.89 ± .14	.28 ± .04	.03 ± .00
Urine	N.C.[b]	12.47 ± .00	21.56 ± .00	65.77 ± .00
Feces	N.C.	1.28 ± .00	3.43 ± .00	32.58 ± .00
Total Percent Recoverable Radioactivity	59.78	84.67	71.53	105.71

[a]BALB/c mice were injected intravenously with 1 m Ci of Na $^{99m}Tc\ 0_4$ and killed at the times indicated.

[b]N.C. indicates that none was collected.

L1210 was strikingly different from that observed with cells given i.v. (Table 3). The greatest amount of radioactivity was found in the GI tract and very small quantities were detected in the plasma suggesting that it was indeed cell-associated rather than cell-free. The lungs had 0.50% of the injected dose at 10 min compared to 37% in animals injected i.v. The liver had a maximum of 6% at 10 min compared to 16% for i.v. injected mice. The total recoverable radioactivity for i.v. compared to i.p. injected cells was greater at 1 hr (46% versus 32%) but very similar at 4 and 24 hrs.

The distribution of C1498 leukemic cells was studied in syngeneic C57BL/6 mice. Compartmentalization differed from that observed for L1210 in BDF_1 mice in that a large amount of radioactivity was detected in the GI tract and blood plasma within 10 min following injection suggesting that it was cell-free rather than cell-associated (Table 4). This most likely was due to the elution of the radioisotope from labeled cells, a problem which can be minimized if post reduction with $SnCl_2$ is carried out following labeling. Fewer numbers of cells initially localized in the lungs when compared to L1210, and a greater number were found with the cellular constituents of

TABLE 2.
Organ Distribution of Lymphocytic Leukemia L1210 in BDF_1 Mice

Organ[a]	Percent Injected Dose of Radioactivity			
	10 min	1 hour	4 hours	24 hours
Thymus	.22 ± .00	.06 ± .00	.02 ± .00	.03 ± .00
Muscle	.04 ± .00	.01 ± .00	.01 ± .00	N.D.[b]
Brain	.12 ± .00	.08 ± .00	.04 ± .00	.02 ± .00
Skin	.09 ± .00	.04 ± .00	.02 ± .00	N.D.
Lymph nodes	.30 ± .02	.06 ± .00	.06 ± .00	.04 ± .00
Heart	.37 ± .03	.21 ± .03	.14 ± .02	.03 ± .00
Spleen	.60 ± .03	.64 ± .02	.72 ± .09	.53 ± .02
Stomach	1.93 ± .07	3.06 ± .08	3.09 ± .13	.75 ± .01
Intestine	2.00 ± .08	3.02 ± .21	7.74 ± .45	2.97 ± .13
Kidney	2.74 ± .12	2.31 ± .14	1.82 ± .21	1.78 ± .07
Liver	16.37 ± .50	12.74 ± .90	12.20 ± .52	10.09 ± .06
Lung	36.91 ± 2.61	17.73 ± 1.04	7.72 ± .16	3.28 ± .03
Bone marrow	.48 ± .04	.46 ± .00	.36 ± .02	.38 ± .01
Blood cells	5.91 ± .00	3.29 ± .00	1.47 ± .00	.51 ± .00
Blood plasma	5.45 ± .00	2.63 ± .00	2.00 ± .00	.48 ± .00
Total Percent Recoverable Radioactivity	73.53	46.34	37.50	20.89

[a]BDF_1 mice were injected i.v. with 10^6 L1210 cells and killed at the times indicated.

[b]N.D. indicates that none was detected.

blood. The total recoverable radioactivity was greater with C1498 but still declined as a function of time suggesting the destruction of cells and/or the elution of radioisotope.

In another experiment mice were injected i.v. with 10^4, 10^5, or 10^6 cells and killed after 1 hr. Percent recoverable injected dose was 99% for 10^4 cells, 68% for 10^5 cells and 42% for 10^6 cells (Table 5).

The lungs and liver accounted for 74% of the injected radioactivity with 10^4 cells, 44% with 10^5 and 33% with 10^6 cells. Thymus, lymph nodes and spleen had 3.1% of the injected dose with 10^4 cells and this decreased to 0.85% with 10^6 cells suggesting that entrapment in the lymphoreticular system may be inversely related to the initial number of circulating tumor cells.

Organ distribution of ^{99m}Tc labeled solid tumor cells. Groups of four A/J mice were injected i.v. with 2.5 X 10^5 ^{99m}Tc labeled Sa I cells and killed after 10 min, 1, 4 and 24 hrs. The liver and lungs accounted for 69% of the injected dose of radioactivity at 10 min, 45% at 1 and 4 hrs, and 35% at 24 hrs (Table 6). The GI tract had 1% of the injected dose at 10 min and this increased to 4% at 24 hrs. In contrast to L1210 and C1498, very few

TABLE 3.
Organ Distribution of Lymphocytic Leukemia L1210 in BDF_1 Mice

Organ[a]	Percent Injected Dose of Radioactivity		
	1 hour	4 hours	24 hours
Thymus	.20 ± .01	.24 ± .01	.03 ± .00
Muscle	.03 ± .00	.01 ± .00	.02 ± .00
Brain	.04 ± .00	.09 ± .01	.02 ± .00
Skin	.01 ± .00	.03 ± .00	.02 ± .00
Lymph nodes	.05 ± .00	.03 ± .00	.03 ± .00
Heart	.13 ± .01	.07 ± .01	.07 ± .01
Spleen	.63 ± .05	.74 ± .04	.53 ± .02
Stomach	2.63 ± .12	5.75 ± .46	5.35 ± .46
Intestine	17.31 ± 1.26	22.39 ± .27	7.32 ± .70
Kidneys	2.58 ± .21	1.86 ± .05	.72 ± .10
Liver	5.52 ± .20	5.09 ± .35	1.67 ± .25
Lung	.50 ± .05	.24 ± .02	.10 ± .02
Bone marrow	.39 ± .01	.37 ± .01	.25 ± .03
Blood cells	.50 ± .00	.74 ± .00	.14 ± .00
Blood plasma	1.52 ± .00	.91 ± .00	.21 ± .00
Total Percent Recoverable Radioactivity	32.04	38.91	16.48

[a]BDF_1 mice were injected i.p. with 10^6 L1210 cells and killed at the times indicated.

TABLE 4.
Organ Distribution of Myeloid Leukemia C1498 in C57BL/6 Mice

Organ[a]	Percent Injected Dose of Radioactivity		
	10 min	1 hour	4 hours
Thymus	.21 ± .01	.17 ± .01	.12 ± .01
Muscle	.11 ± .00	.11 ± .00	.08 ± .01
Brain	.29 ± .01	.27 ± .01	.29 ± .02
Skin	.17 ± .01	.19 ± .04	.14 ± .01
Lymph nodes	.42 ± .02	.25 ± .03	.21 ± .02
Heart	.34 ± .01	.40 ± .06	.32 ± .02
Spleen	.75 ± .01	.87 ± .03	1.81 ± .14
Stomach	5.41 ± .17	5.77 ± .21	4.52 ± .15
Intestine	17.00 ± 1.78	6.56 ± .44	14.18 ± 1.01
Kidneys	2.91 ± .17	2.51 ± .17	2.24 ± .19
Liver	13.94 ± .20	13.37 ± .82	15.66 ± .84
Lung	16.71 ± .38	13.78 ± .75	3.03 ± .43
Bone marrow	1.41 ± .17	1.08 ± .03	.92 ± .03
Blood cells	15.62 ± .00	14.58 ± .00	11.08 ± .00
Blood plasma	7.18 ± .00	4.70 ± .00	.94 ± .00
Total Percent Recoverable Radioactivity	82.47	63.81	55.54

[a]C57BL/6 mice were injected i.v. with 10^6 C1498 cells and killed at the times indicated.

TABLE 5.
Organ Distribution of Myeloid Leukemia C1498 in C57BL/6 Mice

Organ[a]	Percent Injected Dose of Radioactivity		
	10^4	10^5	10^6
Thymus	.26 ± .02	.03 ± .00	.02 ± .00
Muscle	.11 ± .00	.02 ± .00	N.D.[b]
Brain	.29 ± .03	.07 ± .00	.03 ± .00
Skin	.17 ± .01	.03 ± .00	.01 ± .00
Lymph nodes	.33 ± .03	.06 ± .00	.03 ± .00
Heart	.49 ± .06	.19 ± .02	.08 ± .00
Spleen	2.52 ± .12	1.61 ± .04	.80 ± .05
Stomach	1.29 ± .11	.38 ± .05	.18 ± .08
Intestine	5.98 ± .31	3.50 ± .27	1.19 ± .05
Kidneys	5.15 ± .20	2.93 ± .12	1.49 ± .10
Liver	25.73 ± .74	16.02 ± 1.09	8.75 ± .48
Lung	48.44 ± .92	38.43 ± 1.71	24.18 ± .97
Bone marrow	1.00 ± .06	.40 ± .02	.15 ± .08
Blood cells	2.75 ± .00	2.26 ± .00	2.37 ± .00
Blood plasma	4.72 ± .00	2.49 ± .00	2.18 ± .00
Total Percent Recoverable Radioactivity	99.23	68.42	41.46

[a]C57BL/6 mice were injected i.v. with 10^3 to 10^6 cells and killed 1 hr later.
[b]N.D. indicates that none was detected.

radiolabeled cells initially were found in the blood but this increased to 4.8% of the total by 24 hrs. There was a marked increase in the amount of radioactivity localized in the thymus, lymph nodes and spleen between 4 and 24 hours (1.1% increasing to 5.1%), suggesting the transmigration of tumor cells to these lymphoid organs. Total recoverable radioactivity ranged from 72% at 10 min to 48% at 24 hrs.

The compartmentalization of B16 melanoma was studied in syngeneic C57BL/6 mice following the i.v. injection of 5 X 10^5 cells. The liver and lungs had approximately 80% of the injected radioactivity at 10 min and 1 hr, 59% at 4 hrs and 16% at 24 hrs (Table 7). Increased amounts were detected in the kidneys and blood when compared to Sa I. The blood alone accounted for 10% of the injected dose and 25% of the total recovered radioactivity at 24 hrs. Thymus, lymph nodes and spleen had 2% of the injected dose at 10 min and 5% at 24 hrs compared to 0.6% for L1210 and 2% for C1498 at this time.

DISCUSSION

The present series of experiments demonstrate that ^{99m}Tc can be used as a radioisotopic label to study the hematogenous dissemination of malignant cells. The *in vivo* localization of the free radionuclide was markedly different from that of radiolabeled cells thereby delineating cell-assòciated and cell-free

TABLE 6.
Organ Distribution of Sarcoma I in A/J Mice

Organ[a]	Percent Injected Dose of Radioactivity			
	10 min	1 hour	4 hours	24 hours
Thymus	.01 ± .00	.01 ± .00	.04 ± .00	.41 ± .02
Muscle	N.D.[b]	N.D.[b]	.04 ± .00	.17 ± .00
Brain	.03 ± .00	.02 ± .00	.12 ± .00	.19 ± .01
Skin	.01 ± .00	N.D.[b]	.08 ± .00	.47 ± .04
Lymph nodes	.03 ± .00	.03 ± .00	.12 ± .00	1.84 ± .06
Heart	.13 ± .00	.05 ± .00	.10 ± .00	.27 ± .01
Spleen	.07 ± .00	.16 ± .01	.27 ± .00	.75 ± .02
Stomach	.07 ± .00	.46 ± .02	.73 ± .03	1.10 ± .00
Intestine	.37 ± .02	.61 ± .00	1.27 ± .02	2.82 ± .16
Kidneys	.79 ± .03	1.39 ± .00	1.71 ± .05	.47 ± .04
Liver	6.71 ± .04	5.32 ± .16	6.62 ± .22	7.89 ± .19
Lung	62.47 ± 2.04	40.33 ± 1.58	38.68 ± 1.54	26.97 ± 3.42
Bone marrow	.09 ± .00	.08 ± .00	.27 ± .01	.27 ± .02
Blood	1.40 ± .05	2.36 ± .06	3.50 ± .08	4.84 ± .33
Total Percent Recoverable Radioactivity	72.18	50.82	53.55	48.46

[a]A/J mice were injected i.v. with 2.5×10^5 cells and killed at the times indicated.

[b]N.D. indicates that none was detected.

radioactivity from one another. Although ^{99m}Tc is not released from dead or injured cells (21), it is eluted in a non-reutilizable form from viable cells (21). The free radionuclide is rapidly excreted via the gut and kidneys and by 24 hrs over 98% has been eliminated. This is in contrast to ^{51}Cr, ^{3}H-TdR and ^{67}Ga which are extensively reutilized (2,4,6,10). Cellular uptake of ^{99m}Tc occurs rapidly by passive diffusion (22). DNA and protein synthesis are not significantly altered in ^{99m}Tc labeled cells (21) and the biophysical characteristics of the radionuclide are such that the energy deposition per cell is of insufficient magnitude to produce any significant radiation injury (22). Although gamma photons of 140 keV are the primary decay product, Auger electrons in the energy range of 0.4 to 20.2 keV are emitted thereby making ^{99m}Tc suitable for autoradiographic studies (23-25). The short half-life of ^{99m}Tc precludes its use in long term studies of cell migration but its high photon flux should permit gamma imaging to a degree unobtainable with other radionuclides currently used as cellular labels and suggests important clinical applications. Lymphocyte and granulocyte sequestration patterns, for example, could be studied in patients with leukemia, lymphomas and other malignancies. The hematogenous dissemination of malignant cells could be investigated in experimental animals by a non-invasive method which does not

TABLE 7.
Organ Distribution of B16 Melanoma in C57BL/6 Mice

Organ[a]	Percent Injected Dose of Radioactivity			
	10 min	1 hour	4 hours	24 hours
Thymus	.51 ± .02	.21 ± .00	.19 ± .00	1.55 ± .17
Muscle	.16 ± .00	.10 ± .00	.11 ± .00	.35 ± .06
Brain	.35 ± .00	.41 ± .00	.22 ± .01	.78 ± .07
Skin	.14 ± .00	.11 ± .00	.12 ± .00	N.D.[b]
Lymph nodes	.27 ± .00	.37 ± .00	.41 ± .01	1.73 ± .05
Heart	.39 ± .00	.58 ± .00	.39 ± .00	1.91 ± .14
Spleen	1.16 ± .06	1.76 ± .05	1.96 ± .05	1.60 ± .07
Stomach	1.30 ± .01	2.02 ± .09	3.35 ± .16	1.07 ± .05
Intestine	2.02 ± .06	3.11 ± .05	8.50 ± .68	1.53 ± .03
Kidneys	5.80 ± .08	6.98 ± .27	6.67 ± .19	2.08 ± .06
Liver	20.85 ± .63	27.30 ± .72	25.92 ± .42	5.61 ± .15
Lung	60.26 ± 1.60	50.49 ± 2.75	33.39 ± 2.11	10.13 ± .13
Bone marrow	.48 ± .01	.43 ± .03	.42 ± .00	.34 ± .06
Blood	6.25 ± .34	6.00 ± .52	5.86 ± .17	9.66 ± 1.38
Total Percent Recoverable Radioactivity	99.94	99.87	87.51	38.34

[a]C57BL/6 mice were injected i.v. with 5 × 10^5 B16 cells and killed at the times indicated.

[b]N.D. indicates that none was detected.

necessitate sacrificing the host in order to determine distribution patterns by gamma scintillation counting.

Data obtained in the present study confirm previous reports that the distribution patterns of lymphoreticular and solid tumor cells differ from one another (3,8,9,26,27). The data obtained with ^{99m}Tc indicate that either a high percentage of tumor cells has been destroyed within 24 hrs of intravenous injection and/or that there has been a significant degree of elution. With B16 melanoma, for example, 62% of the injected dose of radioactivity had been eliminated by this time. Since the free radionuclide distributes itself in a completely different pattern from that of labeled cells, is not reutilized, and is rapidly excreted, this suggests that the radioactivity was cell-associated rather than cell-free. These findings are similar to those reported with ^{125}I-IUDR labeled B16 melanoma (9), although the number of cells surviving as determined by gamma counting for ^{125}I was considerably less than that which we have observed with ^{99m}Tc.

Tumor cell arrest may be an important factor in determining the subsequent development of metastases (28-31). Recent studies with the B16 melanoma suggest that the arrest of hematogenous tumor cells is not an entirely non-specific process. Intravenously administered B16 cells disaggregated by treatment with EDTA gave rise almost exclusively to lung tumors while cells treated with 0.25% trypsin – 0.02% EDTA gave rise to both pulmonary and extrapulmonary tumors (32). Further support for the concept that unique cell properties are important factors in tumor cell arrest comes from recent findings that B16 variant cell lines which have a propensity to form pulmonary metastases also form heterotypic aggregates with normal cells which parallel their preferred site of organ implantation (33). The nature of this recognition mechanism remains to be determined but its elucidation should help us to understand why certain neoplasms have preferential patterns of metastasis formation. Although ^{99m}Tc still may not be the ideal label to study the arrest patterns of malignant cells, nevertheless, it has a number of advantages which suggest that it should be useful for this purpose.

SUMMARY

The present report describes the applicability of ^{99m}Tc as a label to study the hematogenous dissemination of malignant cells and defines the advantages and limitations of this radioisotope for such studies. The distribution patterns of the lymphocytic leukemia L1210, the myeloid leukemia C1498, Sarcoma I, and the B16 melanoma were studied in BDF_1 C57BL/6, A/J and C57BL/6 mice respectively. Labeled cells were distributed primarily to the liver and lungs with fewer numbers localized in the stomach, intestines, kidneys and blood. The distribution of free ^{99m}Tc was completely different from that of radiolabeled cells and by 24 hrs 98% had been excreted via the GI tract and kidneys. Animals given ^{99m}Tc labeled cells intravenously had retained from 16 to 56% of the injected dose of radioactivity at 24 hrs depending upon the type of tumor cell. These data suggest that either substantial numbers of tumor cells were killed within 24 hrs or alternatively that there was elution of ^{99m}Tc from viable radiolabeled cells. The low levels of radioactivity in the GI tract, kidneys and blood argue against the latter alternative, although it cannot be completely excluded at this time. The short half-life of ^{99m}Tc precludes its use in long-term studies of cell migration but its high photon flux should permit gamma imaging to a degree unobtainable with other radionuclides currently used as cellular labels and suggests important clinical applications.

REFERENCES

1. Selecki, E. E. (1959). A study of metastatic distribution of Ehrlich ascites tumour cells in mice. *Aust. J. Exp. Biol. Med. Sci. 37*:489-498.

2. Vincent, P. C. and A. Nicholls (1964). The fate of Cr^{51} labelled Ehrlich ascites tumour cells. *Aust. J. Exp. Biol. Med. Sci. 42*:569-578.

3. Fisher, B. and E. R. Fisher (1967). The organ distribution of disseminated ^{51}Cr-labeled tumor cells. *Cancer Res. 27*:412-420.

4. Hofer, K. G. and W. L. Hughes (1969). Evaluation of ^{51}Cr-chromate for studying migration and death of tumor cells *in vivo. Fed. Proc. 28*:749.

5. Fliedner, T. M., K. Bremer, F. Pretorius, B. Drücke, E. P. Cronkite and I. Fache (1968). Utilisation de la thymidine et de la cytidine tritiées pour l'etude du turnover et du métabolisme des lymphocytes chez l'homme. *Nouv. Rev. franc. Hemat. 8*:613-624.

6. Bremer, K., T. M. Fliedner and P. Schick (1973). Kinetic differences of autotransfused ^{3}H-Cytidine labeled blood lymphocytes in leukemic and non-leukemic lymphoma patients. *Europ. J. Cancer 9*:113-124.

7. Hofer, K. G., W. Prensky and W. L. Hughes (1968). The measurement of tumor cell death *in vivo* with iodine 125 labelled iododeoxyuridine. *J. Cell. Biol. 39*:62a.

8. Hofer, K. G., W. Prensky and W. L. Hughes (1969). Death and metastatic distribution of tumor cells in mice monitored with ^{125}I-iododeoxyuridine. *J. Natl. Cancer Inst. 43*:763-773.

9. Fidler, I. J. (1970). Metastasis: Quantitative analysis of distribution and fate of tumor emboli labeled with ^{125}I-5-iodo-2'deoxyuridine. *J. Natl. Cancer Inst. 45*:773-782.

10. Hofer, K. G. and D. C. Swartzendruber (1973). ^{67}Ga-citrate and ^{125}I-iododeoxyuridine as markers for *in vivo* evaluation of tumor cell metastasis and death. *J. Natl. Cancer Inst. 50*:1039-1045.

11. Dethlefsen, L. A. (1970). Reutilization of ^{131}I-5-iodo-2'-deoxyuridine as compared to ^{3}H-thymidine in mouse duodenum and mammary tumor. *J. Natl. Cancer Inst. 44*:827-840.

12. Glickson, J. D., R. B. Ryel, M. M. Bordenca, K. H. Kim and R. A. Gams (1973). *In vitro* binding of ^{67}Ga to L1210 cells. *Cancer Res. 33*:2706-2713.

13. Edwards, C. L. and R. L. Hayes (1970). Scanning malignant neoplasma with gallium-67. *JAMA 212*:1182-1190.

14. Higasi, T., Y. Nakayama, A. Murata, K. Nakamura, M. Sugiyama, T. Kawaguchi, and S. Suzuki (1972). Clinical evaluation of ^{67}Ga-citrate scanning. *J. Nucl. Med. 13*:196-201.

15. Barth, R. F., G. Y. Gillespie and A. Gobuty (1972). A new radioisotopic microcytotoxicity assay of cellular immunity utilizing technetium-99m. *NCI Monograph 35*:39-41.

16. Gillespie, G. Y., R. F. Barth and A. Gobuty (1973). Labeling of mammalian nucleated cells with ^{99m}Tc. *J. Nucl. Med. 14*:706-708.

17. Barth, R. F., O. Singla and G. Y. Gillespie (1974). Use of ^{99m}Tc as a radioisotopic label to study the migratory patterns of normal and neoplastic cells. *J. Nucl. Med. 15*:656-661.

18. Barth, R. F. and O. Singla (1975). Organ distribution of ^{99m}Tc- and ^{51}Cr-labeled thymocytes. *J. Nucl. Med. 16*:633-638.

19. Barth, R. F. and O. Singla (1975). Migratory patterns of technetium-99m-labeled lymphoid cells. I. Effects of antilymphocyte serum on the organ distribution of murine thymocytes. *Cell. Immunol. 17*:83-95.

20. Barth, R. F. and O. Singla (1975). Distribution of technetium-99m labeled lymphoid cells in allograft recipients. *Transplant. Proc. 7: Suppl. 1*:287-289.

21. Barth, R. F. and G. Y. Gillespie (1974). The use of technetium-99m as a radioisotopic label to assess cell mediated immunity *in vitro. Cell. Immunol. 10*:38-49.

22. Barth, R. F. and J. M. Pugh (1975). Manuscript in preparation.

23. Tilden, R. L., J. Jackson, Jr., W. F. Enneking, F. H. DeLand and J. T. McVey (1973). ^{99m}Tc-polyphosphate: Histological localization in human femurs by autoradiography. *J. Nucl. Med. 14*:576-578.

24. Dewanjee, M. K. (1974). Autoradiography of live and dead mammalian cells with ^{99m}Tc-tetracycline. *J. Nucl. Med. 16*:315-317.

25. Chaudhuri, T. K., T. C. Evans, and T. K. Chaudhuri (1973). Autoradiographic studies of distribution in the liver of ^{198}Au and ^{99m}Tc-sulfur colloids. *Radiology 109*:633-637.

26. Suemasu, K., M. Katagiri, Y. Shimosato, M. Mikuni and S. Ishikawa (1970). Initial stage of hematogenous metastasis of ^{51}Cr-labeled tumor cells. *GANN 61*:7-15.

27. Boranić, M., M. Radacić, and J. Gabrilovac (1974). Distribution and spread of ^{51}Cr-labeled leukemia cells in mice. *Exp. Hemat. 2*:51-57.

28. Greene, H. S. N. and E. K. Harvey (1964). The relationship between the dissemination of tumor cells and the distribution of metastases. *Cancer Res. 24*:799-811.

29. Fisher, E. R. and B. Fisher (1965). Experimental study of factors influencing development of hepatic metastases from circulating tumor cells. *Acta Cytologica 9*:146-159.

30. Takahashi, T., Y. Okamoto, and R. Nakamura (1973). Influence of vascular permeability on blood-borne metastasis. *GANN 64*:1-5.

31. Liotta, L. A., J. Kleinerman, and G. M. Saidel (1974). Quantitative relationships of intravascular tumor cells, tumor vessels, and pulmonary metastases following tumor implantation. *Cancer Res. 34*:997-1004.

32. Hagmar, B. and K. Norrby (1973). Influence of cultivation, trypsinization and aggregation on the transplantability of melanoma B16 cells. *Int. J. Cancer 11*:663-675.

33. Nicolson, G. L. and J. L. Winkelhake (1975). Organ specificity of blood-borne tumour metastasis determined by cell adhesion? *Nature 255*:230-232.

TUMOR MACROPHAGES IN HOST IMMUNITY TO MALIGNANCIES*

Robert Evans

Department of Tumor Immunology
Chester Beatty Research Institute
Institute of Cancer Research
Clifton Avenue, Belmont,
Sutton, Surrey, SM2 5PX.

Many experimentally induced animal tumors evoke a specific antitumor response in the syngeneic host. This response is presumably stimulated by and directed against tumor specific transplantation antigens (TSTAs) and may be manifested as humoral antibodies and cytotoxic mononuclear cells. A variety of effector mechanisms has been detected by *in vitro* techniques, although these appear to be only of potential relevance *in vivo* since they clearly do not operate optimally, the tumor ultimately overwhelming the syngeneic host.

Several investigators (1,5) have observed that during the growth of syngeneic animal tumors infiltration of mononuclear cells occurs, and this presentation will describe certain consequences of this infiltration, which may be a direct measure of the immune response mounted by the host, as well as being responsible perhaps for the first line of defense against metastatic spread. In particular, the possible involvement of macrophages associated with growing tumors in prevention of metastatic spread will be discussed, and also their presence during regression of tumors following azathioprine therapy.

Macrophage Content of Tumors

Tumor-associated macrophages have been detected in various species such as mouse, rat, hamster and man (1,7). The number of macrophages may vary greatly from one tumor type to another. In mouse and rat fibrosarcomas, for example, the level was reported to vary from 2 – 65% (3). Similar findings have been reported for some human tumors (6). In animal models, the level of macrophages found in a given transplantable tumor is fairly constant during the progressive growth of the tumor and from one animal passage to the next. Changes in content may be seen over long periods, the level tending to fall the

*This research was supported by grants from the Medical Research Council and the British Cancer Campaign.

TABLE 1.*
Tumors Tested for Macrophage Content

Tumor[a]	Passage Nos. Tested	Mean Percentage of Macrophages
Mouse		
FS1 (C57B1)	3,5,9,12,16, 13,24,26,29	33 (25-52)
FS6 (C57B1)	3,4,5,6,7	45 (30-54)
FS9 (CBA)	10,10	20 (21,19)
Rat		
A (hooded)	3,4,5,5,6	53 (38-65)
MC1 (hooded)[b]	6,8,9,12,15 15,17,17	33 (24-42)
HSG (hooded)	87	9
HSH (hooded)	47	11
HSN (hooded)	11,17,18,19, 20,22,24	46 (38-62)
MC3 (hooded)[b]	11,12,13	4 (2-6)
Primary 1 (hooded)	–	55
Primary 2 (hooded)	–	45
Primary 3 (hooded)	–	33

[a]Tumors were excised not earlier than 9 days after implantation of trocar piece.

[b]Tumors induced by methylcholanthrene. All other tumors were induced by benzpyrene.

*From Evans (3).

more the tumor is passaged. There seems to be no doubt that the macrophages are of host origin since injection into the syngeneic host of tumor cells freed of macrophages by treatment with anti-macrophage serum and complement or by prolonged growth in culture gives tumors which have a level of macrophages similar to that seen in the routinely transplanted material (3). Whether the progressive increase in numbers of macrophages within the tumor is due to a steady influx of peripheral blood monocytes or to division of a few or many macrophages *in situ* has not been satisfactorily explored. There is some evidence that macrophage precusors occur in the tumor mass, as judged by the ability of isolated cells to divide *in vitro* (4). The experiments reported by Eccles and Alexander (8) on inflammation and delayed type hypersensitivity reactions in tumor bearing rats strongly suggested that circulating monocytes were sequestered by growing tumors, supporting the notion that a steady influx of monocytes occurs. This aspect will be cursorily explored later in this paper.

Relationship between tumor macrophages, immunogenicity and metastasis.

There is circumstantial evidence to suggest that the level of macrophages found in a particular tumor type may be related to the ability of that tumor to provoke an immune response, which in turn may determine the rate or frequency of tumor metastasis. Preliminary experiments (Evans and Rudenstam – unpublished data) indicated that the longer a tumor was maintained in the syngeneic host by regular transplantation, the lower did its macrophage content become and the more readily did the tumor metastasize. Thus it was found that a methylcholanthrene induced sarcoma, syngeneic for Wistar rats, had a high macrophage content of about 50% at passage 2 and there was very little evidence for metastatic spread. However, when passages 17 and 35 were tested, the macrophage content had decreased to about 5% and metastasis to the lung occurred in all animals. These findings were confirmed and extended by Eccles and Alexander (9). Electron microscopic studies by Birbeck and Carter (1) in a hamster tumor model system, revealed that a non-metastasizing tumor contained large stimulated macrophages with long insinuating processes, while the metastasizing line of tumor contained fewer macrophages, which were small and non-stimulated. Their findings, together with those of Carr and McGinty (10) who observed that large numbers of mature macrophages were found in the draining node of a non-metastasizing tumor bearing host, with very few in the metastasizing tumor bearing host, further support the suggestion that the macrophage content of a tumor and its capacity to metastasize may be related. Immunosuppression by continuous thoracic duct drainage significantly reduced the level of tumor macrophages (9) suggesting that macrophage levels are related to the potency of immune response to the tumor and in particular to the lymphoid arm of the immune response.

As mentioned above the possibility exists that the presence of large numbers of macrophages within a growing tumor is the result of sequestration of circulating monocytes, a process which appears to affect other cell-mediated types of immune response. For example, rats bearing tumors with high macrophage counts tended to lose the capacity to respond both to peritoneal irritation and to a second exposure of antigen (delayed type hypersensitivity reactions) much more quickly than rats bearing tumors with a low macrophage content (8). The latter group in time also lost the capacity to respond presumably because of the stronger attraction of the increasing tumor mass for a greater number of monocytes, which for unknown reasons appear to move preferentially to the tumor site rather than to other sites of reactivity. There was little doubt that the lack of DTH reactions was due to macrophage depletion since injection of peritoneal macrophages into the site restored reactivity, whereas injection of thoracic duct lymphocytes did not.

The relationship between immunogenicity and metastatic spread may be expressed as the incidence of tumors which appear at distant sites following surgical removal of the primary tumor, the implication being that highly immunogenic tumors induce potent defense mechanisms which either prevent dissemination from the localized tumor or kill the released tumor cells during their circulation or at their final resting place. However, a recent report by Eccles and Alexander (11) indicates that this issue may not be that straightforward. In a series of experiments on a tumor which was considered to be highly immunogenic it was shown that if rats were immunosuppressed by x-irradiation or T-cell depletion after surgical removal of the primary tumor there was a high incidence of metastases compared with non-suppressed controls. One interpretation of these results is that metastatic spread had indeed occurred before removal of the primary but a T-cell dependent mechanism prevented growth of the disseminated cells, which remained dormant until immunosuppressive treatment was given. Whether this T-cell dependency is a direct T-cell effect on tumor cells or an indirect effect such as cooperation with macrophages to give growth inhibitory effector cells, as described in other systems (12,13), remains to be investigated. Whether the macrophage content of these tumors appearing at distant sites was similar to or less than that of the primary tumor was not reported but would be of interest to ascertain.

Tumor Macrophage Cytotoxicity

A. Direct Cytotoxicity

This refers to the ability of tumor macrophages to kill or inhibit growth of tumor cells *in vitro* without the addition of specific antibody or agents known to render macrophages cytotoxic. Monolayers of tumor macrophages can be readily isolated from solid tumors as described fully elsewhere (3,14). Monolayers in culture dishes are usually maintained in serum free medium for 24-48 hours to eliminate contaminating tumor cells which usually require serum for adhesion and survival in the initial stages of cultivation. After 24 hours the monolayers are ready for use in a cytotoxic assay system. The cells comprising the monolayers consist of 98-100% cells with the characteristic features of macrophages. They are glass adherent, resistant to detachment by trypsinization, lysed by antimacrophage serum and complement, and have Fc receptors as measured by EA rosettes and phagocytosis of opsinized sheep red blood cells. They do not appear to synthesize DNA under these cultural conditions, as determined by ^{125}IUdR incorporation (37), and they can be maintained in the absence of serum for at least 10 days as long as the culture medium is renewed every 24-48 hours.

Cytotoxicity can be expressed either as growth inhibition or lysis depending on the circumstances (see ref. 15 for definition of cytotoxicity).

Macrophages from a number of different mouse and rat tumor types have been tested for this ability to inhibit growth of or to kill both lymphoma and sarcoma cells in culture in a totally non-specific manner. Such macrophages are termed activated macrophages (16). As shown previously (15,17) tumor macrophages exhibit varying degrees of cytotoxicity depending on the tumor from which the macrophages are isolated. For example, two rat fibrosarcomas, the HSN and ASBPl, syngeneic for hooded and August strains respectively, yielded extremely destructive macrophages, while the mouse FS6 and rat HSBPA fibrosarcomas yielded macrophages whose growth inhibitory capacity could only be detected if used on the same day they were isolated from the tumor. If they were maintained for 24-48 hours before use, cytotoxicity had usually disappeared. When growth inhibition was detectable in such cultures the effect was so weak that the process was reversible and the tumor cells recovered the ability to divide. The reasons for the strong cytotoxicity associated with some tumors and weak with others are not known. The FS6 tumor does not appear to metastasize in C57 Black mice, and of the rat sarcomas tested the HSBPA metastasizes least of all (11). Both of these tumors at the present time have the highest tumor macrophage content of their respective species. Could this low degree or absence of metastatic spread be related to a potent macrophage cytotoxic reaction, which may be dissipated fairly rapidly following the *in vivo* interaction with tumor cells? During isolation and cultivation of these tumor macrophages *in vitro* this "run-down" is completed within 24-48 hours by which the time tumor cells are able to grow at their normal rate on the macrophage monolayers. This explanation would necessarily imply that because the HSN and ASBPl tumors metastasize more readily the tumor macrophages do not exert a strong cytotoxic effect *in vivo*. However, the HSN and ASBPl tumor macrophages both lose their *in vitro* cytotoxic capacity within 3 to 5 days, and after this time they will support growth of all tumor cells tested. Indeed, growth of cells was stimulated by these "aged" macrophages (see macrophage supernatants below).

There are many reports demonstrating that cytotoxic peritoneal macrophages differentiate between tumor cells and non-tumorigenic cell types (18-24) such as embryonic and non-transformed cells. Exceptions to this are reports by (a) Jones *et al.* (25) who showed that adjuvant-induced cytotoxic peritoneal macrophages lysed syngeneic embryo cells, as measured by the release of ^{51}Cr. These authors commented that other investigators not using isotopic-release assays might have missed small but significant amounts of lysis, especially if arbitrary visual assessment of overall damage was used as a measure of cytotoxicity; (b) Gallily (26) was demonstrated by ^{86}Rb uptake destruction of normal peritoneal macrophages by alloimmune macrophages.

We have shown that tumor macrophage monolayers will inhibit growth of and destroy a transformed line of hamster cells but will not affect the growth of the non-transformed counterparts (unpublished data). They also inhibited growth to varying degrees of both C57 Black mouse embryo and FS6 fibrosarcoma cells (Table 2) but over a period of 3 days only the tumor cells were destroyed. The embryo cells remained intact. Whether selective destruction of some embryo cells occurred under these conditions was not tested. Moreover, the embryo cells became less susceptible to growth inhibition by tumor macrophages the longer they were passaged in culture. C57Black embryo cells, passage 1 and 4, were added to tumor macrophage monolayers and the extent of growth inhibition was assayed at 3 days. It is seen in Table 3 that growth inhibition of passage 1 cells occurred but not of passage 4. Since DNA synthesis was only reduced in the susceptible passage 1 cultures and not totally arrested these results suggest that there may be a certain amount of selectivity by the macrophages for some cell types amongst the embryo cells. These cells in time may either disappear or lose those features which the cytotoxic macrophages recognize as different from normal.

The mechanism of macrophage cytotoxicity is far from being understood. Most investigators agree that cell to cell contact is required, although the possible involvement of toxic supernatant factors needs clarification (see below). Hibbs (27) has claimed that the mechanism of action of BCG activated peritoneal macrophages is associated with the transfer of lysosomes to the tumor cells. Inhibition of lysosomal enzymes with trypan blue abrogated the cytotoxic effect, though not the physical transfer. Several attempts using a wide range of trypan blue concentrations (10^{-2} to 10^{-6}M) have been made to block cytotoxicity by this method but in no instance was trypan blue found to abrogate or reduce cytotoxicity. Table 4 shows that at

TABLE 2.
Effect of Tumor Macrophages (TM) on Growth of C57 Black Tumor Cells and Embryo Cells*

Cultures	Total Cell Counts ($\times 10^5$)		^{125}IUdR Incorporation** γ CPM	
Day	1	3	1	3
TM + embryo cells	0.6 ± 0.1	1.1 ± 0.2	687 ± 163	2035 ± 217
Embryo cells alone	0.9 ± 0.2	2.8 ± 0.1	1979 ± 361	3986 ± 392
TM + FS6 cells	0.4 ± 0.1	<0.1	809 ± 93	<500
FS6 cells alone	0.9 ± 0.3	3.9 ± 0.2	2360 ± 111	7536 ± 821

*HSN tumor macrophages 2×10^6 per 3 cm culture dish, maintained for 24 hours in serum-free medium before challenge with 5×10^4 cells in 3 mls RPM1 + 10% fbs.

**Method of Boyle and Ormerod (37) used throughout this presentation to estimate the extent of DNA synthesis. Target cells were incubated for 4 hrs in the presence of 0.1 μCi ^{125}IUdR/ml.

TABLE 3.
Effect on HSN Tumor Macrophages on Growth of and ^{125}IUdR Incorporation by Early and Late Passage Mouse Embryo Cells

Cultures*	Total Cell Counts (X 10^5) on Day 3	γ CPM
TM + Passage 1 embryo cells	1.2 ± 0.3	1987 ± 206
Passage 1 embryo cells alone	3.3 ± 0.1	3935 ± 613
TM + Passage 4 embryo cells	3.5 ± 0.2	4768 ± 962
Passage 4 embryo cells alone	3.3 ± 0.2	4583 ± 623

*5 X 10^4 cells in 3 ml RPM1 + 10% fbs added to each dish. Results from minimum of 5 dishes per sample.

the dose reported by Hibbs, tumor macrophages still reduced uptake of ^{125}IUdR. This was accompanied by a reduction in cell numbers and finally death of target cells. The trypan blue was not toxic directly to the tumor cells when these were incubated with the various dilutions of the vital stain (data not shown).

The mechanism by which either peritoneal or tumor macrophages acquire cytotoxicity *in vivo* has not been adequately explored. Specific immunization of mice yields immune peritoneal macrophages which are rendered non-specifically cytotoxic by contact with the specific antigen (16). Whether cytotoxic macrophages from BCG or *Corynebacterium parvum*–injected mice arise by this pathway is a possibility. It is also possible that bacterial cell products, endotoxin, peptidoglycan may render macrophages cytotoxic *in vivo* (28). Induction of cytotoxicity *in vivo* by reagents such as pyran copolymer

TABLE 4.
Effect of Trypan Blue on the HSN Tumor Macrophage Cytotoxicity*

Culture	γ CPM at 48 Hrs
TM + SL2 cells	801 ± 126
TM + Trypan blue + SL2 cells	639 ± 245
SL2 cells alone	56,809 ± 3,261
TM + HSN cells	926 ± 101
TM + Trypan blue + HSN cells	899 ± 176
HSN cells alone	9,724 ± 1,007

*2 mls of growth medium containing 4.2 X 10^{-4} M trypan blue (Hopkins and Williams Ltd., England) incubated with macrophages for 18 hours followed by washing of monolayers and challenging with 10^5 SL2 cells or 5 X 10^4 HSN cells.

(21) or double stranded RNA (28) appears to occur by an indirect pathway especially since cytotoxic macrophages do not appear until several days after administration of the compound.

B. Indirect Macrophage Cytotoxicity

The transformation of an immune or armed macrophage into a non-specific, growth inhibitory effector cell after contact with specific antigen (16) presupposes the formation of an immune complex on the macrophage surface. Whether this complex is antigen-antibody or antigen-T cell factor (i.e. perhaps a non-immunoglobulin (29)) has yet to be determined. Nevertheless an immunologically specific interaction occurs and leads to activation. A number of cell types (so-called K cells) are known to become specifically cytotoxic on contact with immune complexes, the reaction depending on binding of the target cell-antibody complex to Fc receptors on the effector cells. The cytotoxic reaction is specific and is mediated by immunoglobulin of the IgG class. It is usual to use a lytic assay system but the choice of assay should be dependent on the type of target cell, and whether the assay is used primarily to detect a cytotoxic effect or to demonstrate the presence of antibody. For example, when macrophages are the effectors both lysis and growth inhibition may be detected using a variety of tumor cells as targets (15,31). Tumor macrophages that had lost their cytotoxicity by maintenance *in vitro* were shown to lyse lymphoma cells as measured by ^{125}I-release in the presence of specific allo-antiserum up to a dilution of 10^{-3} to 10^{-4}. Lysis was detected at a ratio of 2.5 macrophages:1 tumor cell. When growth inhibition was measured by the reduction in ^{125}IUdR incorporation antibody could be detected at a dilution of 10^{-6}. The class of antibody responsible was IgG in both cases. Thus as a means of detecting the presence of antibody growth inhibition was at least 100x more sensitive than lysis. Phagocytosis, although seen at low serum dilutions, was not responsible for most of the lysis that occurred within 8 hours. Phagocytosed cells released their ^{125}I only after overnight incubation. Both lysis and growth inhibition were immunologically specific, although after the reaction was initiated macrophages were able to inhibit growth of tumor cells quite non-specifically. Whether other categories of effector cells participating in antibody-dependent cytotoxicity become non-specifically growth inhibitory has not been reported as far as we are aware, and this seems to be the major difference between macrophages and other types of killer (K) cells.

The implications of indirect macrophage cytotoxicity is that macrophage cytotoxicity *in vivo* may depend on such reactions in which antibody directed against TSTAs combines either with the macrophages or monocytes (i.e. arming) or with circulating TSTAs, the complex then binding to the Fc receptors. Since, as suggested above, the potency of the immune response may determine the number of macrophages found associated with growing tumors, the level of circulating or tumor associated cytotoxic macrophages and their cytotoxic capacity might be expected to vary according to the amount of antibody, antigen or immune complex found at any particular phase of tumor growth. Whether excess antigen blocks cytotoxicity as has been suggested for lymphocyte cytotoxicity in the tumor bearing host (32) has yet to be resolved.

Macrophage Culture Supernatants

The ability of macrophage supernatants to induce lysis (33-36), growth inhibition (37,38) or growth stimulation of cells (39) in culture has been the subject of much debate in recent years, mainly because of the difficulty in reproducing such findings from one laboratory to the next. Not only do strains of a particular species vary but also target cells, culture media, culture vessels and methods of assay. Lysis should not be difficult to detect since either a cell disintegrates or it does not. Growth inhibition, however, is variously assayed including cell counting or incorporation of tritiated thymidine or ^{125}IUdR. The use of such isotopically labelled compounds has its problems in that incorporation into DNA is affected if competitive inhibitors occur in the culture supernatants (40,41). Thus for consistent results we find that it is necessary to remove the culture supernatants or wash the target cells before they are exposed to these labels. Without such precautions the apparent failure of cells to incorporate the label in the presence of various supernatants may bear little or no relationship to the true state of DNA synthesis. Growth stimulation by macrophage supernatants is of great interest in that they may enhance or support lymphocyte functions such as stimulation by lectins (42), stimulate proliferation of spleen and thymus lymphocytes or enable spleen cells from nude athymic mice to make plaque forming cells to sheep red blood cells, that is in the absence of T cells (39).

Tumor macrophages, cytotoxic or not, do not appear to synthesize or release lytic or growth inhibitory materials, but they do produce a supernatant activity which stimulates growth of cells. This effect is best seen by adding tumor macrophage supernatants to depleted culture medium in which normal or tumor cells divide only slowly, as measured by cell counts and ^{125}IUdR incorporation. In the presence of complete growth medium, the effect of the supernatant activity is minimal since the cells are dividing at almost maximal rate. Table 5 shows that the cells maintained in culture medium consisting of RPMI + medium 199 (1:1 v/v) and 10% fetal bovine serum (fbs) divide much more slowly than the same cells maintained in RPMI and tumor macrophage supernatant. These incorporate much higher levels of ^{125}IUdR. Medium 199 + 10% fbs itself is not a good growth promoting medium for these cells (not shown). However, normal cells and the tumor cells grow well in this

TABLE 5.
Stimulation of DNA Synthesis by Tumor Macrophage Supernatant

Cultures	Macrophage Supernatant*	γ CPM at 24 Hours
Untransformed	–	1,236 ± 210
Hamster cells	+	10,589 ± 876
Transformed	–	5,336 ± 766
Hamster cells	+	25,329 ± 1,293
SL2 cells	–	11,836 ± 731
	+	27,109 ± 2,382

*Culture medium consisted of RPM1 + 199 (v/v 1:1) + 10% fbs or RPM1 + Conditioned medium from HSN tumor macrophage cultures maintained for 24 hours in serum-free medium 199.

conditioned medium 199 when fetal calf serum is added. The effect of lymphocyte proliferation has yet to be clarified. The stimulating activity is lost if the supernatant is diluted beyond ¼. It does not appear to bind to cells during stimulation of growth suggesting a medium conditioning effect rather than a direct mitogenic effect. Since the activity is present in supernatants of cytotoxic tumor macrophage cultures, cytotoxicity must therefore override the stimulatory activity on the target cell. Table 6 shows an experiment in which a tumor macrophage supernatant prepared in medium 199 was mixed with RPMl containing 10^5 SL2 cells and added to cytotoxic tumor macrophage monolayers.

It is seen that in the absence of macrophages the conditioned medium stimulated growth but on the macrophage monolayers growth inhibition was not affected by its presence.

The synthetic capability of the macrophage is enormous and because of the complexity of culture supernatants in terms of "factors" extreme caution is warranted in the interpretation of data and in making generalizations concerning mechanisms of action of cytotoxic macrophages. Whether growth inhibition or lysis is dependent on cell to cell contact, as most investigators seem to suggest, or mediated by a soluble factor which may be labile and acts only in the vicinity of the contact between macrophage and target cell, as indicated in experiments measuring red cell lysis by macrophages (43) can only be verified by appropriate experimentation. Perhaps one should also consider the possibility that macrophages may not produce lytic or growth inhibitory factors directly but modify or break down components of the culture medium. On this basis, differences in culture medium and serum might explain why some investigators are able to detect such factors while others cannot.

TABLE 6.
The Effect of Tumor Macrophage Supernatant on the Reduction of ^{125}IUdR Incorporation by Lymphoma Cells on HSN Tumor Macrophage Monolayers

Cultures	Supernatant*	γ CPM at 24 Hours
TM + SL2 cells	–	2,106 ± 338
	+	1,985 ± 527
SL2 cells alone	–	10,367 ± 1,761
	+	25,001 ± 2,653

*Culture medium consisted of RPM1 + 199 (v/v 1:1) + 10% fbs or RPM1 + Conditioned medium from HSN tumor macrophage cultures maintained for 24 hours in serum-free medium 199.

Tumor Macrophages During Rejection by Chemotherapy.

The ability of macrophages (or monocytes) to infiltrate growing tumors is of potential value in either immunotherapy or chemotherapy. The major problems would seem to be 1) rendering the macrophages cytotoxic to such a degree that they retain the capacity to destroy while they find their way to the tumor and 2) facilitating migration into the tumor mass.

Agents such as B.C.G. or *C. parvum* may induce either infiltration or division of macrophages, particularly after intralesional injection of tumors, and are known to stimulate the appearance of cytotoxic peritoneal macrophages (18,44). Similarly, compounds such an endotoxin, lipid A, double-stranded RNA (45), pyran copolymer (46) may also induce regressions, as well as stimulate the appearance of cytotoxic peritoneal macrophages. Clinically, intralesional or subcutaneous administration of compounds such as glucan may result in tumor regressions, and on the basis of histological sections it was suggested that macrophages were the main agents responsible for regression (7).

In preliminary experiments we have investigated the changes in cellular composition of a murine fibrosarcoma after azathroprine therapy by both trypsin-dispersal of tumors and histological section. This compound related to the purine analogue 6-mercaptopurine (6-MP) is a known immunosuppressive agent having a direct effect on dividing cells, induces regression of some tumors (47) and at appropriate concentrations in mice will deplete the circulation of monocytes (48). C57Black mice were injected s.c. or i.m. in different experiments with 10^6 syngeneic FS6 fibrosarcoma cells. This dose gives a 100% take and produces a tumor 1 cm in diameter by 10 days, at which time mice received up to 8 daily intraperitoneal doses of azathioprine suspended in saline (150 mg per kilogm. in 0.1 ml); controls received saline. The antitumor effect was noticeable by the 5th day after the beginning of treatment and within 14 days tumors had completely regressed. These mice subsequently were resistant to challenge with 10^6 FS6 tumor cells. Assessment of macrophage content at intervals indicated that the percentage remained fairly constant, perhaps rising slightly after discontinuation of azathioprine treatment. Since the tumor was decreasing in size this constant level indicated that there was no increase and probably a decrease in macrophage numbers during or after therapy. Tumor cells decreased in numbers and looked extremely granular following dissociation of the tumors with trypsin. It was noticeable that as the tumor decreased in size, there was an increase in the percentage of small round, non-adherent cells, probably lymphocytes though their identity has not yet been established. In control tumors, the percentage of these small cells never exceeded 15% of the total but during regression the percentage increased to 40-55%. This probably indicates that as the tumor decreased in size the absolute number of small cells remained fairly constant. There was no direct evidence for an actual infiltration of cells.

The macrophages isolated from the tumor of the azathioprine treated group spread out to a much greater extent than control tumor macrophages but in neither group were the tumor macrophages growth inhibitory when maintained for 24 hours before use. Both produced a growth stimulating supernatant. The tumor cells from the azathioprine-treated mice grew when isolated during therapy but as regression became more evident cultivation of cells became more and more difficult. The small cells were not cytotoxic when mixed with FS6 tumor cells at a ratio of 5 cells to 1 tumor cell although the addition of cultured tumor macrophage supernatant to the mixture induced cytotoxicity. This preliminary result needs clarification but suggests the possibility that these cells are perhaps lymphocytes which transform into cytotoxic blasts in the presence of the macrophage supernatant. The small cells were seen to adhere strongly to the tumor cells, but not to the bare culture surface, and were also seen to extrude a small membrane giving the cell the morphological appearance of a monocyte. However, Fc receptors appear to be absent.

CONCLUSIONS

The presence of host mononuclear cells within the growing mass of tumor suggests that an attempt, albeit inadequate, is being made by the host to reject the neoplasm. That the host does not reject the tumor is not necessarily a reflection of the inadequacy of the pluripotential effector mechanisms but perhaps gives an indication that the tumor itself is an active entity and has its own means of "escape" which will not be discussed here. The overall evidence suggests that the level of macrophages, or monocytes, associated with a given tumor may indicate whether the tumor has a high or low metastatic potential. It would, therefore, follow that the level of macrophages and the immunogenicity of a tumor are related, since highly immunogenic tumors are said to metastasize less readily than the low immunogenic variety. However, in view of the recent report by Eccles and Alexander (11) that latent metastatic foci may be present even with high immunogenic tumors, this generalization may require reviewing.

Current dogma on the basis of *in vitro* studies would indicate that cytotoxic macrophages selectively destroy tumor cells. However, the data are somewhat equivocal since there is evidence that normal cells are lysed by activated or immune macrophages (25,26). Moreover, there is little information on the effect of cytotoxic macrophages on primary syngeneic adult cell cultures, which would seem to be of greater relevance than embryo cells or lines of cells grown in culture for many generations. The possibility that macrophages inhibit DNA synthesis of dividing syngeneic lymphocytes (49) suggests that macrophages recognize certain membrane structures of dividing cells as well as being able to recognize debris, and dead or damaged host cells and tissues, a reaction fundamental to the macrophage system *in vivo*. What the mechanism of recognition is either for tumor cell or for damaged host cell membranes has not been clarified. Indeed, little is known about the mechanism of tumor cell killing, whether by direct cell to cell contact or by a soluble labile factor. The attractive concept of lysosomal transfer proposed by Hibbs (27) would not seem to apply to tumor macrophage cytotoxicity since trypan blue did not abrogate cytotoxic effects.

The preliminary study of azathioprine therapy of the C57Black sarcoma FS6 suggests at least two possibilities for a mechanism of action during rejection. The first possibility is that regression is mediated directly by azathioprine or 6 M-P, which is known to effect DNA synthesis. The presence of mononuclear cells, as detected after enzymic dispersal of the tumor and also by histology, may represent residual cells which remained relatively unaffected by azathioprine. The apparent lack of increase in absolute numbers of mononuclear cells would support this. The second possibility is that azathioprine predisposes the tumor cells to attack by certain effector mechanisms, which in this case might involve either macrophages or lymphocytes, or both cell types. The failure to demonstrate cell-mediated cytotoxicity *in vitro* does not necessarily indicate a lack of effectiveness *in vivo*, and it may be explained on the basis that cytotoxicity in the regressing tumor is relatively short-lived as discussed above. Further experiments are required to elucidate these possibilities.

REFERENCES

1. Birbeck, M.S.C. and R. C. Carter (1972). Observations on the ultrastructure of two hamster lymphomas with particular reference to infiltrating macrophages. *Int. J. Cancer 9*:249-257.

2. Carr, I., J.C.E. Underwood, F. McGinty and P. Wood (1974). The ultrastructure of the local lymphoreticular response to an experimental neoplasm. *J. Path. 113*:175-182.

3. Evans, R. (1972). Macrophages in syngeneic animal tumours. *Transplantation 14*:468-473.

4. Haskill, J., J. W. Proctor and Y. Yamamura (1975). Host responses within solid tumors. 1. Monocytic effector cells within rat sarcomas. *J. Natl. Cancer Inst. 54*:387-393.

5. Van Loveren, H. and W. Den Otter (1974). Macrophages in solid tumours. 1. Immunologically specific effector cells. *J. Natl. Cancer Inst. 53*:1057-1060.

6. Gauci, C. L. and P. Alexander (1975). The macrophage content of some human tumours. *Cancer Letters 1*:29-32.

7. Mansell, P. W. A., H. Ichinose, R. J. Reed, E. T. Kremenz, R. McNamee and N. R. Di Luzio (1975). Macrophage-mediated destruction of human malignant cells *in vivo. J. Natl. Cancer Inst. 54*:571-580.

8. Eccles, S. A. and P. Alexander (1974). Sequestration of macrophages in growing tumours and its effect on the immunological capacity of the host. *Br. J. Cancer. 30*:42-49.

9. Eccles, S. A. and P. Alexander (1974). Macrophage content of tumours in relation to metastatic spread and host immune reaction. *Nature 250*:667-669.

10. Carr, I. and F. McGinty (1974). Lymphatic metastasis and its inhibition: An experimental model. *J. Path. 113*:85-95.

11. Eccles, S. A. and P. Alexander (1975). Immunologically-mediated restraint of latent tumour metastases. *Nature 257*:52-53.

12. Evans, R. and P. Alexander (1970). Cooperation of immune lymphoid cells with macrophages in tumour immunity. *Nature 228*:620-622.

13. Zarling, J. M. and S. S. Trevithia (1973). Transplantation immunity to simian viruses – 40 – transformed cells in tumor-bearing mice. II. Evidence for macrophage participation at the effector level of tumor rejection. *J. Natl. Cancer Inst. 50*:149-158.

14. Evans, R. (1973). Preparation of pure cultures of tumour macrophages. *J. Natl. Cancer Inst. 50*:271-273.

15. Evans, R. (1975). Macrophage mediated cytotoxicity. Its possible role in rheumatoid arthritis. *Ann. N.Y. Acad. Sci. 256*:275-287.

16. Evans, R. and P. Alexander (1972). Mechanism of immunologically specific killing of tumour cells by macrophages. *Nature (New Biology) 236*:168-170.

17. Evans, R. (1973). Macrophages and the tumour-bearing host. *Brit. J. Cancer 28*:19-25.

18. Hibbs, J. B., Jr. (1973). Macrophage non-immunologic recognition: Target cell factors related to contact inhibition. *Science 180*:868-870.

19. Holterman, O. A., E. Klein and G. P. Casale (1973). Selective cytotoxicity of peritoneal leucocytes for neoplastic cells. *Cell. Immunol. 9*:339-352.

20. Keller, R. (1974). Modulation of cell proliferation by macrophages: A possible function apart from cytotoxic tumour rejection. *Br. J. Cancer 30*:401-415.

21. Kaplan, A. M., P. S. Morahan and W. Regelson (1974). Induction of macrophage-mediated tumor-cell cytotoxicity by pyran copolymer. *J. Natl. Cancer Inst. 52*:1919-1921.

22. Cleveland, R. P., M. S. Meltzer and B. Zbar (1974). Tumor cytotoxicity *in vitro* by macrophages from mice infected with Myobacterium bovis strain BCG. *J. Natl. Cancer Inst. 52*:1887-1894.

23. Meltzer, M. S., R. W. Tucker and A. C. Breuer (1975). Interaction of BCG-activated macrophages with neoplastic and non-neoplastic cell lines *in vitro*: Cinemicrographic analysis. *Cell. Immunol. 17*:30-42.

24. Piessens, W. F., W. H. Churchill and J. R. David (1975). Macrophages activated *in vitro* with lymphocyte mediators kill neoplastic but not normal cells. *J. Immunol. 114*:293-299.

25. Jones, J. T., W. H. McBride and D. M. Weir (1975). The *in vitro* killing of syngeneic cells by peritoneal cells from adjuvant-stimulated mice. *Cell. Immunol. 18*:375-383.

26. Gallily, R. (1975). Allogeneic recognition and killing capacity of immune macrophages in mixed macrophage cultures (MMC). *Cell. Immunol. 15*:419-431.

27. Hibbs, J. B., Jr. (1974). Heterocytolysis by macrophages activated by Bacillus Calmette-Guerin: Lysosome exocytosis into tumor cells. *Science 184*:468-471.

28. Evans, R. and P. Alexander (1975). Mechanisms of extracellular killing of nucleated mammalian cells by macrophages. *Immunobiology of the Macrophage.* D. S. Nelson, Ed. Academic Press, in press.

29. Evans, R. (1975). Specific and non-specific activation of macrophages: Significance in tumour immunity. *Modulation of Host Immune Resistance on the Prevention or Control of Induced Neoplasia.* Fogarty International Center Proceedings. U.S. Government Printing Office, Washington D.C., in press.

30. Evans, R., C. K. Grant, H. Cox, K. Steele and P. Alexander (1972). Thymus-derived lymphocytes produce an immunologically specific macrophage-arming factor. *J. Exp. Med. 136*:1318-1322.

31. Evans, R. Cytotoxicity of fibrosarcoma macrophages to mouse lymphoma cells in the presence of alloantibody. *Int. Res. Comm. Syst. 2*:1674.

32. Currie, G. A. and C. Basham (1972). Serum mediated inhibition of the immunological reactions of the patient to his own tumour: A possible role for circulating antigen. *Br. J. Cancer 26*:427-438.

33. Heise, C. R. and R. S. Weiser (1969). Factors in delayed hypersensitivity: Lymphocyte and macrophage cytotoxins in the tuberculin reaction. *J. Immunol. 103*:570-576.

34. Sintek, D. E. and W. B. Pincus (1970). Cytotoxic factor from peritoneal cells: Purification and characteristics. *J. Reticuloendothel. Soc. 8*:508-521.

35. McIvor, K. L. and R. S. Weiser (1971). Mechanism of target cell destruction by alloimmune macrophages. II. Release of a specific cytotoxin from interacting cells. *Immunol. 20*:315-322.

36. Reed, W. P. and Z. J. Lucas (1975). Cytotoxic activity of lymphocytes V Role of soluble toxin in macrophage-inhibited cultures of tumour cells. *J. Immunol. 115*:395-404.

37. Boyle, M. D. P. and M. G. Ormerod (1975). The destruction of tumour cells by alloimmune peritoneal cells: Mechanism of action of activated macrophages *in vitro. J. Reticuloendothel. Soc. 17*:73-83.

38. Calderon, J., R. T. Williams and E. R. Unanue (1974). An inhibitor of cell proliferation released by cultures of macrophages. *Proc. Natl. Acad. Sci., U.S.A. 71*:4273-4277.

39. Calderon, J., J. M. Kiely, J. L. Lefko and E. R. Unanue (1975). The modulation of lymphocyte function by molecules secreted by macrophages. I. Description and partial biochemical analysis. *J. Exp. Med. 142*:151-164.

40. Rubini, J. R., S. Keller, A. Eisentraut and E. P. Cronkite (1961). *Tritium in the Physical and Biological Sciences. Sym. Int. Atomic Energy Agency 2*:247-267.

41. Opitz, H. G., D. Niethammer, H. Lemke, H. D. Flad and R. Huget (1975). Inhibition of ^{3}H-Thymidine incorporation of lymphocytes by a soluble factor from macrophages. *Cell Immunology 16*:379-388.

42. Gery, I. and B. H. Waksman (1972). Potentiation of the T lymphocyte response to mitogens. II. The cellular source of potentiating mediator(s). *J. Exp. Med. 136*:143-155.

43. Melsom, H., G. Kearny, S. Gruca and R. Seljelid (1974). Evidence for a cytolytic factor released by macrophages. *J. Exp. Med. 140*:1085-1096.

44. Olivotto, M. and R. Bomford (1974). *In vitro* inhibition of tumour growth and DNA synthesis by peritoneal and lung macrophages from mice infected with *Corynebacterium parvum. Int. J. Cancer 13*:478-488.

45. Parr, I., E. Wheeler and P. Alexander (1973). Similarities in the anti-tumour actions of endotoxin, lipid A and double stranded RNA. *Br. J. Cancer 27*:370-389.

46. Regelson, W., P. Morahan, A. M. Kaplan, L. G. Baird and J. A. Munson (1974). Synthetic polyanions: Molecular weight, macrophage activation and immunologic response. *Activation of Macrophages* W. H. Wagner and H. Hahn, Eds. *Excerpta Medica, Amsterdam* *2*:97-110.

47. Schlossberg, M. and V. P. Hollander (1973). Imuran-induced regression of plasma cell Tumor MOPC-315. *Cancer Res. 33*:1953-1956.

48. Van Furth, R., A. E. Gassmann and M. M. C. Dieselhoff-den Dulk. The effect of Azathioprine (Imuran) on the cell cycle of promonocytes and the production of monocytes in the bone marrow. *J. Exp. Med. 141*:531-546.

49. Kirchner, H., T. M. Chused, R. B. Herberman, H. T. Holden and D. H. Lavrin (1974). Evidence for suppressor cell activity in spleens of mice bearing primary tumors induced by Moloney sarcoma virus. *J. Exp. Med. 139*:1473-1487.

SESSION II

Macrophage Function and Interaction

Chairman: Dolph O. Adams

INTRODUCTION

Dolph O. Adams, Chairman

To provide a perspective for this session, I shall briefly outline some regulatory aspects of macrophage function and indicate how the interaction of macrophages with other cells can alter the host-tumor balance. Clearly, macrophages interact with other cells in all phases of the immune response, and much of their effector potency derives from such interactions.

The functional malleability of macrophages is inherent in their biology. First, their motility, localization, and proliferation in inflammatory sites are regulated by signals received from other cells (1). Second, their specific recognition function depends primarily upon extrinsically-derived factors such as complement and globulins, although they do possess an intrinsic, non-globulin-mediated recognition system for non-self (2,3). Third, the metabolism of macrophages is readily alterable, so that their functional capacity is governed considerably by their environment. Over several hours, the respiration, lipid metabolism, endocytosis, and motion of macrophages can be markedly increased by appropriate stimulants (3-6). Over several days, the cellular size, content of acid hydrolases, structural complexity and synthetic ability can be enhanced. Concomitantly, phagocytic, degradative and microbicidal abilities increase (3,7). Cellular resistance typifies such interactions, where committed T-cells attract macrophages, stimulate their proliferation, and augment their function (8).

Caution is warranted in considering alterations of macrophage metabolism, since such metabolic changes occur in quite disparate circumstances. Mature macrophages can arise in the normal course of the development of these cells, in certain chronic inflammatory responses, and in culture after the application of surface active molecules (3,9,10). Activated macrophages are taken from animals displaying cellular resistance and have heightened antimicrobial properties (8). Stimulated or elicited macrophages are induced by substances such as peptone or by chronic intracellular parasites and display strong, nonspecific cytotoxicity (11). Although similar in many regards, these three metabolic states are not necessarily synonymous. For example, activated and stimulated macrophages in one experimental model readily engulfed tubercle bacilli, but only the stimulated macrophages actively took up starch granules (12). Too, macrophage hydrolases fall into three separate groups, differing widely in their control mechanisms (13). No biochemical marker has been yet found to identify the various, altered states of macrophage function. My preference is to distinguish sharply between maturation, activation, and stimulation until their interrelationship is clearly defined.

The interaction of macrophages with other cells to regulate their effector function can be demonstrated in tumor immunity. Although the precise mechanisms effecting tumor rejection *in vivo* are far from established (14), macrophages have found to be obligate and to cooperate with T-cells in many experimental models (15-20). The Winn assay, for example, has been shown to require the participation of host macrophages (21). Dr. Gershon will amplify this theme of lymphocyte-macrophage cooperation in mediating rejection. Are such interactions general in the rejection response?

The potential mechanisms of macrophage-lymphocyte cooperation are many, but three deserve strong consideration. First, lymphocytes and other cells could regulate the number of macrophages within tumors (22). Dr. Snyderman will address this point, and Dr. Gershon will implicate mast cells as well as T-cells in governing the inflammatory accumulation of macrophages. Second, lymphocytes could provide specificity to macrophage cytotoxicity (23-26). Third, lymphocytes could alter the metabolism and cytotoxic function of macrophages. Dr. David will discuss in detail the activation of macrophages mediated by soluble products of lymphocytes and the cytotoxic capabilities of such cells. What is the cytotoxic specificity of such cells and what is their role in the specific rejection of tumors?

Not all interactions of macrophages with other cells benefit the host. The presence of a neoplasm is often associated with depressed skin-test reactions and RES clearance (20). Dr. Snyderman will discuss the suppressive effects of human and experimental tumors upon macrophage chemotaxis and present evidence on the mechanism of such suppression. What role does this suppressor play in the development and spread of neoplasms?

We have not considered at all the regulatory effects of macrophages upon other cells, although I should note that such interactions may be of considerable importance to the host (27). The soluble regulatory products secreted by macrophages are particularly relevant here (28).

Obviously, macrophages can interact *in vitro* with a wide variety of other cells in both stimulatory and suppressive modes. Of the twenty-four theoretically possible stimulatory or suppressive interactions between tumor cells, T-cells, B-cells, and macrophages, 21 have now been described *in vitro*. Increased understanding of these complex interrelationships *in vitro* will inevitably focus our attention on the role of such interactions *in vivo*. In constructing models of tumor resistance, comparisons with cellular resistance will be tempting. Cellular resistance, however, is generally nonspecific in effect (8). The destruction of allografts and tumors can be exquisitely specific (29-31), though nonspecific destruction of "innocent bystanders" has been observed in some systems (32,33). Bearing in mind our ultimate goal of establishing which interactions are significant in the intact host, this session will begin with Dr. Snyderman's presentation.

Supported in part by Grants 1 RO1 CA 17684-01 and 1 RO1 CA 14236-03 and by Contract NO1-CP-33313 from the National Cancer Institute.

REFERENCES

1. McGregor, D. D. (1975). Cytokinetics and fate sensitized lymphocytes. *J. Reticuloendothel. Soc. 17*:126-132.

2. Rabinovitch, M. (1970). Phagocytic recognition. *Mononuclear Phagocytes.* R. van Furth, Ed. F. A. Davis Company, Philadelphia.

3. Steinman, R. M., and Z. A. Cohn (1974). The metabolism and physiology of the mononuclear phagocytes. *The Inflammatory Process,* Vol. 1, 2nd edition. B. W. Zweifach, L. Grant and R. T. McClusky, Eds. Academic Press, New York.

4. Dannenberg, A. M., P. C. Walter and F. A. Capral (1963). A histochemical study of phagocytic and enzymatic functions of rabbit mononuclear and polymorphonuclear exudate cells and alveolar macrophages. II. The effect of particle ingestion on enzyme activity; two phases of *in vitro* activation. *J. Immunol. 90*:448-457.

5. Karnovsky, M. L., S. Simons, E. A. Glass, A. W. Shaffer and D'A. Hart (1970). Metabolism of macrophages. *Mononuclear Phagocytes.* R. van Furth, Ed. F. A. Davis Company, Philadelphia.

6. North, R. J. (1968). The uptake of particulate antigens. *J. Reticuloendothel. Soc. 5*:203-229.

7. Blanden, R. V. (1968). Modification of macrophage function. *J. Reticuloendothel. Soc. 5*:179-202.

8. Mackaness, G. B. (1972). Lymphocyte-macrophage interaction. *Inflammation: Mechanisms and Control.* I. H. Lepow and P. A. Ward, Eds. Academic Press, New York.

9. Adams, D. O. (1974). The structure of mononuclear phagocytes differentiating *in vivo*. I. Sequential fine and histologic studies of the effect of *Bacillus Calmette-Guérin* (BCG). *Amer. J. Path. 76*:17-48.

10. Adams, D. O., J. L. Biesecker and L. G. Koss (1973). The activation of mononuclear phagocytes *in vitro*: Immunologically mediated enhancement. *J. Reticuloendothel. Soc. 14*:550-570.

11. Keller, R. (1975). Cytostatic killing of syngeneic tumor cells by activated non-tumor macrophages. *Mononuclear Phagocytes in Immunity and Infection in Pathology.* R. van Furth, Ed. Blackwell Scientific Publications, Oxford.

12. Karnovsky, M. L. (1975). Biochemical aspects of the functions of polymorphonuclear and mononuclear leukocytes. *The Phagocytic Cell and Host Resistance.* J. A. Bellanti and D. H. Dayton, Eds. Raven Press, New York.

13. Gordon, S., J. C. Unkeless and Z. A. Cohn (1974). The macrophage as secretory cell. *Immune Recognition.* A. S. Rosenthal, Ed. Academic Press, New York.

14. Cerottini, J. C. and K. T. Brunner (1974). Cell-mediated cytotoxicity, allograft rejection, and tumor immunity. *Adv. Immunol. 18*:67-132.

15. Ariyan, S. and R. K. Gershon (1973). Augmentation of the adoptive transfer of specific tumor immunity by non-specifically immunized macrophages. *J. Nat. Cancer Inst. 51*:1145-1149.

16. Fidler, I. J. (1974). Inhibition of pulmonary metastases by intravenous injection of specifically activated macrophages. *Cancer Res. 34*:1074-1078.

17. Grant, C. K. and P. Alexander (1974). Nonspecific cytotoxicity of spleen cells and the specific cytotoxic action of thymus-derived lymphocytes *in vitro. Cellular Immunol. 14*:46-51.

18. Kearney, R., A. Basten and D. S. Nelson (1975). Cellular basis for the immune response to methylcholanthrene-induced tumors in mice. Heterogeneity of effector cells. *Internat. J. Cancer 15*:438-450.

19. Hanna, M. G. (1974). Immunologic aspects of BCG-mediated regression of established tumors and metastases in guinea pigs. *Sem. Oncol. 1*:319-335.

20. Levy, M. H. and E. F. Wheelock (1974). The role of macrophages in defense against neoplastic disease. *Adv. Cancer Res. 20*:131-163.

21. Zarling, J. M. and S. S. Tevethia (1973). Transplantation immunity to simian virus 40-transformed cells in tumor-bearing mice. II. Evidence for macrophage participation at the effector level of tumor cell rejection. *J. Nat. Cancer Inst. 50*:149-157.

22. Eccles, S. A. and P. Alexander (1974). Macrophage content of tumours in relation to metastatic spread and host immune reaction. *Nature 250*:667-689.

23. Holm, G. (1974). Mechanisms of antibody-induced hemolytic activity of human blood monocytes. *Activation of Macrophages* W. H. Wagner, H. Hahn and R. Evans, Eds. Excerpta Medica, Amsterdam.

24. Weiser, R., E. Heise, K. McIvor, S. H. Hahn and G. A. Granger (1969). *In vitro* activities of immune macrophages. *Cellular Recognition.* R. T. Smith and R. A. Good, Eds. Appleton Century Crofts, New York.

25. Evans, R. (1975). Macrophage cytotoxicity. *Mononuclear phagocytes in immunity and infection in pathology.* R. van Furth, Ed. Blackwell Scientific Publications, Oxford.

26. Lohmann-Matthes, M.-L. and H. Fisher (1975). Macrophage-mediated cytotoxic induction by a specific T-cell factor. *Mononuclear Phagocytes in Immunity and Infection in Pathology.* R. van Furth, Ed. Blackwell Scientific Publications, Oxford.

27. Unanue, E. R. (1972). The regulatory role of macrophages in antigenic stimulation. *Adv. Immunol. 15*:95-166.

28. Calderon, J., J.-M. Kiely, J. L. Lefko and E. R. Unanue (1975). The modulation of lymphocyte functions by molecules secreted by macrophages. I. Description and partial biochemical analysis. *J. Exp. Med. 142*:151-164.

29. Klein, E. and G. Klein (1972). Specificity of homograft rejection *in vivo*, assessed by inoculation of artificially mixed compatible and incompatible tumor cells. *Cellular Immunol. 5*:201-208.

30. Kearney, R. and D. S. Nelson (1973). Concomitant immunity to syngeneic methylcholanthrene-induced tumors in mice. Occurrence and specificity of concomitant immunity. *Australian J. Exp. Biol. Med. 51*:723-735.

31. Mintz, B. and W. K. Silvers (1970). Histocompatibility antigens on melanoblasts and hair follicle cells. Cell-localized homograft rejection in allophenic skin grafts. *Transplant. 9*:497-502.

32. Prehn, R. T. (1974). Destruction of tumor as an 'innocent bystander' in an immune response specifically directed against nontumor antigens. *Immunological Parameters of the Host Tumor Relationship,* Vol. 2. D. Weiss, Ed. Academic Press, New York.

33. Youdim, S., M. Moser and O. Stutman (1974). Nonspecific suppression of tumor growth by an immune reaction to *Listeria Monocytogenes. J. Nat. Cancer Inst. 52*:193-198.

DEFECTIVE MACROPHAGE MIGRATION PRODUCED BY NEOPLASMS: IDENTIFICATION OF AN INHIBITOR OF MACROPHAGE CHEMOTAXIS[1]

Ralph Snyderman[2]
and
Marilyn C. Pike

Division of Rheumatic and Genetic Disease
Department of Medicine and Division of Immunology
Duke University Medical Center
Durham, North Carolina 27710

INTRODUCTION

The increased incidence of neoplasms in individuals with depressed immune function suggests that immunosurveillance may play some role in protecting a host against the development and spread of cancer. It can indeed be demonstrated that certain types of immune responses to neoplasms can produce tumor destruction and immunologically-mediated tumor killing is frequently associated with the influx of macrophages to the neoplastic site (1-6). If immunological destruction of tumors does normally occur, it would appear to require two processes, the first being the specific recognition of the neoplasm as nonself and the second being the localization of cytotoxic immune effector cells at the tumor site. Since the immune systems of many hosts with neoplasms can be demonstrated to recognize their tumor's presence (7,8), it seems plausible that a deficiency of immune effector function could account for the inability of at least some individuals to destroy tumors.

---

[1] Supported in part by National Cancer Institute Contract No. NO1 CP 33313 and National Institute of Dental Research Grant 5 RO1 DE 03738-03.

[2] Howard Hughes Medical Investigator.

Considering the importance of macrophage accumulation for tumor killing we began the study of monocyte and macrophage migratory function in humans and animals with neoplasms. The present report demonstrates that a large percentage of individuals with cancer have depressed monocyte chemotactic responsiveness *in vitro* and that in such individuals chemotaxis is enhanced by tumor removal. An animal model developed to study macrophage accumulation *in vivo* and chemotaxis *in vitro* permitted the observation that neoplasms or products produced by neoplasms may directly inhibit macrophage migratory function.

MATERIALS AND METHODS

Quantification of Monocyte Chemotactic Responsiveness in Patients with Cancer – Human monocyte chemotactic responsiveness towards a lymphocyte derived chemotactic factor (LDCF) was measured in modified Boyden chambers as previously described (9,10). Briefly, mononuclear leukocytes containing approximately 25% monocytes and 75% lymphocytes were isolated from heparinized blood on Ficoll-Hypaque gradients, extensively washed, then standardized to contain 1.5×10^6 monocytes/ml in serum free RPMI 1640 (Gibco, Grand Island, New York). The cells were placed in the upper compartment of a modified Boyden chamber and a standardized preparation of LDCF placed in the lower compartment. The total number of monocytes which migrated completely through the filter in a 90 minute incubation period were counted in 20 oil immersion fields, and expressed as migrated monocytes per oil immersion field. Normal controls consisted of healthy laboratory personnel, students and University employees. Patient controls consisted of individuals with non-neoplastic disease hospitalized on the medical wards at the Duke University Medical Center. Cancer patients consisted of individuals with various neoplastic diseases not previously treated with chemotherapy or radiation therapy. The preponderance of these patients had newly diagnosed disease and were not debilitated at the time of testing. In the studies concerning the effect of tumor removal on monocyte chemotaxis, patients with suspicious mass lesions in the breast or kidney were tested within 72 hours prior to surgery, and again approximately 10 days thereafter. The patients whose lesions were benign served as controls in this study (11,12).

Mice – Male mice of the lines C3H/HeJ and A/J, aged 5-7 weeks, were purchased from Jackson Laboratories, Bar Harbor, Maine.

Phytohaemagglutinin (PHA) – Purified, lyophilized PHA (Burroughs Wellcome Company, Beckenham, England) was reconstituted to 2.0 mg/ml in sterile saline and kept frozen at –70°C until use. Where indicated, mice were injected with 2 ml of PHA diluted to contain 17.5 μg/ml in sterile non-pyrogenic saline.

Endotoxin – *Salmonella typhosa* 0901 endotoxin was purchased from the Difco Laboratories, Detroit, Michigan.

Malignant and Control Cells – Three tumor lines originating in C3H mice were maintained in the ascitic form until use. These included a benzpyrene induced fibrosarcoma BP8, hepatoma 129 and lymphosarcoma 6C3HED. An allogeneic spontaneous teratocarcinoma tumor line which developed in 129/J mice was also used. Non-neoplastic cells consisted of normal syngeneic (C3H/HeJ) spleen or liver cells or allogeneic (A/J) liver cells. Where indicated, 2.5×10^6 cells contained in 0.15 ml phosphate (0.05 M) buffered (pH 7.2) saline (PBS) were injected subcutaneously in the thighs of C3H/HeJ mice (13).

Malignant and Control Cell Supernatants – Tumor cells of the four malignant lines were suspended in PBS to contain 5×10^7 cells/ml. Normal liver and spleen were used to produce control supernatants. Since the volume of tumor cells far exceeded that of normal cells, control tissue supernatants were made to contain the same packed volume of tissue per ml of PBS as did the tumor cells. The tumor and control cells were then subjected to lytic sonication for two 30 second intervals. Following centrifugation at $1800 \times g$ for 10 minutes, the tumor and control supernatants were aliquoted and stored at −70°C until use. To obtain the low molecular weight fraction (<10,000) of these materials, 2.5 ml of the tumor or control supernatants was dialyzed over night against 5 ml of RPMI 1640, pH 7.0, and used immediately. Where indicated, 0.15 ml of the undialyzed supernatants or 0.2 ml of the dialysates were injected subcutaneously in the thighs of C3H/HeJ mice.

Quantification of Leukocyte Accumulation In Vivo – Experimental and control mice were injected intraperitoneally (i.p.) with either 35 μg of PHA or 100 μg of endotoxin contained in 2 ml of pyrogen free sterile saline. At the indicated times thereafter, animals were sacrificed by cervical dislocation, the peritoneal cavities exposed by abdominal incision, and lavaged vigorously with approximately 10 ml of Gey's balanced salt solution containing 2% bovalbumin (Flow Laboratories, Rockville, Md.), 0.01 M HEPES buffer, pH 7.0 (Gey's BSS) and 10 units of heparin/ml. The peritoneal washings from individual mice were centrifuged at $300 \times g$, 4°C for 10 minutes, washed once, and resuspended in 1 ml of Gey's BSS. The total number of cells present in the individual peritoneal cavities was quantified using a hemacytometer. Individual differential white cell counts were performed using a Shandon cytocentrifuge (Sewickley, Pennsylvania) and Wright's stain.

Quantification of Macrophage Chemotactic Responsiveness In Vitro – The chemotactic ability of peritoneal macrophages recovered from tumor bearing and normal mice was quantified using a modification of previously described techniques (14). Briefly, the peritoneal macrophages were obtained 2 days after i.p. injection of 35 μg of PHA. The washed cells from several tumor or control animals were pooled, standardized to contain 2.2×10^6 macrophages/ml Gey's BSS and 0.4 ml of this suspension was placed in the upper compartment of a modified Boyden chamber. The cells were separated from the chemotactic stimulus, endotoxin activated mouse serum in Gey's BSS, (AMS, 3% v/v) or medium alone by a 5 μ polycarbonate (Nuclepore) filter (Wallabs, San Rafael, California). All assays were performed in triplicate, and the chambers containing cells and stimulants were incubated for 4 hours in humidified air at 37°C. Following incubation, the chambers were emptied, the filters removed, fixed in ethanol and stained in hematoxylin. Chemotaxis was quantified by counting and averaging the number of macrophages per field in 20 oil immersion fields (X1540) that had migrated completely through the filter.

The effect of the various dialysates derived from tumor or control cell supernatants on macrophage chemotactic responsiveness was tested as follows. Extensively washed macrophages (2.2×10^6/ml RPMI 1640) obtained from peritoneal exudates of normal mice injected 2 days previously with PHA were incubated for 30 minutes at 37°C with various doses of the tumor or control dialysates or with medium alone. The cells were then tested for their chemotactic responsiveness to AMS. The effect of these dialysates on the chemotactic factor was also determined. AMS was diluted to 3% v/v in RPMI containing various doses of the tumor or control dialysates or in RPMI alone and incubated for 30 minutes at 37°C. Following incubation, the treated AMS was tested for residual chemotactic activity for macrophages.

RESULTS

Depression of Monocyte Chemotaxis in Patients with Cancer and Effects of Tumor Removal – Monocyte chemotactic responsiveness in 208 patients with a variety of neoplastic diseases was studied and compared with the responses of healthy individuals and patients with non-neoplastic diseases (15). As can be seen in Figure 1, 46 percent of the patients with malignant melanoma, 61 percent of patients with cancer of the breast and 49 percent of patients with a variety of other common neoplasms had depressed monocyte chemotactic responsiveness.

To determine the effect of tumor removal on chemotactic responsiveness, individuals with suspected malignancies were tested within 2 days prior and by three weeks after tumor removal (Table 1) (12). All patients with depressed chemotaxis prior to removal of the malignancy had enhanced responses post-operatively. In contrast, patients who had removal of benign lesions had no enhancement of chemotaxis. These data suggested that the presence of a malignant tumor could itself depress monocyte chemotactic responsiveness.

The Effect of Neoplastic Cell Implantation on Macrophage Accumulation In Vivo and Chemotactic Responsiveness In Vitro – The introduction of an inflammatory agent into the peritoneal cavities of mice is followed by the

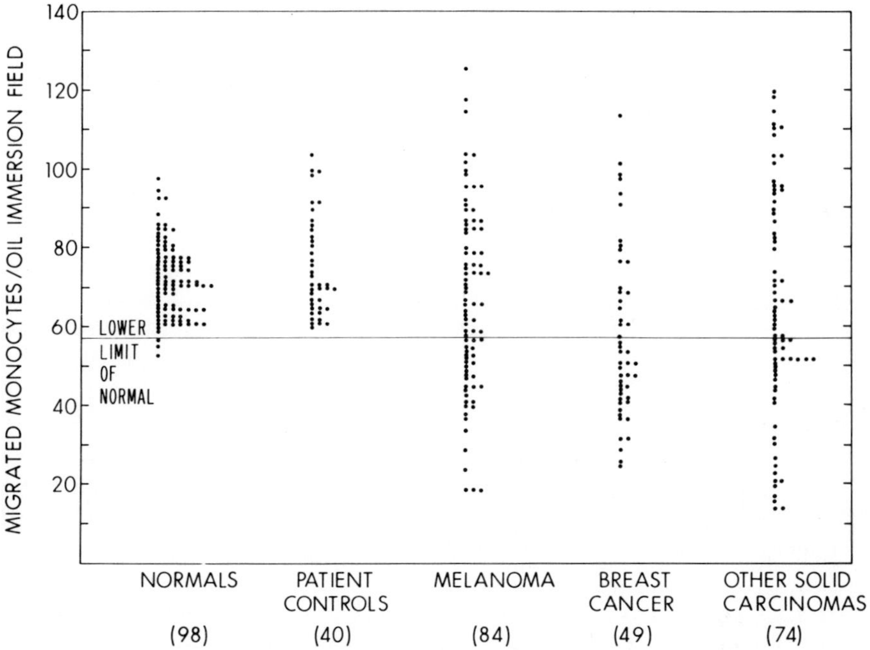

Fig. 1. *Monocyte chemotactic response to lymphocyte derived chemotactic factor in normal individuals, cancer patients and patients with non-neoplastic disease. The other solid carcinomas include predominantly patients with carcinomas of the lung, kidney, and colon.*

influx of leukocytes which can be recovered by peritoneal lavage. The type and number of leukocytes present at various times after the i.p. injection of an inflammatory stimulus can be reproducibly measured and can thus provide a useful tool for the study of the kinetics and quantity of an inflammatory response *in vivo* (13,16). Injection of PHA into the peritoneal cavities of normal mice results in an influx of inflammatory cells, the predominant type being the macrophage (Figure 2). To determine the effect of tumor implantation on macrophage accumulation *in vivo* mice were injected subcutaneously in the thigh with neoplastic cells and at times thereafter injected i.p. with PHA and the inflammatory response measured. Mice were injected with either sarcoma BP8 or hepatoma 129 cells and on the fourth or tenth day after tumor implantation injected i.p. with PHA. Two days after PHA injection, the mice were sacrificed and the number of accumulated peritoneal macrophages determined.

Table 2 illustrates that the number of accumulated macrophages, 6 days after tumor implantation was depressed by 52% in mice which had received the sarcoma and by 45% in mice which had received the hepatoma, when compared to normal mice. Similarly, twelve days after the mice had been

TABLE 1.
Effect of Tumor Removal on Monocyte Chemotactic Responsiveness

Patient	Neoplasm	Chemotactic Response[1] Pre-Op	Post-Op
G. W.	Renal Adenocarcinoma	21.3 ± 4.2	83.3 ± 5.6
A. G.	Renal Adenocarcinoma	20.9 ± 2.6	86.9 ± 7.6
T. W.	Renal Adenocarcinoma	58.2 ± 2.9	74.3 ± 1.7
C. F.	Renal Adenocarcinoma	57.6 ± 5.0	91.9 ± 5.2
M. B.	Carcinoma Breast	49.2 ± 0.9	78.3 ± 1.3
C. M.	Carcinoma Breast	25.9 ± 1.9	54.9 ± 3.6
V. P.	Carcinoma Breast	37.6 ± 5.4	52.6 ± 5.0
M. P.	Carcinoma Breast	32.6 ± 1.7	81.2 ± 0.7
M. S.	Carcinoma Breast	48.2 ± 2.6	69.2 ± 1.9
M. W.	Carcinoma Breast	32.9 ± 3.5	40.6 ± 9.4
M. W.	Carcinoma Breast	46.6 ± 3.6	114.2 ± 3.9
A. W.	Carcinoma Breast	51.9 ± 0.7	69.3 ± 3.6
	Mean ± 1 S.E.M.	40.6 ± 3.7	74.2 ± 5.5
		($p<.0005$)	
Mean of six patients' controls		69.9 ± 10.3	70.9 ± 4.9
		($p>0.2$)	
Normal Mean		71.6 ± 8.2	

[1] Cells per oil immersion field ± S.E.M.

injected with the sarcoma, macrophage accumulation in response to PHA was depressed by 49%.

The chemotactic responsiveness *in vitro* of the peritoneal macrophages recovered from mice implanted with the sarcoma was also measured and found to be depressed by 70% at 6 days after tumor implantation and by 42% at 12 days after tumor implantation.

To eliminate the possibility that depressed macrophage accumulation was the non-specific result of the introduction of cellular debris or antigenic material in the thighs of these mice, animals were injected subcutaneously with either sarcoma cells, hepatoma cells, syngeneic liver cells, syngeneic spleen cells or allogeneic (A/J) liver cells. Four days later, the mice were tested for their ability to mobilize macrophages to the peritoneal cavity in response to an injection of PHA. Table 3 illustrates that, while the injection of non-neoplastic syngeneic or allogeneic material had no effect on macrophage accumulation when compared to untreated animals, the number of macrophages migrating into the peritoneal cavities of mice injected with neoplastic cells was depressed by as much as 60%.

Effect of Tumor Implantation on the Kinetics of Macrophage Accumulation In Vivo – To determine whether the total number of responding macrophages or the kinetics of macrophage migration was depressed in tumor

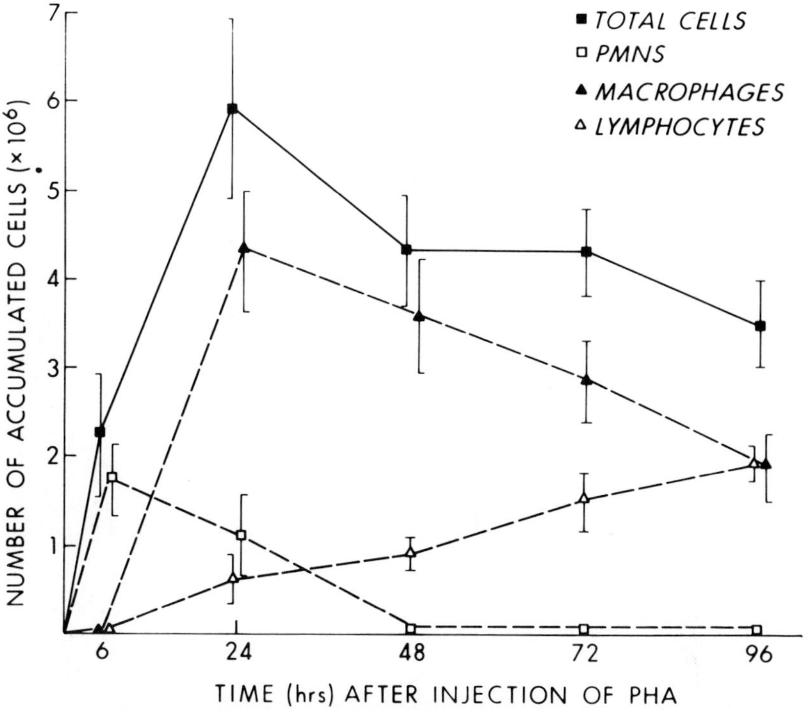

Fig. 2. *Kinetics of inflammatory cell accumulation in the peritoneal cavities of normal mice injected with 35 μg of PHA. Groups of 5 mice were sacrificed at each indicated time after injection, the peritoneal cavities lavaged and the total and differential white cell counts determined for each animal. The indicated values represent the mean ± S.E.M. of each group minus the number of cells present in the peritoneal cavities of untreated mice (approximately 2.2 × 10^6 macrophages, 1.0 × 10^6 lymphocytes and < 1 × 10^5 PMNs). Taken from (13)*

bearing animals, the following experiments were performed. Six days after the subcutaneous injection of sarcoma cells, syngeneic spleen cells or saline, mice were injected i.p. with PHA and the inflammatory response determined at various times thereafter. Figure 3 illustrates the kinetics of macrophage accumulation in tumor bearing or control mice for 4 days following PHA injection. As can be seen, the response of macrophages in the mice implanted with tumors never approached the maximal response of the normal mice.

The Effect of Tumor Implantation on Polymorphonuclear Leukocyte (PMN) Accumulation In Vivo – To determine if the implantation of neoplasms specifically affected macrophage accumulation or more generally affected other inflammatory cells, the following experiments were performed. Seven days after the injection of 2.5 × 10^6 sarcoma BP8 cells subcutaneously in the thigh, tumor bearing and normal animals were injected i.p. with 35 μg

TABLE 2.
Inhibition of Macrophage Accumulation In Vivo and Chemotaxis In Vitro by Tumor Implantation of Mice

Days after tumor implantation:	Number of macrophages ($\times 10^6$) accumulated in the peritoneal cavity[1]			Chemotactic response of macrophages[2]	
	Tumor implanted:[3]			Tumor implanted:	
	Sarcoma	Hepatoma	None	Sarcoma	None
6	3.3 ± 0.2 (52%)[4]	3.8 ± 0.2 (45%)	6.9 ± 0.4	19.1 ± 6.3 (70%)	64.6 ± 4.0
12	2.7 ± 0.3 (49%)	–[5]	5.3 ± 5.0	36.6 ± 5.0 (42%)	63.0 ± 6.0

[1] The values represent the mean (± S.E.M.) number of macrophages accumulated in the peritoneal cavities two days after i.p. injection of 35 μg of PHA into 5 normal mice or 5 mice previously implanted with the indicated tumor.

[2] The recovered cells from tumor bearing or control animals were standardized to contain 2.2×10^6 macrophages/ml and tested for chemotactic ability in response to activated mouse serum. Chemotactic responsiveness is expressed as the average number of macrophages per oil immersion field (×1540) ± S.E.M.

[3] Mice were injected with 2.5×10^6 of the indicated tumor cells subcutaneously in the thigh.

[4] The numbers in parenthesis indicate the percentage inhibition in tumor bearing animals as compared to normals.

$$\% \text{ inhibition} = 1 - \left(\frac{\text{Values obtained from tumor mice}}{\text{Values obtained from normal mice}}\right) \times 100$$

[5] Not done.

Adapted from (13)

PHA or 100 μg *S. typhosa* endotoxin. Six hours later, the mice were sacrificed and the total number and type of cells migrating into the peritoneal cavities was quantified. Table 4 illustrates that the number of PMNs migrating into the peritoneal cavities of tumor bearing mice did not differ significantly ($p > 0.2$) from that of normal mice. These data indicate that implantation of the BP8 sarcoma does not affect the ability of PMNs to accumulate in response to the inflammatory agents, endotoxin or PHA.

Effect of Sonicated Neoplastic Cell Supernatants or Supernatant Dialysates on Macrophage Accumulation In Vivo – To determine if soluble factors contained in neoplastic cells could account for their inhibitory effect on macrophage accumulation, the following experiments were performed. Sarcoma BP8, hepatoma 129, lymphosarcoma 6C3HED, teratocaricinoma cells and normal liver and spleen tissues were sonicated then centrifuged for 10

TABLE 3.
Effect of Neoplastic or Non-Neoplastic Cell Implantation on Macrophage Accumulation In Vivo

Mice injected with:[1]	Number of macrophages ($\times 10^6$) accumulated in the peritoneal cavity[2]	Percent inhibition[3]
C3H Sarcoma BP8 Cells	2.7 ± 0.3	61
C3H Hepatoma 129 Cells	3.8 ± 0.2	43
C3H Spleen Cells	6.5 ± 0.9	3
C3H Liver Cells	7.0 ± 0.3	0
A/J Liver Cells	7.1 ± 0.4	0
No cells	6.7 ± 0.6	–

[1] Groups of 5 C3H mice were injected subcutaneously with 2.5×10^6 of the indicated cells 6 days prior to sacrifice.

[2] The values represent the mean (± S.E.M.) number of macrophages accumulated in the peritoneal cavities, 2 days after i.p. injection of 35 μg of PHA.

[3] Percent Inhibition =

$$1 - \left(\frac{\text{Values obtained from mice injected with cells}}{\text{Values obtained from mice not injected with cells}}\right) \times 100$$

Adapted from (13)

TABLE 4.
Effect of Tumor Implantation on Polymorphonuclear Leukocyte Accumulation In Vivo

Mice[1]	Number of PMNs ($\times 10^6$) migrating into the peritoneal cavity in response to:[2]	
	Endotoxin	PHA
Tumor (BP8)	14.9 ± 1.4 p>0.2	2.5 ± 1.4 p>0.2
Normal	16.7 ± 2.5	2.8 ± 0.3

[1] Groups of 5 mice were implanted with 2.5×10^6 BP8 cells 7 days prior to an i.p. injection of endotoxin or PHA. Five mice not implanted with tumor cells (normal) received only the i.p. injection of either inflammatory agent.

[2] The values represent the mean (± S.E.M.) number of PMNs accumulated in the peritoneal cavities 6 hours after i.p. injection of 100 μg of endotoxin or 35 μg of PHA from 5 normal mice or 5 mice injected with tumor.

Adapted from (13)

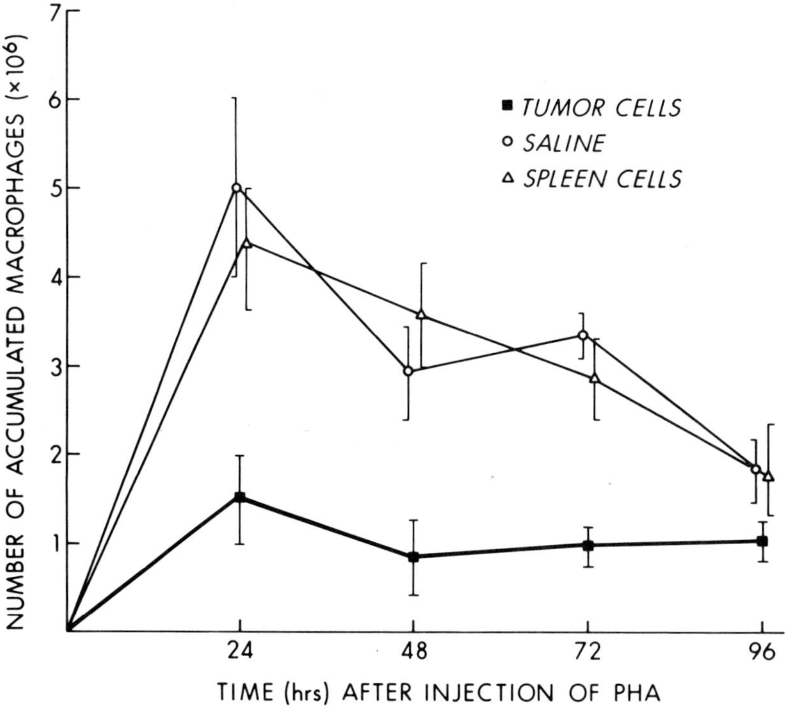

Fig. 3. *Effect of implantation of BP8 sarcoma cells on the kinetics of macrophage accumulation in response to i.p. injection of PHA. Mice were injected with either 2.5 × 10^6 tumor cells, syngeneic spleen cells or saline subcutaneously in the thigh and 7 days later injected with 35 μg of PHA i.p. At the indicated times thereafter groups of 5 mice were sacrificed, the peritoneal cavities lavaged and the total and differential white cell counts determined for each animal. The indicated values represent the mean ± S.E.M. of each group minus the number of macrophages in groups of mice identically treated but not injected with PHA intraperitoneally. (Normal = 2.2 × 10^6, Tumor 2.0 × 10^6). Taken from (13)*

minutes at 1800 × g. The supernatants (0.15 ml) were injected subcutaneously in the thighs of C3H/HeJ mice four days prior to sacrifice. Treated and untreated mice were injected i.p. with 35 μg of PHA, and 48 hours later, the number of macrophages accumulated in the peritoneal cavities was quantified. Table 5 illustrates that the injection of the 4 different tumor supernatants depressed macrophage accumulation by 38 to 73 percent when compared to untreated mice. Injection of supernatants derived from normal tissues, however, had no effect on macrophage accumulation. In order to determine if ultrafiltrates (<10,000 Daltons) of tumor supernatants possessed similar activity, dialysates (0.2 ml) of tumor or control supernatants were injected subcutaneously in the thighs of mice 3 days prior to sacrifice. Table 6

TABLE 5.
Inhibition of Macrophage Accumulation In Vivo by Supernatants of Sonicated Neoplastic Cells

Supernatant injected:[1]	Number of macrophages ($\times 10^6$) accumulated in the peritoneal cavity[2]	Percent inhibition[3]
None	8.5 ± 1.5	–
Sarcoma BP8	2.3 ± 0.3	73
Hepatoma 129	4.1 ± 0.6	52
Teratocarcinoma	5.0 ± 0.2	41
Lymphoma 6C3HED	5.3 ± 0.9	38
Liver	9.1 ± 1.3	0
Spleen	9.5 ± 0.8	0

[1] The indicated tissues (5×10^7 cells/ml PBS) were sonicated, centrifuged ($1800 \times g$ for 10 minutes) and 0.15 ml of the supernatant fluid injected subcutaneously in the thighs of groups of 5 C3H mice 4 days prior to sacrifice.

[2] The values represent the mean (± S.E.M.) number of macrophages accumulated in the peritoneal cavities, 2 days after i.p. injection of 35 μg of PHA.

[3] Percent inhibition =

$$1 - \left(\frac{\text{Values obtained from mice injected with supernatant}}{\text{Values obtained from mice not injected with supernatant}}\right) \times 100$$

Adapted from (18)

TABLE 6.
Inhibition of Macrophage Accumulation by Dialysates of Supernatants of Sonicated Neoplastic Cells

Mice injected with dialysate of:[1]	Number of macrophages ($\times 10^6$) accumulated in the peritoneal cavity[2]	Percent inhibition[3]
Lymphoma 6C3HED	1.8 ± 0.3	73
Hepatoma 129	2.3 ± 0.3	66
Teratocarcinoma	2.4 ± 0.3	64
Sarcoma BP8	3.8 ± 0.3	43
Normal liver	6.6 ± 0.3	1
Normal spleen	6.7 ± 0.6	0
None	6.7 ± 0.4	–

[1] Groups of 5 mice were injected with 0.2 ml of the indicated dialysate 3 days prior to sacrifice. Dialysates were obtained by overnight dialysis of 2.5 ml of the appropriate supernatant of sonicated cells against 5.0 ml RPMI 1640.

[2] The values represent the mean (± S.E.M.) number of macrophages accumulated in the peritoneal cavities, 2 days after i.p. injection of 35 μg of PHA.

[3] Percent inhibition =

$$1 - \left(\frac{\text{Values obtained from mice injected with dialysate}}{\text{Values obtained from mice not injected with dialysate}}\right) \times 100$$

Adapted from (18)

TABLE 7.
Inhibition of Macrophage Chemotaxis In Vitro by Tumor Dialysates

		Dialysate incubated with:			
Dialysate of:[1]	%	Macrophages[2]		Chemotactic factor[3]	
		Response[4]	% Inhibition[5]	Response	% Inhibition
Lymphoma 6C3HED	50	5.0 ± 1.4	93	45.5 ± 5.2	31
	30	18.8 ± 3.1	72	52.8 ± 2.1	23
	10	38.3 ± 0.9	44	64.0 ± 4.0	4
Hepatoma 129	50	39.0 ± 3.8	42	61.7 ± 3.6	6
	30	48.5 ± 5.9	27	64.7 ± 4.0	5
	10	62.4 ± 1.9	9	65.0 ± 1.2	2
Teratocarcinoma	50	36.0 ± 2.1	47	58.7 ± 4.2	11
	30	47.5 ± 2.1	28	65.3 ± 5.2	4
	10	61.4 ± 3.6	10	64.0 ± 2.1	4
Sarcoma BP8	50	31.0 ± 7.8	54	19.1 ± 1.9	71
	30	31.4 ± 3.3	52	23.4 ± 2.1	66
	10	44.9 ± 0.5	34	31.0 ± 2.6	54
Normal spleen	50	70.3 ± 3.6	0	66.3 ± 1.6	0
	30	65.0 ± 4.2	2	65.7 ± 1.9	4
	10	68.0 ± 1.6	0	64.0 ± 1.4	4
Normal liver	50	64.7 ± 1.2	4	63.7 ± 2.4	3
	30	68.6 ± 4.7	0	65.7 ± 3.1	4
	10	68.0 ± 1.4	0	67.7 ± 0.2	0
Medium alone	50	67.7 ± 4.7	–	66.0 ± 1.9	–
	30	66.0 ± 2.9	–	68.3 ± 1.9	–
	10	68.3 ± 5.9	–	66.7 ± 0.2	–
No dialysate[6]			63.7 ± 3.1		
Negative control[7]			8.9 ± 2.1		

[1] 2.5 ml of the indicated tumor cell supernatant, control cell supernatant or medium alone was dialyzed overnight against 5 ml RPMI 1640 pH 7.0.

[2] Peritoneal macrophages (2.2×10^6/ml) from normal mice injected with PHA were incubated for 30 minutes at 37°C with RPMI 1640 containing the indicated amount (% v/v) of the appropriate dialysate and tested for chemotactic responsiveness to activated mouse serum (AMS).

[3] AMS was incubated for 30 minutes at 37°C with RPMI 1640 containing the indicated amount (% v/v) of the appropriate dialysate and tested for chemotactic activity for macrophages.

[4] Chemotactic response is expressed as the average number of macrophages per oil immersion field (×1540) ± S.E.M.

demonstrates that while dialysates of supernatants of normal cells had no effect on macrophage accumulation, dialysates of the 4 neoplastic cell supernatants depressed macrophage accumulation in response to PHA by 43 to 73 percent. These results demonstrated that tumor cells, but not normal tissues contain a low molecular weight substance capable of depressing macrophage accumulation *in vivo* (17,18).

Effect of Dialysates of Neoplastic Cell Supernatants on Macrophage Chemotaxis In Vitro – To better define the mechanism by which tumor supernatants depress macrophage accumulation *in vivo*, we sought to determine if these substances directly affected the chemotactic responsiveness of macrophages *in vitro*. In these studies, macrophages from normal mice were incubated with various amounts of dialysates from tumor or control tissue supernatants or of dialyzed medium RPMI 1640. Treated and control cells were then tested for their chemotactic responsiveness to AMS in modified Boyden chambers. Table 7 demonstrates that the chemotactic responsiveness of macrophages incubated with doses of tumor dialysates ranging from 10 to 50 percent v/v, were depressed by as much as 93 percent when compared to that of macrophages incubated with the dialysate of medium alone. Normal spleen or liver dialysates had no significant effect on the chemotaxis of normal macrophages. When various doses of the dialysates were incubated with AMS itself, rather than with the cells, the chemotactic responsiveness was also depressed but to a lesser extent.

These results indicated that dialysates of tumor cell supernatants are capable of depressing the chemotactic responsiveness of normal macrophages *in vitro*. In addition, the majority of the inhibitory activity appears to be exerted on the macrophage itself, since incubation of three of the four tumor dialysates with the chemotactic factor resulted in less inhibition of chemotactic activity than did incubation of the dialysates with the cells (17,18).

---

[5] % Inhibition =

$$1 - \left(\frac{\text{Chemotactic activity of cells or AMS incubated with experimental dialysates}}{\text{Chemotactic activity of cells or AMS incubated with the dialysate of medium alone}} \right) \times 100$$

[6] Macrophages incubated with undialyzed RPMI 1640 and tested for chemotactic responsiveness to AMS.

[7] Macrophages incubated with undialyzed RPMI 1640 and tested for response to RPMI 1640 medium alone.

Adapted from (18)

DISCUSSION

The importance of immunosurveillance in protecting a host against the development and spread of cancer is as yet uncertain but there is abundant evidence which indicates that the accumulation of macrophages in a tumor may result in its destruction (1-6). Since the depressed ability of a host to localize macrophages at a site of a developing neoplasm could conceivably render that host less likely to destroy the tumor, it became important to determine if patients with cancer had depressed monocyte chemotactic responsiveness. Several years ago, we developed methodology which allowed quantification of human monocyte chemotactic responsiveness *in vitro* (9). Using this methodology, several investigators and ourselves have noted depressed monocyte chemotactic responsiveness in a sizable percentage of patients with cancer (15,19,20). To the present time, we have studied 204 individuals with cancer, and have found 51 percent to have depressed chemotaxis when compared to normal or patient controls. A potentially exciting observation made during the course of these studies was that surgical removal of malignant neoplasms resulted in a rapid enhancement of chemotactic responsiveness in those individuals who had depressed chemotaxis prior to surgery (11,12). Since in other studies we have found that patients with depressed chemotaxis had a poorer prognosis than individuals whose chemotaxis was normal (21), we hypothesized that depressed monocyte chemotaxis could render a host less likely to contain a neoplasm and that once established, neoplasms could produce inhibitory effects on monocyte migratory function. We therefore sought to develop an animal model to permit the study of the effects of neoplasms on macrophage accumulation *in vivo* and chemotaxis *in vitro* (13,14,16).

Following the injection of PHA into the peritoneal cavities of mice, an inflammatory reaction ensues and is characterized by the accumulation of predominantly macrophages, the peak influx of which occurs 24 hours after injection and persists for 72 to 96 hours. By vigorously lavaging the peritoneal cavities of mice at various times after the injection of PHA, one can accurately measure the number and type of cells which have accumulated and thereby quantify a delayed type inflammatory response *in vivo* (13). In addition, the macrophages recovered from the peritoneal cavities can be tested *in vitro* for their responsiveness to various chemotactic factors. Using these methods, it was found that macrophage accumulation *in vivo* and chemotactic responsiveness *in vitro* was depressed in animals implanted with two types of malignant cells. The latter findings have also been reported by Stevenson and Meltzer (22). The implantation of syngeneic or allogeneic non-neoplastic tissues did not depress macrophage accumulation, therefore the mechanism of depressed macrophage accumulation in tumor bearing animals is not a nonspecific phenomenon produced by the local deposition of cellular elements or antigenic materials (13).

The generalized debilitating effects of tumors could not explain these findings since depressed macrophage accumulation was present before the neoplasms became palpable and weeks before the mice displayed any signs of illness. Circulating white blood cell and monocyte counts were not depressed in the tumor bearing mice so it is unlikely that our findings are due to sequestration of many monocytes at the tumor site rendering them unavailable for migration elsewhere. It is also important to note that the accumulation of neutrophils in response to endotoxin or PHA was not diminished in tumor bearing animals when accumulation of macrophages in response to PHA was profoundly depressed (13).

The mechanism by which neoplasms depress macrophage accumulation *in vivo* in response to PHA is not fully understood but there is some evidence which indicates that it is mediated at least in part by a low molecular weight factor (between 500 and 10,000 Daltons) contained in the four murine tumors thus far studied (17,18). Subcutaneous injections in mice of the low molecular weight material but not injection of ultrafiltrates of non-neoplastic tissues produced a similar depression of macrophage accumulation as did injection of viable neoplastic cells. The effect of the dialysates, however, did not last as long as did the effect produced by a growing tumor (17,18). The fact that the effect of tumors could be reproduced by a low molecular weight filtrate thereof indicates that the tumor effect cannot be attributed to a contaminating virus.

There are several possible explanations for depressed macrophage accumulation in tumor bearing animals. These possibilities include the ability of neoplasms to produce factors capable of 1) depressing macrophage chemotactic responsiveness, 2) inhibiting chemotactic factor production or 3) retarding the production or maturation of mononuclear leukocytes capable of migrating chemotactically. Graham and Graham and Fauve *et. al.* have described an anti-inflammatory product contained in neoplasms capable of interfering with allograft rejection, PMN accumulation *in vivo* and the "lining up" of macrophages at the surface of tumor cells *in vitro* (23,24). The factor described by Fauve, *et. al.* had a low molecular weight (between 1,000 and 10,000 Daltons) and may be similar to the factor described herein. However, in contrast to their findings, the neoplasms we have studied did not depress PMN accumulation *in vivo.* Ward *et. al.* described higher molecular weight factors (>68,000 Daltons) present in the plasma of patients with neoplasms capable of inactivating chemotactic factors (25). These chemotactic factor inactivators could not explain our data because their molecular weight is far greater than the factor described herein. In addition, the chemotactic factor inactivators were reported to destroy C5a activity and should therefore have depressed the C5a mediated PMN response to endotoxin *in vivo* (26). Our *in vitro* data are most compatible with the hypothesis that products produced by neoplasms have their major effects directly on macrophage migratory function. Incubation of macrophages from normal mice with the low molecular weight factors greatly depressed their chemotactic responsiveness to AMS. Only the filtrate of one of the four tumors tested produced a greater depression of chemotaxis when incubated with the chemotactic factor rather than directly with the cells. We cannot discount the possibility, however, that the filtrates affect the chemotactic factor's interaction with the macrophage. We have also not eliminated the possibility that the tumor could also affect the activation or maturation of mononuclear leukocytes into chemotactically responsive cells *in vivo*.

In sum, these studies clearly demonstrate that a sizable percentage of humans with cancer have depressed monocyte chemotactic responsiveness *in vitro* and that the depression is at least partially reversed by tumor removal. In addition, murine neoplasms contain factors capable of depressing macrophage accumulation *in vivo* and chemotaxis *in vitro*. The biological consequences of depressed chemotaxis produced by neoplasms has yet to be determined. It could explain, however, how the immune system, while able to recognize the presence of a neoplasm, may still be unable to mobilize sufficient numbers of macrophages to the tumor site to produce its destruction.

REFERENCES

1. Shin, H. S., M. Hayden, S. Langley, N. Kaliss and M. R. Smith (1975). Antibody-mediated suppression of grafted lymphoma III. Evaluation of the role of thymic function, non-thymus derived lymphocytes, macrophages, platelets, and polymorphonuclear leukocytes in syngeneic and allogeneic hosts. *J. Immunol. 114*:1255-1263.

2. Lala, P. K. (1974). Dynamics of leukocyte migration into the mouse ascites tumor. *Cell Tissue Kinet. 7*:293-304.

3. Levy, M. H. and E. F. Wheelock (1974). The role of macrophages in defense against neoplastic diseases. *Adv. Cancer Res. 20*:131-163.

4. Nelson, D. S. (1972). Macrophages as effectors of cell-mediated immunity pp. 45-76 in *Macrophages and Cellular Immunity.* A. I. Laskin and H. LeChevaliner, eds. CRC Press, Cleveland.

5. Cerottini, J. C. and K. T. Brunner (1974). Cell mediated cytotoxicity, allograft rejection, and tumor immunity. *Adv. Immunol. 18*:57-132.

6. Zbar, B., H. T. Wepsic, H. J. Rapp, L. C. Stewart and T. Borsos (1970). Two step mechanism of tumor graft rejection in syngeneic guinea pigs. II. Initiation of reaction by a cell fraction containing lymphocytes and neutrophils. *J. Nat. Can. Inst. 44*:710-717.

7. Bernstein, I. D. (1973). Immunologic defenses against cancer. *J. of Pediatrics 83*:906-918.

8. Hellstrom, K. E. and I. Hellstrom (1970). Immunologic enhancement as studied by cell culture technique. *Ann. Rev. Microbiol. 24*:373-398.

9. Snyderman, R., L. C. Altman, M. S. Hausman and S. E. Mergenhagen (1972). Human mononuclear leukocyte chemotaxis: A quantitative assay for mediators of humoral and cellular chemotactic factors. *J. Immunol. 108*:857-860.

10. Altman, L. C., R. Snyderman, J. J. Oppenheim and S. E. Mergenhagen (1973). A human mononuclear leukocyte chemotactic factor: Characterization, specificity and kinetics of production by homologous leukocytes. *J. Immunol. 110*:801-810.

11. Snyderman, R., L. Meadows, S. Wells and G. Hemstreet (1975). Depression of monocyte chemotaxis in patients with carcinoma of the breast or kidney: Effect of tumor removal. Manuscript in preparation.

12. Snyderman, R., M. C. Pike, L. Meadows, G. Hemstreet and S. Wells (1975). Depression of monocyte chemotaxis by neoplasms. *Clin. Res. 23*:297A.

13. Snyderman, R., M. C. Pike, B. L. Blaylock and P. Weinstein (1975). Effects of neoplasms on inflammation: Depression of macrophage accumulation following tumor implantation. Submitted for publication.

14. Snyderman, R., M. C. Pike, D. McCarley and L. Lang (1975). Quantification of mouse macrophage chemotaxis *in vitro*: Role of C5 for the production of chemotactic activity. *Infection and Immunity 11*:488-492.

15. Synderman, R. and C. Stahl (1975). Defective immune effector function in patients with neoplastic and immune deficiency diseases. pp. 267-281. *In* The Phagocytic Cell in Host Resistance, J. A. Bellanti and D. H. Dayton, eds., Raven Press, New York.

16. Snyderman, R., M. C. Pike and B. L. Blaylock (1975). Depression of macrophage chemotaxis *in vivo* in tumor bearing mice. *Fed. Proc. 34*:991.

17. Snyderman, R. and M. C. Pike. Anti-inflammatory effects of neoplasms: Identification of an inhibitor of macrophage chemotaxis. *Clin. Res.*, In press.

18. Snyderman, R. and M. C. Pike (1975). Effect of neoplasms on inflammation. Isolation of a factor which inhibits macrophage accumulation *in vivo* and chemotaxis *in vitro*. Manuscript in preparation.

19. Boetcher, D. A. and E. J. Leonard (1974). Abnormal monocyte chemotactic response in cancer patients. *J. Nat. Cancer Inst. 52*:1091-1099.

20. Hausman, M. S., S. Brosman, R. Snyderman, M. R. Mickey and J. Fahey (1973). Defective monocyte function in patients with genitourinary carcinoma. *Clin. Res. 21*:646A.

21. Snyderman, R., L. Meadows and H. F. Siegler. Monocyte chemotactic responsiveness in patients with malignant melanoma and the effect of BCG immunotherapy. Manuscript in preparation.

22. Stevenson, M. M. and M. S. Meltzer (1975). Defective macrophage chemotaxis in tumor bearing mice. *Fed. Proc. 34*:991.

23. Fauve, R. M., B. Hevin, H. Jacob, J. A. Gaillard and F. Jacob (1974). Anti-inflammatory effects of murine malignant cells. *Proc. Nat. Acad. Sci. 71*:4052-4056.

24. Graham, J. B. and R. M. Graham (1964). Tolerance agent in human cancer. *Surg. Gynecol. Obstet. 118*:1217-1222.

25. Ward, P. A. and J. L. Berenberg (1974). Defective regulation of inflammatory mediators in Hodgkin's disease. Supranormal levels of chemotactic factor inactivator. *New Eng. J. Med. 290*:76-80.

26. Snyderman, R., J. K. Phillips and S. E. Mergenhagen (1971). Biological activity of complement *in vivo*: Role of C5 in the accumulation of polymorphonuclear leukocytes in inflammatory exudates. *J. Exp. Med. 134*:1131-1143.

MACROPHAGE ACTIVATION BY LYMPHOCYTE MEDIATORS AND TUMOR IMMUNITY: A BRIEF REVIEW

John R. David
Willy F. Piessens[1]
W. Hallowell Churchill, Jr.[2]

Department of Medicine
Harvard Medical School
Robert B. Brigham Hospital
Boston, Massachusetts 02120

There are numerous studies indicating that macrophages play a crucial role both in the induction of the immune response and as a powerful effector cell. In the latter capacity macrophages ingest and dispose of a variety of microorganisms, kill tumor cells and participate in a number of immunopathologic processes. For some time, it has been known that macrophages obtained from immunized animals have altered morphology and metabolism and exhibit an enhanced ability to deal with a number of microorganisms (1-4). Such macrophages have been called activated. More recent studies suggest that *in vivo* activation of macrophages requires the interaction of specifically sensitized T lymphocytes with appropriate antigen (5,6).

How does the interaction of lymphocytes with antigen lead to activation of macrophages? Ever since the discovery that sensitized lymphocytes produced a soluble material, migration inhibitory factor (MIF) which affects the behavior of macrophages (7,8), we have considered the possibility that lymphocyte mediators might also activate macrophages. In the past few years, our laboratory and others have accumulated considerable evidence which supports this hypothesis. The following is a brief review of studies which demonstrate that macrophages activated by lymphocyte mediators have an enhanced ability to kill tumor cells.

Most of the studies described below have been carried out using guinea pig peritoneal exudate macrophages. The macrophages were usually incubated

---

[1] Recipient of a Cancer Research Scholar Award, American Cancer Society, Massachusetts Division, Inc.

[2] Recipient of a Research Career Development Award, K04 CA00116.

as monolayers for varying periods of time with tissue culture media containing lymphocyte mediators; more recently, macrophages have been activated in suspension culture (9). The mediators were produced by incubating lymph node lymphocytes from guinea pigs sensitized to o-chlorobenzoyl gamma globulin (OCB-BGG) with that antigen for 24 hours (10). Control cultures were not stimulated by antigen; after incubation, the cells were removed by centrifugation, and antigen was added to the control supernatant. In some studies, lymphocytes were stimulated by the plant lectin concanavalin A (Con A) instead of antigen (11). In most experiments, the supernatants were chromatographed on Sephadex G-100 columns, and fractions rich in mediators and their control counterparts were used (11). In some experiments, human monocytes and human lymphocyte mediators were used (12). For the sake of convenience, the mediator(s) involved will be referred to as macrophage activating factor (MAF); this does not imply that there is necessarily only one factor that activates macrophages nor that MAF is different from MIF. Indeed, there is some evidence that suggests that MIF and MAF are the same.

Macrophage Activation by Lymphocyte Mediators

Macrophages which have been incubated with MAF-rich lymphocyte supernatants or MAF-rich Sephadex fractions exhibit a number of changes which appear to reflect alterations in the macrophage membrane. They stick better to culture vessels (13,14), and show a marked increase in ruffled membrane movement after three days of culture using time-lapse cinematography (14). Such macrophages also spread out more than controls; similar spreading was observed when the periphery of a fan of cells inhibited from migrating from capillary tubes was examined (15). Increased ameboid movement has been reported (13). On the other hand, early after incubation with mediators, it has been found that cells may spread less (16,17).

Enhancement of both the rate and extent of phagocytosis of dead mycobacteria and starch has been observed (14). However, it should be noted that this is not seen with all particles. For example, Remold and Mednis (18) found a decrease in the phagocytosis of denatured aggregated hemoglobin by macrophages preincubated in MAF-rich Sephadex fractions compared to controls, and that the amount of denatured hemoglobin sticking to the macrophages was also less on activated than control cells. Decrease in phagocytosis of *C. Albicans* by mediator activated macrophages has been reported by Neta and Salvin (19). Hoff noted that mouse macrophages which have been activated *in vivo* by injection of mice with BCG or *T. cruzi* showed a decreased ability to take up *T. cruzi* compared to control macrophages (20). These results suggest that the membrane of the activated macrophage is altered leading to increased or decreased phagocytosis depending on the surface properties of the particle ingested.

Alterations of macrophages incubated with MAF which also appear to reflect membrane changes include the enhanced pinocytosis of radioactive gold (21), increase in levels of the membrane enzyme adenylate cyclase (22), increase in glucosamine incorporation (23) and decrease in electron-dense surface material (24). Other metabolic changes in mediator activated macrophages include increased glucose oxidation through the hexose monophosphate shunt (14), increased cytoplasmic enzyme lactic dehydrogenase (25), production of collagenase (26), and a decrease in several lysosomal enzymes (25) despite an increase in the number of cytoplasmic granules (David and Remold, unpublished observation).

In addition to the morphologic and metabolic changes described above, mediator activated macrophages show important functional changes. They exhibit enhanced bacteriostasis for a number of organisms (27-31) and enhanced tumoricidal capacity. This latter function will now be dealt with in more detail. The alterations seen when macrophages are activated by lymphocyte mediators are summarized on Table I.

Tumor Killing by Macrophages Activated by Lymphocyte Mediators

The tumoricidal capacity of macrophages activated by MAF was studied in a syngeneic strain 2 guinea pig tumor system (32,33). Monolayers of normal strain 2 macrophages were incubated for three days in unfractionated MAF-rich and control supernatants from OCB-BGG stimulated guinea pig lymphocytes. Tumor cells labeled with ^{3}H-thymidine were then added, and, after 24 hours of co-cultivation, cytotoxicity was determined by comparing the numbers of adherent tumor cells remaining in dishes containing similar

Table 1.

Activation of Macrophages by Lymphocyte Mediators

1) Increase in adherence to glass
2) Increase in ruffled membrane activity
3) Increase in phagocytosis of some particles (dead mycobacteria) but decrease in others (aggregated hemoglobin)
4) Increase in membrane enzyme adenylate cyclase
5) Increase in incorporation of glucosamine
6) Decrease in electron-dense surface material
7) Increase in pinocytosis of colloidal gold
8) Increase in glucose oxidation through hexose monophosphate shunt
9) Increase in cytoplasmic enzyme lactic dehydrogenase
10) Decrease in lysosomal enzyme acid phosphatase, cathepsin D, β-glucuronidase
11) Increase in number cytoplasmic granules
12) Production of collagenase
13) Enhanced bacteriostasis to Listeria
14) Enhanced tumoricidal activity

numbers of activated and control macrophages. This is a true reflection of cytotoxicity as 90% of the radioactivity which is released from the monolayers is non-cell associated, and thus must have come from dead cells.

The macrophages which were incubated with MAF-rich supernatants were toxic for Line 1 hepatoma cells in 23 of 29 experiments. The cytotoxicity ranged from 13-72% with a mean of 38% (p for each pair <0.05). Such macrophages were also cytotoxic to MCA-25 fibrosarcoma in 5 of 5 experiments; the degree of cytotoxicity ranged from 14-74% (mean 28% with p <0.05). On the other hand, such activated macrophages did not kill either syngeneic fibroblasts or kidney cells. Tumor cells adhered equally well to both activated and control macrophages when measured after just two hours of co-cultivation (see Figure 1). It should be noted that macrophages could be activated by supernatants devoid of lymphotoxin activity suggesting that the effect was not due to this mediator absorbed to macrophages.

The observation that macrophages activated by MAF kill syngeneic tumor cells but not normal cells is consistent with the previous findings of Hibbs *et al.* who reported that activated macrophages obtained from mice immunized with a number of different microorganisms kill transformed cells but not their

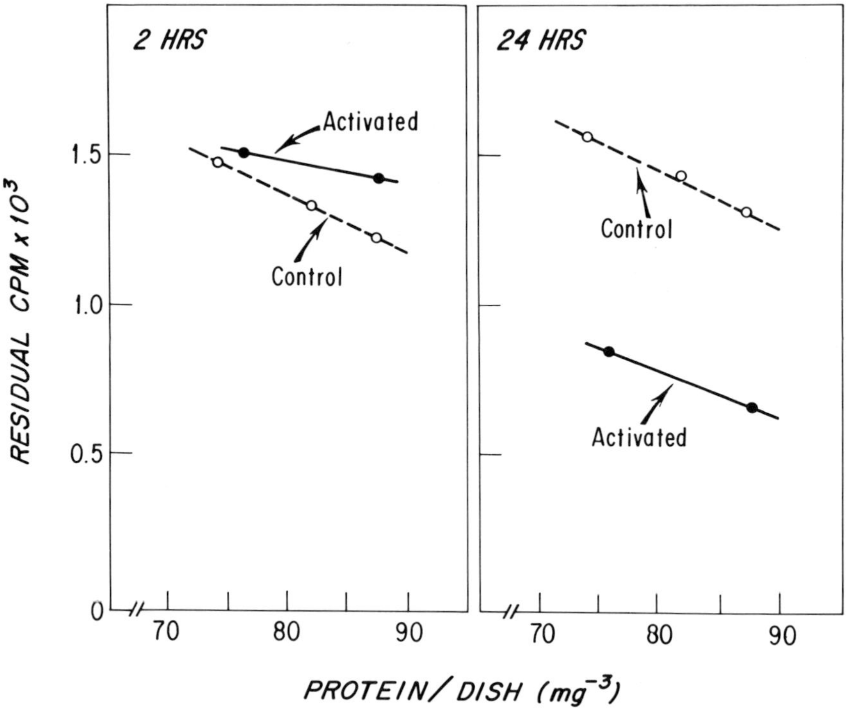

Figure 1

normal counterparts, whereas macrophages from non-immunized mice kill neither cell type (34,35). Since activated macrophages exhibit certain membrane changes discussed above, it is tempting to speculate that membrane alterations possibly analogous to those found between normal and transformed cells might be present between normal and activated macrophages. Such surface changes might lead activated macrophages to recognize or have a greater affinity for altered tumor cell membranes leading to interaction and subsequent killing of the tumor cell.

In more recent studies, it was shown that macrophages incubated for 24 hours with MAF in suspension culture also showed an enhanced capacity to kill syngeneic tumor cells (9) (see Figure 2). MAF-rich Sephadex G-100 fractions free of antigen were capable of enhancing macrophage cytotoxicity. MAF was not cytophilic for macrophages. Further, trypsinization of the activated macrophages did not diminish their cytotoxic potential (9).

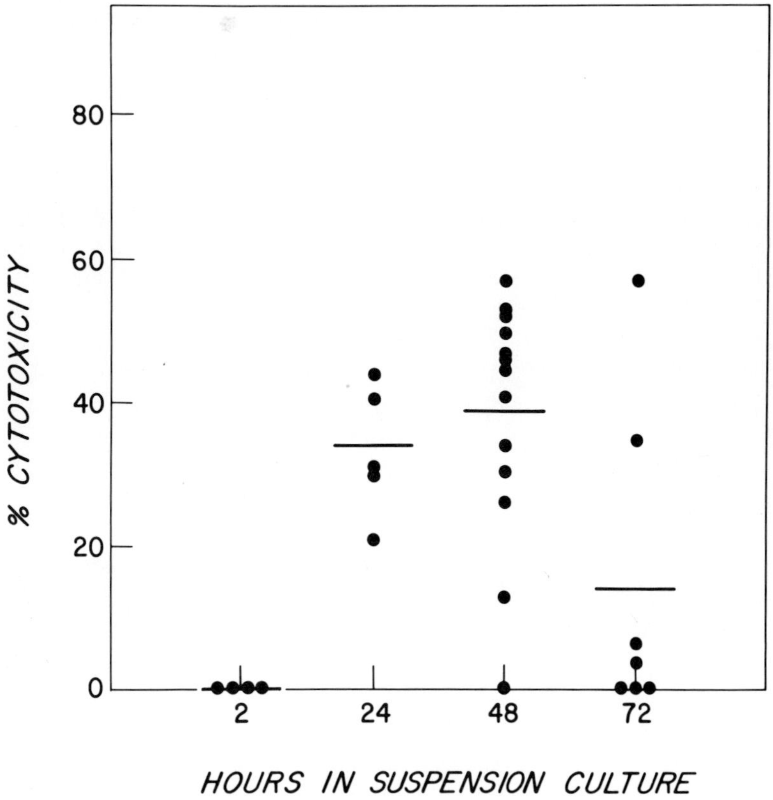

Figure 2

What is known about the physicochemical characteristics of MAF? When assessed in terms of enhancing macrophage ability to kill tumors, or of macrophage sticking, or of enhancement of glucose oxidation, MAF elutes in the same fractions which contain MIF and several other mediators in the range between 68,000-25,000 daltons (9). When MAF is assessed in terms of enhanced adherence or glucose oxidation, it is destroyed by neuraminidase, which also destroys MIF but not chemotactic factor or lymphotoxin, and is recovered after isopycnic centrifugation on CsCl is a band with a buoyant density slightly greater than albumin, as in MIF but not the other two mediators (36). In preliminary studies in collaboration with H. Remold, MAF, as assessed by its ability to enhance macrophage tumor cytotoxicity, has the same pI as MIF on isoelectric focusing. It is of interest that human MAF as assessed by ability to enhance cell adherence and glucose oxidation has the same size as human MIF, and differs from human chemotactic factor, lymphotoxin and leukocyte inhibitory factor (LIF) in this respect (37-39). Thus, at present, there is an increasing amount of evidence that suggests that MAF and MIF are the same, but more studies will be required to be certain about this.

It is of interest at this juncture to compare tumor killing by activated macrophages with killing by "armed macrophages." Evans and Alexander described cytotoxicity by macrophages armed with a product of activated lymphocytes called "specific macrophage arming factor" or SMAF (40). SMAF has the following characteristics: It is a product of thymus-dependent lymphocytes stimulated by antigen (41,42). SMAF produced by stimulating specifically immune lymphocytes with one tumor specifically arms macrophages to kill that tumor but not others. SMAF produced by stimulating sensitive lymphocytes with antigen unrelated to the tumor target usually requires the presence of that specific antigen to arm the macrophage for cytotoxicity (43). The arming factor is cytophilic, i.e., it can render macrophages cytotoxic after short periods of incubation and is absorbed out by the macrophages. It can also be absorbed out by the specific tumor used to produce it. It has been postulated that it may be a cytotoxic receptor shed into the culture medium by activated lymphocytes (42) or a cytophilic antibody (44). Trypsinization of armed macrophages abolishes their cytotoxic capacity (44,45).

It is clear from the above that the mechanism of SMAF is different from that involved in macrophage activation by MAF. In the latter, mediators induced by antigens not cross-reacting with the tumor antigen are effective and the antigen need not be present. MAF is not cytophilic, and further, trypsinization of activated macrophages does not alter their cytotoxic capabilities. There must exist at least two different mechanisms by which normal macrophages can be rendered cytotoxic for tumor cells, one by "arming" and one by "activation."

In addition to specific killing by armed macrophages, direct T cell mediated cytotoxicity is also specific (46,47). *In vivo*, both specific killing and nonspecific immunity have been reported. A classical requirement for specificity is seen in studies of G. Klein who showed that an immune mouse would reject a lymphoma to which it was immune but not an antigenically different lymphoma mixed in the inoculum (48,49). On the other hand, with the hepatoma system, nonspecific immunity can be demonstrated: when two antigenically unrelated hepatomas are injected together into an animal immune to only one, both tumors fail to grow (50). Thus, it would appear that the degree of specificity or nonspecificity of tumor killing will depend on the type of tumor and on the predominant type of cellular immune mechanisms that are operating.

ACKNOWLEDGEMENTS

This work was supported by U.S. Public Health Grants AI-07685, AI-10921, and Contract NIH-N01-CB-33896.

REFERENCES

1. Metchnikoff, E. (1905). *Immunity in Infective Disease.* Cambridge Univ. Press, London and New York.

2. Lurie, M. B. (1964). *Resistance to Tuberculosis: Experimental Studies in Native and Acquired Defensive Mechanisms.* Harvard Univ. Press, Cambridge, Massachusetts.

3. Suter, E. and H. Ramseier (1964). Cellular reactions in infection. *Adv. Immunol. 4*:117-173.

4. Mackaness, G. B. (1964). The immunological basis of acquired cellular resistance. *J. Exp. Med. 120*:105-120.

5. Mackaness, G. B. (1969). The influence of immunologically committed lymphoid cell on macrophage activity *in vivo. J. Exp. Med. 129*:973-992.

6. Lane, F. C. and E. R. Unanue (1972). Requirement of thymus (T) lymphocytes for resistance to Listeriosis. *J. Exp. Med. 135*:1104-1112.

7. David, J. R. (1966). Delayed hypersensitivity *in vitro*. Its mediation by cell-free substances formed by lymphoid cell-antigen interaction. *Proc. Nat. Acad. Sci., Wash. 56*:72-77.

8. Bloom, B. R. and B. Bennett (1966). Mechanism of a reaction *in vitro* associated with delayed-type hypersensitivity. *Science 153*:80-82.

9. Churchill, W. H., Jr., W. F. Piessens, C. A. Sulis and J. R. David (1975). Macrophages activated as suspension cultures with lymphocyte mediators devoid of antigen become cytotoxic for tumor cells. *J. Immunol. 115*:781-786.

10. Remold, H. G., A. B. Katz, E. Haber and J. R. David (1970). Studies on migration inhibitory factor (MIF). Recovery of MIF activity after purification by gel filtration and disc electrophoresis. *Cellular Immunol. 1*:133-145.

11. Remold, H. G., R. A. David and J. R. David (1972). Characterization of migration inhibitory factor (MIF) from guinea pig lymphocytes stimulated with concanavalin A. *J. Immunol. 109*:578-586.

12. Rocklin, R. E., C. T. Winston and J. R. David (1974). Activation of human blood monocytes by products of sensitized lymphocytes. *J. Clin. Invest. 53*:559-564.

13. Mooney, J. J. and B. H. Waksman (1970). Activation of normal rabbit macrophage monolayers by supernatants of antigen-stimulated lymphocytes. *J. Immunol. 105*:1138-1145.

14. Nathan, C. F., M. L. Karnovsky and J. R. David (1971). Alterations of macrophage functions by mediators from lymphocytes. *J. Exp. Med. 133*:1356-1376.

15. David, J. R. and E. Haber (1969). Delayed hypersensitivity *in vitro*. Preliminary fractionation of a soluble migration inhibitory factor formed by antigen-stimulated lymphocytes. *Cellular Recognition. 4th Developmental Workshop 1968.* Appleton-Century-Crofts, New York.

16. Fauve, R. M. and D. Dekaris (1968). Macrophage spreading. Inhibition in delayed hypersensititivy. *Science 160*:795-796.

17. Salvin, S. B., S. Sell and J. Nishio (1971). Activity *in vitro* of lymphocytes and macrophages in delayed hypersensitivity. *J. Immunol. 107*:655-662.

18. Remold, H. G. and A. Mednis (1972). Alterations of macrophage lysosomal enzyme levels induced by MIF-rich supernatants from lymphocytes. *Fed. Proc. 31*:753.

19. Neta, R. and S. B. Salvin (1971). Cellular immunity *in vivo*: Migration inhibition and phagocytosis. *Infec. Immunity 4*:697-702.

20. Hoff, R. (1975). Macrophage killing of *Trypanosoma cruzi. J. Exp. Med. 142*:299-311.

21. Meade, C. J., P. J. Lachmann and S. Brenner (1974). A sensitive assay for cellular hypersensitivity based on the uptake of radioactive colloidal gold. *Immunology 27*:227-239.

22. Remold-O'Donnell, E. and H. G. Remold (1974). The enhancement of macrophage adenylate cyclase by products of stimulated lymphocytes. *J. Biol. Chem. 249*:3622-3627.

23. Hammond, M. E. and H. F. Dvorak (1972). Antigen-induced stimulation of glucosamine incorporation by guinea pig peritoneal macrophages in delayed hypersensitivity. *J. Exp. Med. 136*:1518-1532.

24. Dvorak, A. M., M. E. Hammond, H. F. Dvorak and M. J. Karnovsky (1972). Loss of cell surface material from peritoneal exudate cells associated with lymphocyte-mediated inhibition of macrophage migration from capillary tubes. *Lab. Invest. 27*:561-574.

25. Remold, H. G. and A. Mednis. Decrease of three lysosomal enzymes in guinea pig macrophages activated by lymphocyte mediators. *Inflammation,* in press.

26. Wahl, L., S. M. Wahl, S. E. Mergenhagen and G. R. Martin (1975). Collagenase production by lymphokine-activated macrophages. *Science 187*:261-263.

27. Fowles, R. E., I. M. Fajardo, J. L. Leibowitch and J. R. David (1973). The enhancement of macrophage bacteriostasis by products of activated lymphocytes. *J. Exp. Med. 138*:952-964.

28. Patterson, R. J. and G. P. Youmans (1970). Demonstration in tissue culture of lymphocyte-mediated immunity to tuberculosis. *Infec. Immun. 1*:600-603.

29. Godal, T., R. J. W. Rees and J. O. Lamvik (1971). Lymphocyte-mediated modification of blood-derived macrophage function *in vitro;* inhibition of growth of intracellular Mycobacteria lesprae with lymphokines. *Clin. Exp. Immunol. 8*:625-637.

30. Krahenbuhl, J. L. and J. S. Remington (1971). *In vitro* induction of nonspecific resistance in macrophages by specifically sensitized lymphocytes. *Infec. Immunity 4*:337-343.

31. Anderson, S. E. and J. S. Remington (1974). Effect of normal and activated human macrophages on *Toxoplasma gondii. J. Exp. Med. 139*:1154-1174.

32. Rapp, H., W. H. Churchill, B. S. Kronman, R. T. Rolley, W. G. Hammond and T. Borsos (1968). Antigenicity of a new diethylnitrosamine-induced transplantable guinea pig hepatoma: Pathology and formation of ascites variant. *J. Natl. Cancer Inst. 41*:1-11.

33. Piessens, W. F., W. H. Churchill and J. R. David (1975). Macrophages activated *in vitro* with lymphocyte mediators kill neoplastic but not normal cells. *J. Immunol. 114*:293-299.

34. Hibbs, J. B. (1972). Activated macrophage immunologic recognition. Target cell factors related to contact inhibition. *Science 180*:868-870.

35. Hibbs, J. B., L. H. Lambert and J. S. Remington (1972). Control of carcinogenesis: A possible role for activated macrophages. *Science 177*:998-1000.

36. Nathan, C. F., H. G. Remold and J. R. David (1973). Characterization of a lymphocyte function which alters macrophage function. *J. Exp. Med. 137*:275-290.

37. Kolb, W. P. and G. A. Granger (1968). Characterization of human lymphotoxin. *Proc. Nat. Acad. Sci., Wash. 61*:1250-1255.

38. Altman, L. C., R. Snyderman and J. J. Oppenheim (1973). A human mononuclear leukocyte chemotactic factor: Characterization, specificity and kinetics of production by homologous leukocytes. *J. Immunol. 110*:801-810.

39. Rocklin, R. E. (1974). Products of activated lymphocytes: Leukocyte inhibitory factor (LIF) distinct from migration inhibitory factor (MIF). *J. Immunol. 112*:1461-1466.

40. Evans, R. and P. Alexander (1970). Cooperation of immune lymphoid cells with macrophages in tumor immunity. *Nature (Lond.) 228*:620-622.

41. Evans, R., C. K. Grant, H. Cox, K. Steele and P. Alexander (1972). Thymus derived lymphocytes produce an immunologically specific macrophage-arming factor. *J. Exp. Med. 136*:1318-1322.

42. Lohmann-Matthes, M. L., F. G. Zigler and H. Fischer (1973). Macrophage cytotoxicity factor. A product of *in vitro* sensitized thymus dependent cells. *Eur. J. Immunol. 3*:56-68.

43. Evans, R., H. Cox and P. Alexander (1973). Immunologically specific activation of macrophages armed with the specific macrophage arming factor (SMAF). *Proc. Soc. Exp. Biol. Med. 143*:256-259.

44. Pels, E. and W. Den Otter (1974). The role of a cytophilic factor from challenged immune peritoneal lymphocytes in specific macrophage cytotoxicity. *Cancer Res. 34*:3089-3094.

45. Lohmann-Matthes, M. L., H. Schipper and H. Fischer (1972). Macrophage-mediated cytotoxicity against allogeneic target cells *in vitro*. *Eur. J. Immunol.* 2:45-49.

46. Cerottini, J. C., A. A. Nordin and K. T. Brunner (1970). Specific *in vitro* cytotoxicity of thymus-derived lymphocytes sensitized to alloantigens. *Nature 228*:1308-1309.

47. Henney, C. S. (1974). Mechanisms of cytolysis by thymus-derived lymphocytes. Implications in tumor immunity. *Progr. Exp. Tumor Res.* Karger, Basel. pp. 203-216.

48. Klein, G. and E. Klein (1956). Genetic studies of the relationship of tumour-host cells. *Nature 178*:1389-1391.

49. Klein, E. and G. Klein (1972). Specificity of homograft rejection *in vivo* assessed by inoculation of artificially mixed compatible and incompatible tumor cells. *Cell. Immunol. 5*:201-208.

50. Zbar, B., T. Wepsic, T. Borsos and H. J. Rapp (1970). Tumor graft rejection in syngeneic guinea pigs: Evidence for a two-step mechanism. *J. Natl. Cancer Inst. 44*:473-481.

DISCUSSION

Dolph O. Adams, Chairman

The mechanisms producing tumor-induced depression of monocyte chemotaxis were extensively discussed. Snyderman suggested sequestration of mononuclear phagocytes within tumors was not responsible, since peripheral monocyte counts of the tumor bearing animals were not significantly altered. He emphasized the depression was tumor-specific, in that tumors produced the effect while neither large allografts nor extensive pneumococcal pneumonia could. Synderman pointed out that the chemotactic depression, produced by one hour of incubation with sonicates of the tumors, could be reversed by vigorous washing of the monocytes. The failure to achieve such reversal by washing human monocytes might be ascribed to their prolonged contact with an inhibitor *in vivo*. Tumor antigens were thought an unlikely candidate for the inhibitor, whose molecular weight was less than 10,000. It was suggested that recognition of the tumor by serum substances, such as recognition factor or cytophilic antibody, might mediate the chemotactic attraction of macrophages.

The significance of the chemotactic depression in humans was considered at length. Snyderman stated that preliminary observations indicated an inhibitor of chemotaxis was present in the sera of many tumor bearing patients. He suggested such an inhibitor, rather than a lack of chemotactic factor, could account for the depression of chemotaxis and for the depression of the MLC reaction in tumor bearing patients (mediated by generalized depression of macrophage function). It was pointed out that tumor cells produce both chemotactic factors and inhibitors of chemotaxis and could thus potentially enhance or depress mononuclear chemotaxis. Snyderman concurred and noted that in his study only extremely-high or extremely-low levels of chemotactic ability offered any clue to patient prognosis (both indicating a poor outcome).

Initial discussion of Gershon's presentation* centered on the cellular mechanisms involved in murine delayed-hypersensitivity. Gershon stressed the obligate role of T-cells, by pointing out delayed responses were conferred upon naive mice only by transfers of theta-positive cells. He supported the contention that basophils were not involved, by observing that mice possess

*Editor's Note: Dr. Gershon presented a paper during Session II but did not submit a manuscript for publication in this volume.

very few basophils. A lively comparison of basophils and mast cells followed, emphasizing that basophils were marrow-derived granulocytes while mast cells were mesenchymal elements (see *Prog. Immunol. II 3*:171, 1974). These observations led to the prediction that strains of mice giving good delayed responses in the flank should have large numbers of mast cells there (see *Adv. Immunol. 20*:197, 1975). In conclusion, Gershon pointed out that the interaction *in vivo* between antigen T-cells, mast cells, and monocytes to produce delayed responses was a minimal model and that other cells, such as regulator T-cells, might also be involved.

The precise pharmacologic mediators involved and the potential of interaction with the sympathetic nervous system were considered. Gershon pointed out that, while these questions were still to be resolved, the data to date did clearly indicate that mediators such as vasoactive amines were involved in mononuclear inflammatory responses. Since injection of serotonin into the footpads of sensitized mice blocked delayed swelling, he suggested temporary refractoriness of the endothelial cells to vasoactive amines produced this effect and noted he had not been able to demonstrate serotonin receptors on murine T-cells.

The conferees pointed out several other immune responses *in vivo*, where mast cells might play an important role. For example, mice adoptively immunized against *Listeria monocytogenese* expressed strong cellular resistance to an intravenous challenge of bacteria but not to an aerosol challenge unless inflammation had been previously induced in the lungs. Likewise, the tumoricidal effects of Lentinan were stated to depend upon both T-cell function and alterations in vasoactive amines. It was suggested that Gershon's model of delayed sensitivity involving mast cells might explain the prevalence of specific rejection responses in mice, as opposed to the prevalence of nonspecific rejection responses in other species such as the guinea pig.

David first discussed the role of cyclic nucleotides in the regulation of migration-inhibition, pointing out that the stimulation of cAMP blocked the effect of MIF (i.e., lead to normal degrees of migration). He added that Higgins had not found depressed levels of cyclic AMP within macrophages treated with MIF.

Vigorous discussion on the nature of the activated macrophage ensued. Several conferees noted that activated macrophages of cellular resistance and stimulated macrophages of various sorts generally had an increased content of acid hydrolases. David pointed out that the number of granules within the macrophages increased considerably, though the biochemical content of three lysosomal enzymes was depressed in his system. Amos indicated that the macrophages of rejecting murine tumors contained macrophages richly-laden with acid phosphatase, while immunologically-enhanced (progressing) tumors contained macrophages bearing little phosphatase. David emphasized the paradoxical nature of these observations and stated that, in his experimental system, the lysosomal enzymes were neither unstable, inhibited, nor leaked into the medium. He pointed out that the macrophages of guinea pigs differed considerably from those of mice in both elicitation and behavior in culture. It was pointed out that certain eliciting agents, thioglycolate and perhaps casein as well, were retained within elicited macrophages and could thus serve as lysosomal "sinks," into which newly-synthesized lysosomes could be poured and destroyed. Other disassociations between lysosomal content and macrophage function were pointed out, as typified by cellular resistance to *Salmonella,* where macrophages had essentially no acid phosphatase but expressed vigorous antimicrobial function. It was then emphasized that macrophage lysosomes were dynamic, increasing or decreasing rapidly depending on endocytic events and external stimulants. The conferees pointed out that macrophages stimulated in various ways could differ significantly in function and that reliable biochemical markers to distinguish these various modes of stimulation and various alterations in functions were needed.

Papermaster discussed some of his current work on macrophage activating factors (MAF). These were partially purified from the supernatant culture

Effect of α-2 Macroglobulin on Adherent Murine Peritoneal Cells in an In Vitro Cytotoxicity Assay Against Syngeneic L1210 Target Cells

	% Cytotoxicity (±95% Confidence Limits)
1. ^{3}H L1210 cells in culture medium only	
2. ^{3}H L1210 adherent cells only in medium	8 ± 5
3. Adherent peritoneal cells cultured for three days with α-2 macroglobulin from fresh medium (1.0 mg/ml)	8 ± 5
4. Adherent peritoneal cell cultured for three days with G-200 void volume peak from culture supernate of cell line 1788 (0.06 mg/ml)	26 ± 12
5. Adherent peritoneal cells cultured for three days with α-2 macroglobulin from 1788 culture supernate (0.03 mg/ml)	27 ± 10

Acid Phosphatase Activity of Murine Peritoneal Cells Stimulated by Culture for 3 Days with Partially Purified MAF-Containing Fractions

	Acid Phosphatase μM/10^6 cells/60 min × 10^{-6}
α-2 macroglobulin from control culture medium	0.64
α-2 macroglobulin from 1788 culture medium	1.64

medium of the long-term human lymphoid cell line RPMI 1788 by gel filtration on Sephadex G-200 and preparative acrylamide slab gel electrophoresis. Macrophage activation properties were shown to be associated with α-2 macroglobulin isolated from the cell culture medium in two assays utilizing *in vitro* activation: 1) cytotoxicity in an adherent population of DBA/2 mouse peritoneal cells against the syngeneic L1210 lymphoma, and 2) measurement of acid phosphatase in adherent cells.

The level of acid phosphatase was raised in the macrophages activated by cultured lymphoid cell fractions. The fact that these macrophages were activated, but not phagocytosing, at the time of measurement may account for the level of acid phosphatase increasing to, at most, four-fold over background levels. Further work will be necessary before definitive positive or negative correlation can be established between enzyme levels and macrophage activity, and particularly for the role of macrophage lysosomal hydrolases in tumor cell toxicity.

It should be emphasized that the MAF activity associated with α-2 macroglobulin was acquired during incubation with cultured lymphoid cells, since human serum albumin and α-2 macroglobulin from fresh culture medium or normal serum were inactive in our assays. The results suggest that α-2 macroglobulin may act as serum carriers for mediators of cellular immunity. (See Papermaster, B. W., O. A. Holtermann, E. Klein, S. Parmett, D. Dobkin, R. Laudico and I. Djerassi, *Clin. Immunol. Immunopathol.*, in press; and McDaniel, M. C., R. Laudico, and B. W. Papermaster, *Clin. Immunol. Immunopathol.*, in press). Supported in part by DHEW 1PO1 CA 16964-01 and DHEW 5SO1 RR 05427-12.

SESSION III

Mechanisms of Macrophage Mediated Cytotoxicity

Chairman: D. Bernard Amos

THE MACROPHAGE AS A TUMORICIDAL EFFECTOR CELL: A REVIEW OF *IN VIVO* AND *IN VITRO* STUDIES ON THE MECHANISM OF THE ACTIVATED MACROPHAGE NONSPECIFIC CYTOTOXIC REACTION*

John B. Hibbs, Jr., M.D.

INTRODUCTION

In vitro studies have demonstrated that macrophages can destroy target cells by both specific and nonspecific cytotoxic mechanisms (for reviews see references 1-3). Do specific or nonspecific cytotoxic mechanisms have significance in the control of neoplastic growth in animals? A conclusive answer to this question is still elusive and must await more time and much work in many laboratories. The purpose of this paper is to review the work of several investigators focusing on the nonspecific tumoricidal effect of activated macrophages and to make a case for the possible role of the activated macrophage cytotoxicity system in the economy of metazoans.

To acquire nonspecific tumoricidal potential, normal macrophages must undergo functional modification.

Normal mouse peritoneal macrophages are not tumoricidal under usual or unstressed physiologic conditions as determined by their interaction with tumor cells *in vitro* (4). Indeed, modification of macrophage function is a fundamental aspect of the development of tumoricidal potential by activated macrophages. Our early studies demonstrated that chronic infection with a variety of phylogenetically unrelated micro-organisms including *Toxoplasma gondii, Besnoitia jellisoni, Listeria monocytogenes,* and Bacillus Calmette-Guérin (BCG) induced in mice a population of activated peritoneal macro-

*This work was supported by the Veterans Administration, Washington, D.C., and by National Institutes of Health Grants CA14045 and CA15811.

phages that were tumoricidal when tested *in vitro* (4-8). These results suggested that stimuli induced by the host reaction to infection were important in the acquisition of tumoricidal potential by activated macrophages.

Independently, Alexander and Evans, as well as Keller and Jones, provided similar experimental evidence showing that tumoricidal activated macrophages were produced in response to heterologous inducing agents—endotoxin or polyinosinic-polycytidylic acid (poly I:C) and the nematode, *Nippostrongylus brasiliensis,* respectively (9,10). It has since been shown that the administration of other agents to experimental animals will likewise induce the mobilization of a population of activated macrophages that are nonspecifically cytotoxic for tumor cells *in vitro*. Included are complete Freund's adjuvant (6), allogeneic tumor cells (11), *Corynebacterium parvum* (12), *Corynebacterium granulosum* (13), and pyran copolymer (14).

In the mouse at least, merely inducing a sterile inflammatory exudate in the peritoneal cavity with agents such as starch, mineral oil, thioglycollate, or peptone is not sufficient stimulus to convert macrophages into tumoricidal cells (4,15-17). This suggests a requirement for a specific chemical signal(s), produced in response to the inducing agent, which mediates the acquisition of the cytotoxic state by macrophages. The work of Piessens and his colleagues has helped us to functionally bridge the gap between the inducing agent and the recruitment of a population of tumoricidal activated macrophages by providing experimental evidence of a source for the chemical signal (18). These workers demonstrated that normal guinea pig macrophages become cytotoxic for syngeneic tumor cells after they have been activated *in vitro* by mediator-rich supernatants prepared from lymphocytes sensitized to an antigen unrelated to the tumor cells.

Under certain circumstances host cells other than T-lymphocytes may be the source of mediators inducing tumoricidal activated macrophages. For example, Kaplan *et al.* have shown that pyran copolymer can induce tumor regression and a population of cytotoxic activated macrophages in thymectomized, irradiated, bone-marrow-reconstituted mice (14). In addition, BCG administration to athymic nude mice has induced the regression of tumor xenographs (19), also suggesting that macrophage activation occurred in the absence of functional T-lymphocytes.

A possible conclusion to be drawn from these results is that other cells, in addition to T-lymphocytes, produce the mediator that converts normal macrophages to tumoricidal activated macrophages. A recent report by Chess *et al.* (20) suggests that this may be the case. These workers demonstrated that sensitized B-lymphocytes stimulated with specific antigen secreted large amounts of migration inhibitory factor (MIF). If MIF and the mediator which induces the potential for nonspecific macrophage tumoricidal activity are identical, this finding would explain why T-lymphocyte-depleted mice can be induced to express nonspecific tumor resistance.

Finally, Fidler has shown that normal macrophages, as well as macrophages from tumor bearing mice, can be converted into cytotoxic activated macrophages by mediators released from sensitized syngeneic, allogeneic, or xenogeneic lymphocytes *in vitro* (21).

The maintenance of nonspecific tumoricidal potential by activated macrophages during prolonged in vitro culture requires interaction between inducing antigen and sensitized lymphocytes.

When mice are infected with BCG or toxoplasma by the intraperitoneal route, a chronic infection is established. Mediators produced by the ongoing interaction between BCG or toxoplasma antigens with sensitized lymphocytes in the peritoneal cavity induce and maintain a population of activated macrophages. When activated macrophages are removed from the peritoneal cavity of mice with chronic BCG infection, they are isolated from the mediator-rich environment. In order to express a significant nonspecific cytotoxic effect *in vitro* they must be challenged with tumor cells within 24 hours of being placed in culture. For example, within 48-72 hours of *in vitro* culture the macrophages from BCG-infected mice are no longer cytotoxic for tumor cells (22). It seems reasonable to assume that this lack of cytotoxicity is due to withdrawal of the mediator that induces and maintains the activated state. To test this we added purified peritoneal lymphocytes to the macrophages plus specific antigen (tuberculin protein) and removed nonadherent cells as well as antigen prior to tumor cell challenge. Results showed that if macrophages were in contact with specific antigen and sensitized lymphocytes, they retained significant cytotoxic effect (22). Tuberculin protein alone or sensitized lymphocytes alone were not effective. This suggests a need for the interaction of specific antigen and sensitized lymphocytes to maintain cytotoxic activated macrophages for prolonged periods in culture and is compatible with the notion that a lymphocyte-derived mediator induces and maintains the nonspecific cytotoxic potential of activated macrophages as has been suggested by the study of Piessens *et al.* (18).

Nonspecific tumor resistance tends to be restricted anatomically because the inducing agent or antigen is not a structural component of the tumor. It is expressed when the heterologous inducing agent, the cytotoxic activated macrophages mobilized in response to the heterologous inducing agent, and the tumor graft are in intimate contact in the same anatomical compartment.

The studies of Zbar *et al.* showed that the nonspecific rejection of syngeneic tumor grafts in guinea pigs requires several steps (23-24). Recognition, the first step, resides in sensitized lymphocytes and is specific, but tumor cell destruction, the second step, is nonspecific. These investigators demonstrated that close contact among sensitized cells, sensitizing antigen, and the antigenically unrelated tumor cells was required to suppress nonspecifically the growth of antigenically unrelated tumor cells.

Subsequently, we provided strong circumstantial evidence that the nonspecific component in mediating tumor resistance in mice is due to a population of activated macrophages (4-6,25). A more recent investigation has further defined the requirements for the *in vivo* expression of nonspecific resistance and has provided further evidence that the nonspecific effector cell in the expression of this resistance is the cytotoxic activated macrophage (22,26).

We found that there is a requirement for local persistence of inducing antigen for the continued presence of a population of cytotoxic activated macrophages in an anatomical compartment, e.g., in mice high levels of BCG tend to remain localized in the anatomical compartment(s) into which they were administered. Likewise, the presence of cytotoxic activated macrophages in the tissue tends to be a local phenomenon, also confined to the anatomical compartment(s) that contain high levels of inducing antigen (22) (See Table 1).

TABLE 1.
Correlation of BCG in peritoneal lymph nodes with the in vitro cytotoxic effect of peritoneal macrophages and resistance to i.p. grafts of S180

Group	Route of administration of BCG[c]	Colonies of BCG cultured from peritoneal lymph nodes[a]	Cytotoxic effect of peritoneal macrophages for 3T12 target cells[b]	Result of i.p. graft of 4 × 10^5 S180 cells; No. of mice dead of tumor growth/ No. of mice tested
A	Control	0	0	20/20
B	BCG i.p.	3 to 4+	4+	9/20 (P<0.001)
C	BCG i.v.	0 to 1+	0	20/20
D	BCG i.m.R.	0 to 1+	0	19/20

[a]Quantitation of BCG growth: 0, no growth; 1+, 1–5 colonies per Petri dish; 2+, 6–20 colonies per Petri dish; 3+, 21–50 colonies per Petri dish; 4+, 51–100 colonies per Petri dish.

[b]Cytotoxic effect of macrophages for 3T12 cells: 0, multilayer of 3T12 cells among macrophages (no cytotoxic or cytostatic effect); 1+, patchy areas of confluent 3T12 growth among macrophages (slight cytostatic effect); 2+, 10–20 3T12 cells per 430× field among macrophages (cytostatic effect); 3+, 3–9 3T12 cells per 430× field among macrophages (cytotoxic effect); 4+, 2 or fewer 3T12 cells per 430× field among macrophages (marked cytotoxic effect). The results are given as the range obtained from three separately performed experiments.

[c]Intraperitoneal (i.p.), intravenous (i.v.), and right gastrocnemius muscle (i.m.R).

For example, the number of viable BCG organisms present in the peritoneal cavity was related to the route of BCG administration. Between 21 and 100 BCG colonies were cultured from peritoneal lymph nodes from mice receiving BCG intraperitoneally, while none of the mice that received BCG in the right gastrocnemius muscle or by the lateral tail vein grew more than two colonies of BCG from peritoneal lymph nodes. Furthermore, *in vitro* cytotoxicity test results showed that mice infected with BCG by the intraperitoneal route had peritoneal macrophages that were highly cytotoxic to tumorigenic cells, while peritoneal macrophages from mice infected with BCG by the lateral tail vein or in the right gastrocnemius muscle were not cytotoxic. In this same study we also noted that the *in vivo* expression of nonspecific resistance to tumor growth in the peritoneal cavity correlated with the presence of high levels of inducing antigen (BCG) and with activated macrophages with nonspecific cytotoxic effect for tumorigenic cells *in vitro.*

In nonspecific tumor cell destruction the cytotoxic activated macrophages induced by a heterologous antigen, e.g., BCG or toxoplasma, were present in the tissues before grafting the tumor cells and could be detected after the tumor cells had been rejected (22). This continuing presence may be due to the fact that the specific antigen (BCG or toxoplasma) which induced the production of cytotoxic activated macrophages remains in the tissues and provides a continuing stimulus for elaboration of a chemical signal that maintains macrophage activation.

Specific tumor resistance is not restricted anatomically and is expressed regardless of the location of the graft because the inducing antigen is a structural component of the tumor target. However, cytotoxic activated macrophages are restricted to the anatomical compartment(s) containing high levels of inducing antigen.

In contrast to our results with the induction of nonspecific resistance with BCG, the specific rejection of lymphoma L1210 cells was not restricted anatomically. CBA mice immunized with L1210 cells i.m.R rejected secondary L1210 grafts (2×10^7 cells) i.p., as can be seen in Table 2.

We noted that the specific rejection of secondary grafts of the allogeneic L1210 lymphoma in immunized CBA mice (inducing antigens are present on the lymphoma cell surface) produces activated macrophages with nonspecific cytotoxic effect for antigenically unrelated SV_{40} transformed W1-38 cells. However, we found that the nonspecifically cytotoxic activated macrophages rapidly revert to normal when the antigen that induced their mobilization (allogeneic L1210 cells) is cleared from the tissues and are not cytotoxic for tumorigenic 3T12 cells which share common $H\text{-}2^d$ antigens. It is important to note that the population of cytotoxic activated macrophages was confined to the anatomical compartment containing the inducing antigen (the tumor

TABLE 2.
Correlation of the presence of viable L1210 cells in the peritoneal cavity of CBA mice with the cytotoxic effect of peritoneal macrophages in vitro

Group	Site of primary L1210 graft	Site of secondary L1210 graft	Time interval between secondary L1210 graft and collection of peritoneal cells for the cytotoxicity test (hr)	Cytotoxic effect[a]	
				3T12	VA-13
A	i.m.R	i.p.	24	4+	4+
B	i.m.R	i.p.	48	4+	4+
C	i.m.R	i.p.	72	2 to 3+	2 to 3+
D	i.m.R	i.p.	96	0	0
E	i.m.R	i.m.R	24	0	0
F	i.m.R	i.m.R	48	0	0
G	i.m.R	i.m.R	72	0	0
H	i.m.R	–	–	0	0
I	L1210 i.p.[b]	–	–	0	0
J	–	–	–	0	0

[a]See footnotes to Table 1 for interpretation of symbols used.

[b]The primary immunizing dose of L1210 cells was 2×10^6.

allograft). When the secondary graft of L1210 cells was administered i.m.R, cytotoxic activated macrophages did not appear in the peritoneal cavity (See Table 2).

It is interesting that activated macrophages with nonspecific cytotoxic effect for tumor cells comprise 70 to 85 percent of the peritoneal exudate cells in CBA mice 48-72 hours after a secondary graft of L1210 cells (Hibbs, unpublished data). These results clearly show that activated macrophages with nonspecific cytotoxic effect for tumorigenic cells are produced in large numbers during the specific rejection of allogeneic lymphoma cells in mice. Whether or not cytotoxic activated macrophages are significant effector cells in clearing allogeneic L1210 cells from the tissues was not determined in this study. Other effector mechanisms are certainly not excluded and it is probable that they have a major role in the destruction of L1210 cells in immunized allogeneic mice.

To summarize up to this point, it is our opinion that activated macrophages participate as cytotoxic effector cells in both nonspecific and specific tumor destruction. A major difference between the two mechanisms of tumor resistance is the source of the stimulus for lymphocytes to produce a mediator that converts normal macrophages into cytotoxic activated macrophages. In nonspecific tumor resistance the inducing agent is unrelated (BCG, toxoplasma, etc.), and in specific tumor resistance it is an antigen specific to the tumor.

Significant points include:

1. Injected inducing agent or antigen tends to remain in the anatomical compartment into which it was injected.
2. Cytotoxic activated macrophages also tend to be local. They are found in the same anatomical compartment as the inducing antigen and are associated with the expression of both nonspecific and specific tumor resistance.
3. Cytotoxic activated macrophages disappear in parallel with the clearance of inducing antigen from the tissues. In nonspecific tumor resistance the heterologous inducing antigen and the cytotoxic activated macrophages can still be detected after a tumor graft has been nonspecifically rejected by the host. However, in specific tumor resistance since the antigen inducing the cytotoxic macrophages is a component of the tumor cell, the population of cytotoxic activated macrophages disappears after the inducing antigen (tumor cell) is removed from the tissues by the host response.
4. There appears to be a requirement for a mediator produced by the interaction between sensitized lymphocytes and specific antigen to maintain a state of macrophage activation *in vitro*. This may be analogous to the *in vivo* situations described above.
5. The host response could be viewed as a focusing and amplifying process for mobilization of cytotoxic activated macrophages. If this is the case, the tumor target cell will be less likely to escape destruction if the antigen inducing the mobilization is a component of the tumor cell. However, if the heterologous inducing agent has immunologic adjuvant action, in addition to the ability to directly recruit cytotoxic activated macrophages, then increased sensitization to tumor antigens may occur. In this case, lymphocytes sensitized to tumor antigens will cooperate with lymphocytes secreting mediator in response to the heterogous inducing agent and markedly improve the focusing and amplifying of mobilization of cytotoxic activated macrophages in areas of tumor growth.

Neoplastic cells are destroyed by cytotoxic activated macrophages under in vitro conditions in which nonneoplastic target cells are spared and grow to confluency.

In our initial studies we made the observation that the cytotoxic effect of activated macrophages was selective (4). Activated peritoneal macrophages from mice with chronic toxoplasma, besnoitia, listeria, or BCG infection did not destroy contact-inhibited allogeneic fibroblast or kidney cell strains that have surfaces of high immunogenic potential, but were markedly cytotoxic to both syngeneic and allogeneic tumorigenic cell lines. These experiments suggest that normal cells may acquire a property in parallel with neoplastic transformation that elicits nonimmunologic recognition and subsequent destruction by activated macrophages.

To test this hypothesis, we studied the cytotoxic activity of activated mouse macrophages against mouse embryo fibroblasts before and after spontaneous transformation of the fibroblasts *in vitro* (7). We found that activated C3H HeJ macrophages did not destroy two allogeneic fibroblast cell strains differing from them at a strongly antigenic H-2 locus. In contrast, these macrophages were markedly cytotoxic for the same allogeneic fibroblasts (and also for syngeneic fibroblasts) after the fibroblasts had spontaneously developed abnormal growth properties that included loss of contact inhibition of cell division. Because H-2 antigens are more immunogenic than tumor specific transplantation antigens or fetal antigens expressed on tumor cells, this study strongly suggests that a change associated with the acquisition of abnormal growth properties by target cells, rather than a change in antigens, is responsible for the increased susceptibility of tumor cells to destruction by activated macrophages.

To show the importance of cell-surface factors in the nonimmunologic cytotoxic reaction between activated macrophages and target cells, the following cell lines were evaluated: BALB/3T3 fibroblasts (a contact-inhibited, nontumorigenic cell line), BALB/3T12 fibroblasts (a non-contact-inhibited, tumorigenic cell line from the same original pool of mouse cells as the BALB/3T3 line), and BALB/SV-3T3 fibroblasts (a non-contact-inhibited, tumorigenic cell line). The results show that under the conditions of the experiment BALB/3T3 fibroblasts were not destroyed whereas BALB/3T12 and BALB/SV-3T3 fibroblasts were destroyed by syngeneic and allogeneic activated macrophages (8). This suggests that surface alterations related to loss of contact inhibition, a property of the BALB/3T12 and BALB/SV-3T3 lines, are important factors in target cell recognition and destruction. Abnormal characteristics of the BALB/3T3 fibroblast line seeming not to be factors in nonimmunologic recognition and destruction by activated macrophages include 1) loss of normal cell morphology, 2) hypotetraploid karyotype, 3) maximum growth *in vitro* to confluency from a low inoculum, and 4) continuous multiplication *in vitro*.

These results indicate that surface modification of non-contact-inhibited cells may be so extensive that it can evoke nonimmunologic recognition and response by activated macrophages even without specific sensitization to the target cell.

The cell surface is extensively modified after loss of contact inhibition (27-32). Others working with the BALB/3T3, BALB/3T12, and BALB/SV-3T3 series of mouse fibroblasts showed that tumorigenicity (27) and cell agglutination after plant lectin binding (28) correlate with loss of contact inhibition. Likewise, we demonstrated that nonimmunologic destruction by activated macrophages is also associated with loss of contact inhibition by these target cells. All these findings may be related to extensive biochemical and topographic differences (or both) in the surface membrane of non-contact-inhibited (BALB/SV-3T3) fibroblasts.

Figure 1 shows the effect of normal and BCG-activated BALB/c macrophages on BALB/3T3 contact-inhibited fibroblasts, BALB/SV-3T3 non-contact-inhibited fibroblasts, and a mixture of the same BALB/3T3 and BALB/SV-3T3 fibroblasts (Hibbs, unpublished data). (A) No destruction of BALB/SV-3T3 cells by normal macrophages. A thick multilayer of BALB/SV-

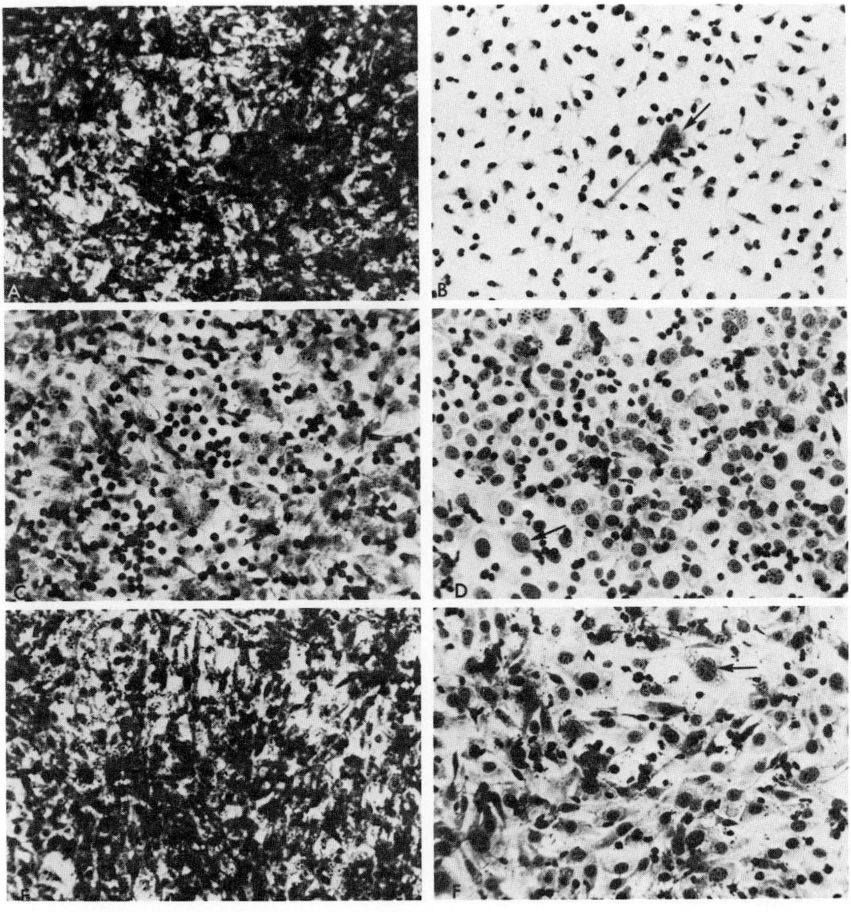

Figure 1

3T3 cells covers the normal macrophages. (B) Marked destruction of BALB/SV-3T3 fibroblasts by BCG-activated macrophages. The arrow points to the one remaining BALB/SV-3T3 cell in the microscopic field. (C) Shows a mixed monolayer of normal macrophages and BALB/3T3 fibroblasts. (D) BALB/3T3 fibroblasts are not destroyed by BCG-activated macrophages. Arrow points to a BALB/3T3 cell. Note the distinct "cobble stone" appearance of the BALB/3T3 cells. (E) A thick mixed multilayer of BALB/SV-3T3 and BALB/3T3 fibroblasts covers a monolayer of normal macrophages. (F) BCG-activated macrophages selectively destroy BALB/SV-3T3 cells when challenged with a mixture of BALB/SV-3T3 and BALB/3T3 fibroblasts. The predominant BALB/3T3 cell can be identified by its larger size and polygonal shape. Arrow points to a BALB/3T3 fibroblast.*

The observation of selective cytotoxic effect of activated macrophages for neoplastic target cells has been confirmed in several laboratories (13,14,17,18,33-35). In addition, using a mixture of neoplastic and non-neoplastic cell lines prelabeled with ^{3}H-thymidine, Meltzer *et al.* demonstrated that BCG-activated macrophages selectively destroyed neoplastic cells. The nonneoplastic cells were not affected as "innocent bystanders" (34). Meltzer and his colleagues have made an additional interesting observation using cinemicrographic analysis (35). They noted that the translational movement rate of BCG-activated macrophages among neoplastic cells was four times that observed among nonneoplastic cells. At 46 hours of *in vitro* culture, when no viable tumor cells remained, the translational movement of BCG-activated macrophages had decreased and had become identical to that observed in BCG-activated macrophages without tumor target cells. They reported that this phenomenon was not observed with normal macrophages.

Intimate cell contact appears to be an absolute requirement for the destruction of target cells by cytotoxic-activated macrophages.

We have not been able to identify a soluble cytotoxic mediator (SCM) elaborated by cytotoxic-activated macrophages. No cytopathic effect was noted when supernatant media, taken from cultures in which activated

*It is important to note that the studies reviewed here were performed in 1972 with the first group of BALB/3T3 cells supplied to us by Dr. George Todaro. However, after approximately six months of *in vivo* culture in our laboratory, these BALB/3T3 fibroblasts spontaneously lost density dependent inhibition of growth. Coincidently, we noted that they became quite susceptible to destruction by cytotoxic activated macrophages. Since then Dr. Todaro has sent us replacement BALB/3T3 cells on four occasions. We have consistently found that, unlike the first BALB/3T3 fibroblasts used in our studies, the replacement cells were all quite susceptible to destruction by cytotoxic activated macrophages when compared to normal mouse embryo fibroblasts. In addition, these replacement BALB/3T3 cells all grew to significantly higher saturation densities then the original BALB/3T3 cells.

macrophages had mediated target cell destruction, was added to target cell monolayers growing alone (4). Further studies were done to determine if evidence for an SCM could be implicated in the destruction of target cells by cytotoxic-activated macrophages (36).

Figure 2 shows a thick multilayer of tumorigenic BALB/3T12 cells surrounding a central monolayer of BCG-activated macrophages. The destruction of BALB/3T12 cells occurred only where they were in contact with activated macrophages. This is evidence that the cytotoxic mechanism does not involve a soluble SCM. To further test for a possible SCM elaborated by activated macrophages, we removed culture medium every three hours and each time replaced it with fresh medium warmed to 36.5°C. The cytotoxic effect was identical to that of control cultures (where the medium was not changed), suggesting that destruction was independent of an SCM whose effect could be diminished by dilution. To promote the thorough distribution of an SCM, we mixed the culture medium with a sterile Pasteur pipette every 60 minutes during the 72-hour incubation period. This did not interfere with BALB/3T12 cell destruction among activated macrophages, nor did it produce inhibition of BALB/3T12 cell growth on the periphery of the cover slip which was free of activated macrophages. It was also possible that an SCM was present but active only in cooperation with macrophages. To test this, we removed the supernatant medium after 24, 48, and 72 hours of incubation from monolayers of activated macrophages or from activated macrophages that had been challenged with BALB/3T12 cells. Both types of activated-macrophage-conditioned medium were added to normal macrophages that had been challenged with BALB/3T12 cells one hour earlier, and the cultures were evaluated for cytotoxic effect after a 72-hour incubation period. Activated-macrophage-conditioned medium did not render normal macrophages cytotoxic.

Other studies further underline the requirement for intimate activated macrophage target cell contact (Hibbs, unpublished data). The cytotoxicity

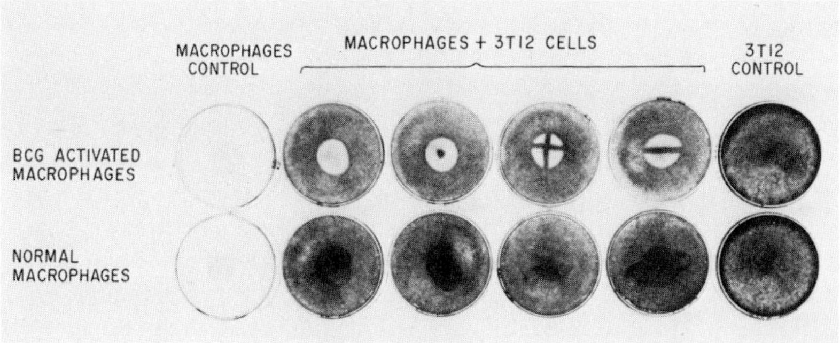

Figure 2

test was performed as previously described (36) with several minor modifications. Briefly, peritoneal cells from BCG-infected or normal BALB/c mice (6 × 10^5) in 0.1 ml of Dulbeco's modification of Eagle medium with 10 percent fetal bovine serum, streptomycin (100 μg/ml), and penicillin (100 unit/ml) (complete medium) were added to the center of 35 mm Falcon plastic petri dishes for one hour at 37°C in air with 5 percent CO_2 to allow for adherence of macrophages. Each petri dish was then washed with Hanks' balanced salt solution to remove nonadherent cells so that the central monolayer of adherent macrophages was restricted to the size of the 0.1 ml drop in which they were added to the petri dish. The peripheral portion of the petri dish remains free of macrophages. A rubber policeman was then used to remove a narrow strip of adherent macrophages from the centrally located monolayer and several varieties of macrophage-free areas were produced on different macrophage monolayers. Target cells (tumorigenic BALB/3T12 cells, 1 × 10^5) were added in 2 ml of complete medium and attached evenly to the bottom of the petri dish.

Results are shown in Figure 2. In all situations, the BALB/3T12 cells have completely overgrown and formed a multilayer over the normal macrophages. On the other hand, wherever the BALB/3T12 cells come into contact with BCG-activated macrophages, there is a marked cytotoxic effect. Furthermore, it can be seen that wherever a narrow strip of adherent macrophages was removed from the petri dish with a rubber policeman prior to BALB/3T12 cell challenge, the macrophage-free substrate is overgrown with a multilayer of target cells, even though they are surrounded by viable fully cytotoxic BCG-activated macrophages. Microscopically, the BALB/3T12 cells grew to the immediate edge of the macrophage-free areas.

In another experiment, we added peritoneal cells from BCG-infected or normal BALB/c mice (6 × 10^6) in 2 ml of complete medium. The remainder of the procedure was as described above. The difference in this experiment was that the macrophages adhered to the entire surface of the petri dish rather than to a small central area only. A rubber policeman was then used to remove adherent macrophages from two narrow strips in the macrophage monolayer, and 1 × 10^5 BALB/3T12 cells were added in 2 ml of complete medium.

Again results showed, even though there was an order of magnitude larger number of peritoneal cells added to the petri dishes, the BALB/3T12 cells formed a multilayer on the narrow strips of BCG-activated macrophage-free surface. On the other hand, BALB/3T12 cells formed a multilayer over both the normal macrophages and the areas of normal macrophage-free substrate.

Finally, we added peritoneal cells from BCG-infected or normal BALB/c mice (8 × 10^4) in 0.01 ml of complete medium using a micropipette. The macrophages were allowed to adhere as described above. Each petri dish was then washed to remove nonadherent cells so that the monolayer of macrophages was restricted to the size of the very small 0.01 ml drop in which they were added to the petri dish surface. In this case, virtually the entire surface of the petri dish is macrophage free except for the monolayer of macrophages which has the diameter of the 0.01 ml drop. The monolayer of macrophages was washed as described above to remove nonadherent cells, and 1×10^5 3T12 cells were added in 2 ml of complete medium. Results showed that microscopically the small monolayer of BCG-activated macrophages were fully cytotoxic for the BALB/3T12 cells that they contacted. In addition, a grossly small circumscribed plaque was formed on the petri dish surface that was otherwise covered with a multilayer of BALB/3T12 cells. The normal macrophages were not cytotoxic, and a multilayer of BALB/3T12 cells covered the entire petri dish surface.

These results suggest that tumorigenic target cells will not be destroyed when they are growing in the midst of a large number of cytotoxic activated macrophages if the activated macrophages cannot directly contact them. In addition, very few BCG-activated macrophages cultured among an excess of tumorigenic target cells remain fully cytotoxic for the small number of target cells that they contact.

The cytotoxic effect of activated macrophages against tumorigenic target cells appears to be mediated by lysosomal enzymes of activated macrophage origin. Lysosomes of activated macrophages appear to be secreted directly into the cytoplasm of susceptible target cells, which subsequently undergo heterolysis.

Nonenzymatic agents that accumulate and are stored in the vacuolar system of macrophages were used to study the nonphagocytic contact-dependent mechanism or mechanisms of target cell destruction. Normal and activated macrophages readily take up dextran sulfate which is concentrated in secondary lysosomes (37). Dextran sulfate is indigestible and nontoxic, and it stains metachromatically with toluidine blue 0 (37). Normal and activated macrophages were labeled with dextran sulfate (see Table 3 below) (36).

The transfer of the dextran sulfate secondary lysosome marker to target cells paralleled their susceptibility to destruction by activated macrophages (see Figure 3 below).

For example, after a 24-hour incubation period, 68 ± 8 percent of BALB/3T12 cells but only 10 ± 9 percent of BALB/MEF in contact with BALB/c BCG-activated macrophages had metachromatic cytoplasmic vacuoles. Similar results were obtained with the same target cells with the use of C3H/He macrophages activated by chronic toxoplasma infection. Transfer of dextran sulfate to BALB/3T12 cells from BCG- or toxoplasma-activated macrophages could be detected at 6 hours and was increased at 12 hours. Normal BALB/c

TABLE 3.[1]

Treatment of activated macrophages used as effector cells*		Target cells and cytotoxic effect†			
		Nontumorigenic		Tumorigenic	
Lysosomal label	Concentration (*M*)	BALB/c MEF	C3H MEF	BALB/c 3T12	BALB/c 3T3 SV40 trans-formed
Dextran sulfate‡	2×10^{-8} or 4×10^{-8}	0–1+	0–1+	4+	4+
Dextran sulfate + hydrocortisone‡	2×10^{-8} or 4×10^{-8} 3.6×10^{-6}	0	0	0–1+	0–1+
Neutral red	1.2×10^{-4}	0–1+	0–1+	4+	4+
Trypan blue	4.2×10^{-4}	0	0	0–1+	0–1+
Sucrose	2.9×10^{-3}	0–1+	0–1+	4+	4+
Ficoll	2.5×10^{-5}	0–1+	0–1+	4+	4+
None		0–1+	0–1+	4+	4+
None + hydrocortisone	3.5×10^{-5}	0	0	0–1+	0–1+

*Control normal BALB/c and C3H/He macrophages were exposed to the same lysosomal markers as activated macrophages in each of the above experiments. Normal macrophages never inhibited the growth of or were cytotoxic for target cells. †The results are given as the range obtained from four separately performed experiments. ‡Macrophages from C3H/He female and BALB/c female mice activated *in vitro* with endotoxin as described (2) produced similar results to those listed above except that the cytotoxic effect and the transfer of dextran sulfate markers was not as great as in equivalent experiments when macrophages activated *in vivo* by immunologic mechanisms were used.

macrophages transferred dextran sulfate to 5 ± 2 percent of BALB/3T12 cells and 2 ± 2 percent of BALB/MEF. Similar results were obtained with normal C3H/He macrophages and the same target cells. It was found that BALB/3T12 cells growing on the cover slip periphery and not in contact with macrophages did not contain metachromatic granules. Results similar to those with dextran sulfate were obtained with normal and activated macrophages labeled in the dark with neutral red, which also accumulates in lysosomes (38).

These results suggest that activated macrophages directly transfer the contents of secondary lysosomes into susceptible target cells. Such a process of exocytosis involved membrane fusion which should be partially inhibited by membrane stabilization (39). Hydrocortisone, a known membrane stabilizing agent (40), was added to normal and activated macrophages for 6 to 24 hours before the target cells were challenged. Preliminary treatment of activated macrophages with hydrocortisone inhibited their cytotoxic effect (shown above in Table 3). Maximum inhibitory effect was seen with doses as

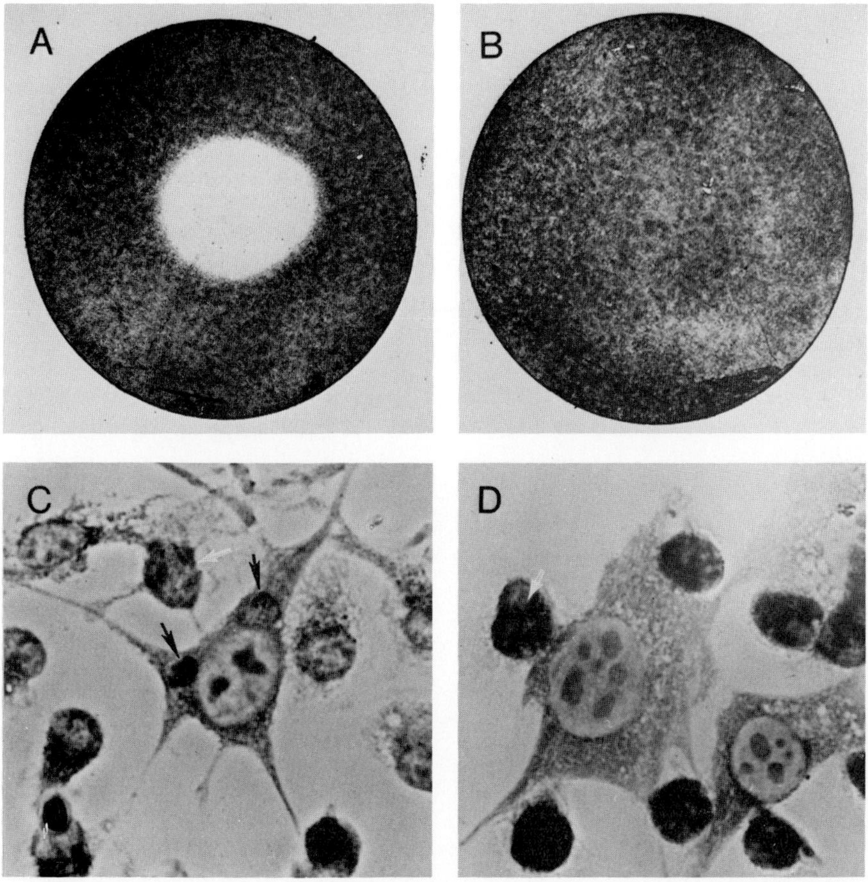

Fig. 3 *Macroscopic and microscopic views of the interaction of BCG-activated and normal BALB/c macrophages with 3T12 target cells. The cytotoxicity test is described in the caption to Table 1. (A) and (B) were stained with Giemsa 72 hours after 3T12 cell challenge. In (C) and (D), macrophages were first labeled with dextran sulfate, challenged with 3T12 cells, and 24 hours later were stained with toluidine blue O. Macrophages are marked with white arrows. (A) A thick multilayer of 3T12 cells grows to the immediate edge of a central monolayer of activated macrophages, which have destroyed the 3T12 cells (0.4 3T12 cells per field at ×400) with which they were in initial contact. (B) The central monolayer of normal macrophages has been completely overgrown by a thick multilayer of 3T12 cells. (C) A 3T12 cell in contact with activated macrophages is undergoing degenerative changes which include clumping of nuclear chromatin, vacuolation, and partial retraction of cytoplasm. The vacuoles (black arrows) of the 3T12 cell contain large dark dextran sulfate particles, which were strongly metachromatic when viewed with bright-field microscopy. (D) Healthy 3T12 cells, which are in contact with normal macrophages, contained no metachromatic granules when viewed with bright-field microscopy. Darker staining normal macrophages were strongly metachromatic [(A) and (B), ×2; (C) and (D), ×790].*

low as 2.8 $\times 10^{-7}$ M if maintained in the culture medium throughout the 72-hour incubation period. Hydrocortisone also inhibited the transfer of dextran sulfate to BALB/3T12 target cells. After a 24-hour incubation period 23 ± 7 percent of BALB/3T12 cells in contact with labeled BALB/c BCG-activated macrophages had metachromatically cytoplasmic vacuoles. The reduction in the transfer of dextran sulfate to BALB/3T12 cells was significant at $P \leq .001$. These results provide evidence that transfer of the contents of activated macrophage lysosomes is associated with target cell destruction.

Experiments were done to determine whether lysosomal hydrolases of activated macrophages could be the effectors of target cell heterolysis. Trypan blue, an inhibitor of lysosomal hydrolases (41), is readily taken up by macrophages, is nontoxic, and is stored in secondary lysosomes (42). Normal and activated macrophages were vitally stained *in vitro* by incubation with 4.2 $\times 10^{-4}$ M trypan blue in culture medium for 18 hours to challenge with target cells. Peritoneal macrophages were also labeled *in vivo* by inoculation of 4 mg of trypan blue intraperitoneally 48 hours before the mice were used as a source of macrophages for the cytotoxicity test. The cytotoxic effect of BCG- and toxoplasma-activated macrophages containing trypan blue in their vacuolar system was inhibited (Table 3). However, there was abundant transfer of trypan blue from activated macrophages to BALB/3T12 cells. For example, after a 24-hour incubation period 62 ± 10 percent of BALB/3T12 cells in contact with BCG-activated macrophages had vacuoles containing trypan blue when viewed in Sykes-Moore chambers with bright-field microscopy. These results suggest that lysosomal enzymes of activated macrophage origin may be the final molecular effectors of target cell destruction in this cytotoxicity system.

The inhibitory effect of trypan blue is not shared by the other tested nonenzymatic agents stored in secondary lysosomes. Dextran sulfate and neutral red had no inhibitory effect on the cytotoxic reaction, and similar results were found with sucrose and Ficoll (average molecular weight, 400,000) – carbohydrates not digested by macrophages – that are taken up by macrophages and stored in secondary lysosomes (43). Normal macrophages with large secondary lysosomes containing sucrose or Ficoll were not cytotoxic for BALB/3T12 cells. Activated macrophages containing sucrose and Ficoll were cytotoxic for BALB/3T12 cells (Table 3 above).

The interaction of macrophages and target cells in Sykes-Moore chambers maintained at 37°C was observed by phase contrast microscopy. Initial contact between macrophages and target cells began as the target cells were spreading on the cover slip among the macrophages. Long thin extensions of macrophage cytoplasm (pseudopods) made contact with the target cell surface (Figure 3 above). Activated macrophages were more active in extending pseudopods than were normal macrophages. Phase-dense granules could be seen to move from the macrophage perinuclear region to the pseudopod which they entered and slowly traversed centrifugally toward the target cell.

Phase-dense granules were observed to be transferred from activated macrophages into the cytoplasm of BALB/3T12 cells. Activated macrophages vitally stained with neutral red or trypan blue were observed to transfer secondary lysosomes containing dye to BALB/3T12 cells. The cytoplasmic bridges between activated macrophages and target cells were always temporary, lasting several minutes to many hours. Activated macrophages were only rarely seen to transfer phase-dense granules or vitally stained secondary lysosomes to normal target cells. Normal macrophages were not observed to transfer phase-dense granules or vitally stained secondary lysosomes to either normal or tumorigenic target cells.

The findings suggest that the critical modification underlying the destruction of tumorigenic cells by activated macrophages may be local or general membrane destabilization in both cells, which favors focal and temporary membrane fusion (38,44). The apparent universal susceptibility of tumorigenic cells to destruction by activated macrophages (4-18) suggests that decreased membrane stability (increased membrane fluidity) may be fundamental to expression of the neoplastic phenotype. In addition to morphologic (45) and biochemical modifications (46), the results suggest that destabilization of macrophage membranes may occur in parallel with activation. Therefore, normal macrophages may not be cytotoxic because their stable membranes do not participate in the fusion reactions required for target cell heterolysis. Likewise, activated macrophages may have little or no cytotoxic effect for normal target cells because the stability of the latter's membranes does not favor the temporary cell fusion reaction required for heterolysis.

Inhibition of specific and nonspecific tumor resistance by trypan blue.

Our experiments with trypan blue began during studies on the mechanism(s) of the activated macrophage cytotoxic effect. We were asking ourselves the question of whether or not lysosomal hydrolases of activated macrophages could be the effectors of target cell heterolysis. We made use of trypan blue as an experimental tool to help find the answer. The results showed that activated macrophages which had been exposed to trypan blue and, consequently, had accumulated the dye in their vacuolar system by pinocytosis prior to *in vitro* contact with tumor target cells had a markedly diminished cytotoxic effect (36). Because trypan blue is not ingested by viable lymphocytes, neutrophils, basophils, or eosinophils (47), it seems to be a useful experimental tool for the evaluation of the role of macrophages and macrophage-derived lysosomal enzymes in the *in vivo* as well as the *in vitro* destruction of tumor cells. We then administered trypan blue to mice and found it to suppress the rejection of tumor allografts and to reverse toxoplasma- and BCG-induced nonspecific resistance to tumor growth (26).

To test the effect of trypan blue in suppressing BCG-induced resistance to allografts of S180 cells, ICR mice were pretreated with the dye 24 hours and

3 hours before the tumor graft. A maintenance dose of trypan blue was given twice weekly.

The timing and location of the S180 graft in relation to the administration of BCG was as follows. Schedule 1, no BCG (saline-Tween 80 controls); schedule 2, BCG and S180 cells mixed together before inoculation; schedule 3, BCG administered 25 days before the graft of S180 cells (but at the same anatomical site); schedule 4, BCG administered 25 days before a graft of S180 cells mixed with BCG (both inoculations were at the same anatomical site); schedule 5, BCG and S180 cells administered simultaneously but at different sites; schedule 6, BCG administered 25 days before the graft of S180 cells (but at a different anatomical site); schedule 7, BCG administered 25 days before the inoculation of a second dose of BCG at the same site (S180 grafted at the same time as the second dose of BCG but at a different anatomical site); and schedule 8, no S180 (BCG control).

The results show that when BCG and the graft of S180 cells were in the same anatomical compartment (Table 4, Groups C-F), there was a significant increase in resistance to S180 growth. Trypan blue treatment of the mice markedly abrogated the nonspecific resistance induced by BCG (Table 4, Groups C-F). Control mice and BCG-infected mice treated with trypan blue developed progressively growing tumors. The effect of trypan blue in suppressing nonspecific resistance to S180 was not attributable to an antibacterial effect of the trypan blue on the viability of BCG. BCG could be readily

TABLE 4.
Effect of trypan blue and site of BCG administration on nonspecific resistance to S180

Group	Site of BCG adminis-tration	No. of S180 cells and site of graft	Schedule of S180 graft and BCG administration	No. of mice dead of tumor growth/No. of mice tested		p^b
				No trypan blue	Trypan blue	
A	–	2×10^5 i.m.R	1	10/10	10/10	NS
B	–	4×10^5 i.p.	1	19/20	20/20	NS
C	i.m.R	2×10^5 i.m.R	2	0/10	10/10	<0.001
D	i.m.R	2×10^5 i.m.R	3	4/10	10/10	<0.005
E	i.m.R	2×10^5 i.m.R	4	0/10	10/10	<0.001
F	i.p.	4×10^5 i.p.	3	9/20	19/20	<0.001
G	i.m.R	2×10^5 i.m.L	5	9/10	10/10	NS
H	i.m.R	2×10^5 i.m.L	6	8/10	10/10	NS
I	i.m.R	2×10^5 i.m.L	7	9/10	10/10	NS
J	i.m.R	4×10^5 i.p.	6	19/20	20/20	NS
K	i.m.R	–	8	0/10	0/10	NS

[a] See text for information concerning schedules.

[b] NS, not significant.

cultured from the tissues of mice that had been treated with trypan blue. In addition, BCG grew well in *in vitro* culture (described above) supplemented with trypan blue. The requirement for intimate contact between the tumor target cell and the population of activated macrophages produced in response to the BCG infection is also demonstrated in this experiment. When BCG and S180 cells were in a different anatomical compartment, no significant nonspecific resistance was induced by the BCG injection (Table 4, Groups G-J). Trypan blue administration also inhibited the expression of increased nonspecific resistance to S180 in ICR mice with chronic toxoplasma infection (26).

The above results demonstrate that trypan blue is an inhibitor of nonspecific resistance induced by chronic infection with BCG or toxoplasma. It was, therefore, of interest to determine the effect of trypan blue on the growth of an allogeneic lymphoma rejected by immunologically specific mechanisms. L1210 cells ($H\text{-}2^d$) were used in this study. CBA mice ($H\text{-}2^k$) tested for the effect of trypan blue on the rejection of primary grafts of L1210 cells were given the dye before the graft of L1210 cells, followed by a maintenance dose twice weekly (Table 5, Groups A-F).

The allografts of L1210 cells in normal CBA mice grew for about 7-10 days, at which time the tumor nodule began to regress. All normal CBA mice completely rejected primary allografts of L1210 cells. However, in mice that received trypan blue treatment, the primary L1210 allografts grew progressively, the tumor in the gastrocnemius muscle reaching a diameter of 20-34 mm before death. Histopathological sections of autopsy material from these

TABLE 5.
Effect of trypan blue and site of immunization on allograft immunity to leukemia L1210

Group	Mouse strain	No. of cells and site of administration: Primary L1210 graft	Secondary L1210 graft	No. of mice dead of tumor growth/No. of mice tested: No trypan blue	Trypan blue	*P*
A	CBA	1×10^7 i.m.R	–	0/20	20/20	<0.001
B	CBA	1×10^6 i.m.R	–	0/20	20/20	<0.001
C	CBA	1×10^5 i.m.R	–	0/20	20/20	<0.001
D	CBA	1×10^4 i.m.R	–	0/20	20/20	<0.001
E	CBA	1×10^3 i.m.R	–	0/20	20/20	<0.001
F	CBA	1×10^2 i.m.R	–	0/20	20/20	<0.001
G	CBA	–	–	–	0/20	–
H	DBA 2	1×10^2 i.m.R	–	10/10	10/10	–
I	CBA	1×10^7 i.m.R	1×10^7 i.m.R	0/20	13/20	<0.001
J	CBA	1×10^7 i.m.R	1×10^7 i.m.L	0/20	12/20	<0.001
K	CBA	–	–	–	0/10	–

mice showed that L1210 cells had infiltrated distant organs as well as the graft site. It is remarkable that an inoculum of as few as 1×10^2 cells (the smallest number tested) produced progressive and fatal tumor growth in all trypan-blue-treated mice grafted (Table 5, Group F).

We also studied the effect of trypan blue on the rejection of secondary grafts of L1210 cells in CBA mice. Trypan blue also had an effect on the rejection of L1210 allografts. However, the ability of trypan blue to inhibit secondary tumor allograft rejection was much less marked than that seen with the primary response (26).

The following discussion is a brief review of the known biologic effects of the azo dye trypan blue.

1. Early studies on the effect of trypan blue on tissue rejection.

In 1931 Ludford reported that trypan blue lowers the resistance of mice to the growth of transplantable tumors (48). Saphir and Appel in 1943 investigated the secondary rejection of the Brown-Pearce carcinoma in previously immunized rabbits. They found that prolonged administration of trypan blue resulted in abrogation of immunity in 7 of 9 tumor-immune rabbits tested (49). Another report of the ability of trypan blue to interfere with resistance to tumor growth occurred in 1951 when Cohen and Cohen noted that a transplantable rat hepatoma grew vigorously and progressively in all animals that were treated with trypan blue. In rats not treated with trypan blue they noted a high percentage of spontaneous regressions (50).

2. The teratogenic effect of trypan blue.

Gillman *et al.* first observed the teratogenic effect of trypan blue in 1948 (51). Since then, trypan blue has become a useful tool in experimental teratology. Several widely applicable principles have been demonstrated with this agent; these include the changing susceptibility of the fetus with stage of gestation (52), the association between embryonic malformation and increased incidence of intrauterine death (53), and the changing pattern of response with varying dosage (54). A large number of animal species has been found susceptible to the teratogenic action of trypan blue. The considerable literature available on the teratogenic effects of trypan blue mentioned above has been reviewed (55).

3. Evidence that trypan blue may largely exert its biologic effects by affecting the vacuolar system of cells.

Trypan blue administered parenterally to animals combines with albumin and other proteins of extracellular fluids and then enters the vacuolar system of mononuclear phagocytes (56) and certain types of epithelial cells by endocytosis. The first clear demonstration that trypan blue is stored in lysosomes was made by Schmidt (57) and Trump (58) in electron microscopic studies of renal proximal tubules from rats and mice previously injected with the dye. In 1968 Lloyd *et al.* described a biochemical study on the distribution of dye among fractions obtained by differential centrifugation of liver and visceral yolk sac cells from dye-treated rats. The results obtained are consistent with a lysosomal location for trypan blue (59).

While searching for the molecular basis for the teratogenic effects of trypan blue, Lloyd, Beck, and their colleagues examined the effect that intralysosomal trypan blue could have on lysosome function. They found the dye to be a strong inhibitor of lysosomal hydrolases and postulated that congenital malformations caused by administration of the dye to pregnant rats might be due to loss of intracellular digestive capacity of the yolk sac cells with consequent nutritional deprivation of the embryo (41,60).

Evidence for a possible selective in vivo immunosuppressive effect of trypan blue.

The results described above implicate trypan blue as a suppressor of activated macrophage cytotoxic function. It was shown that trypan blue pretreatment of peritoneal macrophages harvested from mice with chronic BCG or toxoplasma infection caused a loss of the macrophage's ability to destroy tumor target cells *in vivo* (36). Further, trypan blue treatment of mice suppressed the rejection of tumor allografts and reversed toxoplasma- and BCG-induced nonspecific resistance to tumor growth (26). Since this azo dye is taken up only by macrophages and not by other viable lymphoid cells (47), these findings suggested that trypan blue might selectively inhibit macrophage effector functions, without altering the immunologic reactions of lymphocytes. Such a selective inhibitor would provide a useful tool for determining the contribution of cytotoxic macrophages in the *in vivo* rejection of normal and neoplastic tissues.

In collaboration with Dr. Margaret Kripke, we have initiated studies to test the effect of trypan blue treatment on a variety of immunologic responses in mice. Our preliminary findings are as follows (Kripke, Gruys, and Hibbs, unpublished data):

1. The effect of trypan blue treatment on skin allograft rejection.

Full-thickness, circular, abdominal skin grafts (15 mm in diameter) from strain A (H-2^a) female donors were transplanted to the thorax of CBA of C3Hf (H-2^k) recipients by the method of Billingham and Medawar (61). Plaster casts were removed after 8 days, using light ether anesthesia, and the grafts were inspected daily for gross signs of rejection. Complete destruction of the epidermis was used as the rejection endpoint. We tested several doses and regimens of trypan blue for their ability to delay the rejection of skin allografts across a major histocompatibility barrier. The results are summarized in Table 6.

A single dose of 1 mg of trypan blue caused a modest delay in graft rejection, while a single dose of 4 mg nearly doubled the median graft survival time. Treatment of the graft donor with 4 mg of trypan blue 24 hours before grafting did not influence graft survival, even though the grafts had absorbed enough dye to be dark blue in color (Group 4). Chronic treatment with a low dose of trypan blue also delayed graft rejection from a median time of 11.5 days to 15 days.

These results confirm the earlier observation of Brent and Medawar (62) that trypan blue treatment retards skin allograft rejection and suggest that trypan blue is effective in inhibiting the host response to normal as well as neoplastic tissue.

2. The effect of trypan blue administration on hemagglutinin titer.

Mice were injected intravenously (iv) with 5×10^7 sheep red blood cells (SRBC) in 0.5 ml of saline, on days 0 and 12. The mice were bled from the tail vein at intervals following each immunization. Sera were collected and stored at –20°C prior to testing. Serum samples from each animal were assayed individually for hemagglutinating antibodies in micro-titer plates. All sera were tested on the same day.

Three groups of C3Hf males were immunized with SRBC. Twenty-four hours prior to the first immunization, one group was given 4 mg of trypan blue sc, followed by 0.4 mg twice per week, beginning in the second week. Another group was given the same regimen of trypan blue

TABLE 6.
Effect of trypan blue treatment on skin allograft rejection

Donor → Recipient	Group	Treatment	Number of Mice	Rejection Time (days) Median (range)	P[a]
A → CBA	1	None	6	9(9-11)	
A → CBA	2	1 mg trypan blue to recipient, day 0	5	11(9-22)	<0.05
A → CBA	3	4 mg trypan blue to recipient, day 0	6	17.5(13-23)	=0.001
A → CBA	4	4 mg trypan blue to graft donor, –24 hours	6	10(9-12)	>0.05
A → C3Hf	5	saline 3X/week for 4 weeks	8	11.5(10-15)	
A → C3Hf	6	0.1 mg trypan blue 3X/week for 4 weeks	7	15(13-19)	=0.005

[a]p = probability of no difference between control and treated groups, determined by a 1-tailed Mann-Whitney U test

beginning 24 hours before the second SRBC immunization. This dose and regimen of trypan blue was effective in delaying tumor rejection (see Table 7).

The third group received 0.5 ml saline sc twice per week. As is illustrated in Table 7, trypan blue treatment had no effect on either the primary or the secondary hemagglutinin response against SRBC. Further, adding as much as 0.16 mg/ml of trypan blue to the serum dilutions did not reduce the antibody titer, indicating that trypan blue does not interfere with the interaction between antibody and cellular antigens.

3. The effect of trypan blue administration on *in vitro* lymphocyte stimulation.

Stimulation of mouse lymph node cells *in vitro* by Con A was carried out as described by Williams (63). Briefly, single cell suspensions were prepared in RPMI 1640 tissue culture medium containing penicillin (100 unit/ml), streptomycin (100 μg/ml), and 10 percent fetal bovine serum. Cell viability, determined by trypan blue exclusion, was >99 percent. The cells were cultured at a concentration of 5×10^5 cells in 0.15 ml in Falcon microtiter plates. Con A (0.25 μg in 0.05 ml of medium) was added to half the cultures at time zero. Cells from each trypan-blue-treated or control mouse was cultured in triplicate with and without Con A. After 24 hours of culture at 37°C in air with 5 percent CO_2, 2 μCi of ^{3}H-thymidine were added to each chamber in 0.05 ml of medium. The cultures were harvested after an additional 20 hours of incubation; radioactivity was determined by liquid scintillation counting. Table 8 summarized the results of experiments on the effect of trypan blue treatment on lymphocyte stimulation by Con A. C3H mice were injected

BLE 7
ect of trypan blue treatment on the hemagglutinin response to SRBC

		Hemagglutinin Titers[a]					
	Number	Primary Response			Secondary Response		
atment[b]	of Mice	Day: 5	7	10	14	17	21
ne	10	10(9-11)	9(8-10)	9(7-10)	9(8-11)	12(10-13)	11(10-13)
g trypan blue, −1 0.4 mg week thereafter	10	10(9-12)	9(8-10)	10(9-11)	10(9-10)	12(9-13)	11(9-13)
g trypan blue, +11 0.4 mg week thereafter	10	10(8-11)	9(7-9)	9(8-9)	9(8-11)	12(10-13)	12(10-13)

g_2 of reciprocal of highest serum dilution showing complete agglutination. Median (range).
l groups were immunized with 5×10^7 SRBC iv on days 0 and 12.

with trypan blue sc at various intervals prior to removal of their lymph node cells for culturing. The doses of trypan blue used in these experiments were sufficient to prolong skin allograft survival (see Table 6 above), or impair resistance to an allogeneic lymphoma (26). As can be seen in Table 8, the trypan-blue-treated groups did not differ significantly from non-treated controls.

In the studies reported here we have not examined all the possibilities for the suppressive effect of trypan blue on tissue rejection. For example, trypan blue could prevent the generation of cytotoxic T-lymphocytes or inhibit the secretion or action of one or more lymphokines. However, our results do show that doses of trypan blue that prolonged the survival of normal and neoplastic tissue transplants (Table 6 above) (26) did not decrease other immune responses tested. The primary and secondary serum hemagglutinin responses to SRBC, a T-cell dependent antigen (64-65), were unaffected by trypan blue treatment (Table 7 above). In addition, trypan blue treatment of mice did not interfere with the ability of lymphocytes to be stimulated *in vitro* by Con A (Table 8 above). These results imply that the mode of action of trypan blue *in vivo* probably is not mediated through an effect on antigen recognition, T-lymphocyte helper function in the induction of antibody synthesis, or through immunologic amplification produced by the proliferation of B-lymphocytes to specific antigen (SRBC). In addition, the formation and

TABLE 8.
Effect of in vivo trypan blue treatment on lymphocyte stimulation by Con A

Treatment	Average CPM – Con A	Average CPM + Con A	Average of Increments in CPM ± SEM[a]
saline, –24 hours	2,538 (4)[b]	250,456 (4)	195,513 ± 8,557
4.0 mg trypan blue, –24 hours	4,076 (4)	229,331 (4)	203,021 ± 9,665
saline, –48 hours	1,960 (3)	176,312 (3)	174,352 ± 9,554
4.0 mg trypan blue, –48 hours	4,431 (4)	203,898 (4)	199,467 ± 17,066
saline, –72 hours	677 (3)	176,080 (3)	175,403 ± 18,448
4.0 mg trypan blue, –72 hours	3,863 (4)	195,551 (4)	191,688 ± 6,961
saline, –96 hours	2,517 (3)	215,714 (3)	213,197 ± 26,757
4.0 mg trypan blue, –96 hours	8,607 (4)	209,597 (4)	200,990 ± 10,901
saline, 7 days	1,880 (3)	201,476 (3)	199,596 ± 15,787
4.0 mg trypan blue, –7 days	7,820 (2)	238,778 (2)	230,958 ± 5,578

[a]SEM = Standard Error of the Mean

[b]number of mice in each group in parenthesis

secretion of immunoglobulins remain intact in mice whose ability to control tumor growth or reject allografts of normal skin has been reduced by trypan blue treatment. However, it should be reemphasized that caution must be exercised in attributing prolonged survival of normal skin or neoplastic grafts in trypan-blue-treated mice entirely to the effect of trypan blue on final cytotoxic effector functions of activated macrophages. A more extensive evaluation of trypan blue will be necessary to rule out additional mechanisms for the observed *in vivo* immunosuppression.

CONCLUSION

I believe there is now good evidence that macrophages have an important role as cytotoxic effector cells in host resistance to cancer. The histopathologic study of Hanna *et al.* supplements the work I have discussed and underlines the possible biologic significance of cytotoxic activated macrophages. These workers demonstrated the BCG-induced regression of a transplanted syngeneic hepatocarcinoma in guinea pigs was associated with massive infiltration of macrophages into the tumor site and regional lymph nodes (66). In the absence of BCG there was progressive tumor growth associated with a lymphoproliferative response in the regional lymph nodes but without infiltration of macrophages.

Finally, the observation that most tumors may contain a large number of macrophages is highly significant (67,68). What chemical signals attracted them to the tumor? What are the macrophage-tumor cell interactions that occur in progressively growing lesions? What is the nature of this interaction in regressing lesions? These are the questions for future work.

ACKNOWLEDGEMENTS

I thank Read R. Taintor, C. C. Moore, James E. Brisbay, and John F. Elsholz for technical assistance; and Martha S. Knowlton for secretarial help.

REFERENCES

1. Hibbs, J. B., Jr. (1975). Role of macrophages in host defense against cancer. *Immunologic Aspects of Neoplasia.* (The University of Texas M.D. Anderson Hospital and Tumor Institute at Houston, 26th Annual Symposium on Fundamental Cancer. Research, 1973). The Williams and Wilkins Company, Baltimore, Maryland.

2. Remington, J. S., J. L. Krahenbuhl and J. B. Hibbs, Jr. (1975). A role for the macrophage in resistance to tumor development and tumor destruction. *Mononuclear Phagocytes in Immunity, Infection, and Pathology*. Ralph Van Furth, Ed. Blackwell Scientific Publishers, London.

3. Levy, M. H. and E. F. Wheelock (1974). The role of macrophages in defense against neoplastic disease. *Advances in Cancer Research 20*:131-163.

4. Hibbs, J. B., Jr., L. H. Lambert, Jr. and J. S. Remington (1972). Possible role of macrophage mediated nonspecific cytotoxicity in tumour resistance. *Nature New Biology 235*:48-50.

5. Hibbs, J. B., Jr., L. H. Lambert, Jr. and J. S. Remington (1971). Resistance to murine tumors conferred by chronic infection with intracellular protozoa, *Toxoplasma gondii* and *Besnoitia jellisoni. Journal of Infectious Diseases 124*:587-592.

6. Hibbs, J. B., Jr., L. H. Lambert, Jr. and J. S. Remington (1972). *In vitro* nonimmunologic destruction of cells with abnormal growth characteristics by adjuvant activated macrophages. *Proceedings of the Society for Experimental Biology and Medicine 139*:1049-1052.

7. Hibbs, J. B., Jr., L. H. Lambert, Jr. and J. S. Remington (1972). Control of carcinogenesis: A possible role for the activated macrophage. *Science 177*:998-1000.

8. Hibbs, J. B., Jr. (1973). Macrophage nonimmunologic recognition: Target cell factors related to contact inhibition. *Science 180*: 868-870.

9. Alexander, P. and R. Evans (1971). Endotoxin and double stranded RNA render macrophages cytotoxic. *Nature New Biology 232*:76-78.

10. Keller, R. and V. E. Jones (1971). Role of activated macrophages and antibody in inhibition and enhancement of tumour growth in rats. *The Lancet*, October 16, 1971:847-849.

11. Evans, R. and P. Alexander (1972). Mechanism of immunologically specific killing of tumour cells by macrophages. *Nature 236*:168-170.

12. Scott, M. T. (1975). *In vivo* cortisone sensitivity of nonspecific antitumor activity of *Corynebacterium parvum* – activated mouse peritoneal macrophages. *Journal of the National Cancer Institute 54*:789-792.

13. Basic, I., L. Milas, D. J. Grdina and H. R. Withers (1974). Destruction of hamster ovarian cell cultures by peritoneal macrophages from mice treated with *Corynebacterium granulosum. Journal of the National Cancer Institute 52*:1839-1841.

14. Kaplan, A. M., P. S. Morahan and W. Regelson (1974). Induction of macrophage-mediated tumor-cell cytotoxicity by pyran copolymer. *Journal of the National Cancer Institute 52*:1919-1921.

15. Hibbs, J. B., Jr. (1974). Discrimination between neoplastic and nonneoplastic cells *in vitro* by activated macrophages. *Journal of the National Cancer Institute 53*:1487-1492.

16. Krahenbuhl, J. L. and J. S. Remington (1974). The role of activated macrophages in specific and nonspecific cytostasis of tumor cells. *Journal of Immunology 113*:507-516.

17. Cleveland, R. P., M. S. Meltzer and B. Zbar (1974). Tumor cytotoxicity *in vitro* by macrophages from mice infected with *Mycobacterium bovis* strain BCG. *Journal of the National Cancer Institute 52*:1887-1894.

18. Piessens, W. F., W. H. Churchill, Jr. and J. R. David (1975). Macrophages activated *in vitro* with lymphocyte mediators kill neoplastic but not normal cells. *Journal of Immunology 114*:293-299.

19. Pimm, M. V. and R. W. Baldwin (1975). BCG immunotherapy of rat tumours in athymic nude mice. *Nature 254*:77-78.

20., Chess, L., R. P. MacDermott, P. M. Sondel and S. F. Schlossman (1974). Isolation and characterization of cells involved in human cellular hypersensitivity. *Progress in Immunology II, 3*:125-132.

21. Fidler, I. J. (1975). Activation *in vitro* of mouse macrophages by syngeneic, allogeneic, or xenogeneic lymphocyte supernatants. *Journal of the National Cancer Institute 55*:1159-1163.

22. Hibbs, J. B., Jr. (1975). Activated macrophages as cytotoxic effector cells. II. Requirement for local persistence of inducing antigen. *Transplantation 19*:81-87.

23. Zbar, B., H. T. Wepsic, T. Borsos and H. J. Rapp (1970). Tumor-graft rejection in syngeneic guinea pigs: Evidence for a two-step mechanism. *Journal of the National Cancer Institute 44*:473-481.

24. Zbar, B., H. T. Wepsic, H. J. Rapp, L. C. Stewart and T. Borsos (1970). Two-step mechanism of tumor graft rejection in syngeneic guinea pigs. II. Initiation of reaction by a cell fraction containing lymphocytes and neutrophils. *Journal of the National Cancer Institute 44*:701-717.

25. Hibbs, J. B., Jr., L. H. Lambert, Jr. and J. S. Remington (1972). Adjuvant induced resistance to tumor development in mice. *Proceedings of the Society for Experimental Biology and Medicine 139*:1053-1056.

26. Hibbs, J. B., Jr. (1975). Activated macrophages as cytotoxic effector cells. I. Inhibition of specific and nonspecific tumor resistance by trypan blue. *Transplantation 19*:77-81.

27. Aaronson, S. A. and G. Todaro (1968). Basis for the acquisition of malignant potential by mouse cells cultivated *in vitro. Science 162*:1024-1026.

28. Pollack, R. E. and M. M. Burger (1969). Surface-specific characteristic of a contact-inhibited cell line containing the SV_{40} viral genome. *Proceedings of the National Academy of Sciences USA 62*:1074-1076.

29. Sanford, K. K. (1965). Malignant transformation of cells *in vitro. International Review of Cytology 18*:249-311.

30. Wu, H. C., E. Meezan, P. H. Black and P. W. Robbins (1969). Comparative studies on the carbohydrate containing membrane components of normal and virus transformed mouse fibroblasts. I. Glucosine-labeling patterns in 3T3 cells. *Biochemistry* labeling patterns in 3T3, and SV-40 transformed 3T3 cells. *Biochemistry 8*:2509-2517.

31. Nicolson, G. L. (1971). Difference in topology of normal and tumour cell membranes shown by different surface distributions of ferritin-conjugated concanavalin A. *Nature New Biology 233*:244-246.

32. Sheinin, R. and K. Onodera (1972). Studies of the plasma membrane of normal and virus-transformed 3T3 mouse cells. *Biochimica Biophysica Acta 274*:49-63.

33. Holtermann, O. A., E. Klein and G. P. Casale (1973). Selective cytotoxicity of peritoneal leucocytes for neoplastic cells. *Cellular Immunology 9*:339-352.

34. Meltzer, M. S., R. W. Tucker, K. K. Sanford and E. J. Leonard (1975). Interaction of BCG-activated macrophages with neoplastic and nonneoplastic cell lines *in vitro*: Quantitation of the cytotoxic reaction by release of tritiated thymidine from prelabeled target cells. *Journal of the National Cancer Institute 54*:1177-1184.

35. Meltzer, M. S., R. W. Tucker and A. C. Breuer. Interaction of BCG-activated macrophages with neoplastic and nonneoplastic cell lines *in vitro*. Cinemicrographic analysis. *Cellular Immunology 17*:30-42.

36. Hibbs, J. B., Jr. (1974). Heterocytolysis by macrophages activated by Bacillus Calmette-Guérin: Lysosome exocytosis into tumor cells. *Science 184*:468-471.

37. Gordon, S. and Z. Cohn (1970). Macrophage-melanocyte heterokaryons. I. Preparation and properties. *Journal of Experimental Medicine 131*:981-1003.

38. Allison, A. C. and M. R. Young (1964). Uptake of dyes and drugs by living cells in culture. *Life Science 3*:1407-1414.

39. Poste, G. and A. C. Allison (1971). Membrane fusion reaction: A theory. *Journal of Theoretical Biology 32*:165-184.

40. Weissmann, G. and J. T. Dingle (1961). Release of lysosomal protease by ultraviolet irradiation and inhibition by hydrocortisone. *Experimental Cell Research 25*:207-210.

41. Beck, F., J. B. Lloyd and A. Griffiths (1967). Lysosomal enzyme inhibition by trypan blue: A theory of teratogenesis. *Science 157*:1180-1182.

42. Beck, F. and J. B. Lloyd (1969). Histochemistry and electron microscopy of lysosomes. *Lysosomes in Biology and Pathology*. North-Holland Publishing Co., Amsterdam.

43. Cohn, Z. A. and B. A. Ehrenreich (1969). The uptake, storage, and intracellular hydrolysis of carbohydrates by macrophages. *Journal of Experimental Medicine 129*:201-225.

44. Lucy, J. A. (1970). The fusion of biological membranes. *Nature (London) 227*:815-817.

45. Mackaness, G. B. (1970). The monocyte in cellular immunity. *Seminars in Hematology* 7:172-184.

46. Stubbs, M., A. V. Kuhner, E. A. Glass, J. R. David and M. L. Karnovsky (1973). Metabolic and functional studies on activated mouse macrophages. *Journal of Experimental Medicine 137*:537-542.

47. Padawer, J. (1973). The peritoneal cavity as a site for studying cell-cell and cell-virus interactions. *Journal of the Reticulo-endothelial Society 14*:462-512.

48. Ludford, R. J. (1931). Resistance to the growth of transplantable tumours: (2) The influence of dyestuffs and of colloids on natural resistance. *British Journal of Experimental Pathology 12*:108-113.

49. Saphir, O. and M. Appel (1943). Attempts to abrogate immunity to the Brown-Pearce Carcinoma. *Cancer Research 3*:767-769.

50. Cohen, A. and L. Cohen (1951). Analogous effects of radiation and trypan blue on rats resistant to transplanted hepatoma. *Nature 167*:1063.

51. Gillman, J., C. Gilbert, T. Gillman and I. Spence (1948). A preliminary report on hydrocephalus, spina bifida, and other congenital anomalies in the rat produced by trypan blue. *South African Journal of Medical Science 13*:47-90.

52. Wilson, J. G., A. R. Beaudoin and H. J. Free (1959). Studies on the mechanism of teratogenic action of trypan blue. *Anatomical Record 133*:115-128.

53. Beck, F. and J. B. Lloyd (1963). An investigation of the relationship between foetal death and foetal malformation. *Journal of Anatomy* (London) 97:555-564.

54. Beck, F. and J. B. Lloyd (1964). Dosage – response curves for the teratogenic activity of trypan blue. *Nature 201*:1136-1137.

55. Beck, F. and J. B. Lloyd (1966). The teratogenic effects of azo dyes. *Advances in Teratology I.* Logos Press, London.

56. Padawer, J. (1971). Phagocytosis of particulate substances by mast cells. *Laboratory Investigation 25*:320-330.

57. Schmidt, W. (1960). Electron microscopic studies on the uptake of trypan blue in the cells of the main segment of the kidney. *Z. Zellforsch. Mikroskop. Anat. 52*:598-603.

58. Trump, B. F. (1961). An electron microscope study of the uptake, transport, and storage of colloidal materials by the cells of the vertebrate nephron. *Journal of Ultrastructure Research 5*:291-310.

59. Lloyd, J. B., F. Beck, A. Griffiths and L. M. Parry (1968). The mechanism of action of acid bisazo dyes. *The Interaction of Drugs and Subcellular Components of Animal Cells.* J. & A. Churchill Ltd., London.

60. Davies, M., J. B. Lloyd and F. Beck (1971). The effect of trypan blue, suramin and aurothiomalate on the breakdown of 125I-labelled albumin within rat liver lysosomes. *Biochemical Journal 121*:21-26.

61. Billingham, R. E. and P. B. Medawar (1951). The technique of free skin grafting in mammals. *Journal of Experimental Biology 28*:385-403.

62. Brent, L. and P. B. Medawar (1961). Quantitative studies on tissue transplantation immunity. V. The role of antiserum in enhancement and desensitization. *Proceedings of the Royal Society B 155*:392-416.

63. Williams, R. M. (1973). DNA synthesis by cultured lymphocytes: A modified method of measuring ^{3}H-thymidine incorporation. *Cellular Immunology 9*:435-444.

64. Miller, J. F. A. P. and G. P. Mitchell (1968). Cell to cell interactions in the immune response. I. Hemolysin-forming cells in neonatally thymectomized mice reconstituted with thymus of thoracic duct lymphocytes. *Journal of Experimental Medicine 128*:801-820.

65. Schimpl, A. and E. Wecker (1970). Inhibition of *in vitro* immune response by treatment of spleen cell suspensions with anti-θ serum. *Nature (London) 226*:1258-1259.

66. Hanna, M. G., Jr., B. Zbar and H. J. Rapp. (1972). Histopathology of tumor regression after intralesional injection of *Mycobacterium bovis.* I. Tumor growth and metastasis. *Journal of the National Cancer Institute 48*:1441-1455.

67. Evans, R. (1973). Preparation of pure cultures of tumor macrophages. *Journal of the National Cancer Institute 50*:271-273.

68. Eccles, S. A. and P. Alexander (1974). Macrophage content of tumours in relation to metastatic spread and host immune reaction. *Nature 250*:667-669.

MORPHOLOGIC ASPECTS OF TUMOR CELL CYTOTOXICITY BY EFFECTOR CELLS OF THE MACROPHAGE-HISTIOCYTE COMPARTMENT: *IN VITRO* AND *IN VIVO* STUDIES IN BCG-MEDIATED TUMOR REGRESSION[1]

M. G. Hanna, Jr., Corazon Bucana,
Barbara Hobbs and I. J. Fidler

Basic Research Program
NCI-Frederick Cancer Research Center
Frederick, Maryland 21701

INTRODUCTION

Histopathological and ultrastructural studies of BCG-mediated regression of regional skin tumors in guinea pigs have suggested that infiltrating cells of the macrophage-histiocyte compartment are primary effector cells of the antitumor response of the host (1-3). Both at the tumor site and in the regional lymph node, tumor cell destruction occurs within a BCG-induced granulomatous reaction characterized by proliferation of stromal reticuloendothelial components and infiltrating cells of the macrophage-histiocyte compartment. In contrast, an induced nonspecific lymphoproliferative response or an induced inflammatory reaction does not destroy the localized tumor or eliminate regional lymph node metastases.

The role of lymphocytes *in vivo* in the host response to BCG antigen has been clearly demonstrated for effective BCG-mediated immunotherapy in the syngeneic guinea pig model (4). An indirect role of lymphocytes *in vivo* as a source of "arming" or "activating" soluble factors for macrophages has also been proposed (5,6). Therefore, although it is assumed that there is a

[1] Research supported by the National Cancer Institute under Contract NOI-CO-25423 with Litton Bionetics, Incorporated.

synergistic response of lymphocytes and macrophages in BCG-mediated tumor regression, the *in vitro* and *in vivo* data that exist to date suggest that the primary cytotoxic cells are from the macrophage-histiocyte compartment.

The cytopathic mechanism by which such "activated" cells destroy tumor cells is not completely understood. At present there is little evidence to support the involvement of a cytotoxin or a cytophilic antibody, although each may be necessary for contact or binding of activated macrophages with target cells. It has been suggested that protuberances of the target cell may be pinched off and engulfed by the macrophage, resulting eventually in irreparable membrane damage that leads to the degeneration of the target cell (7). Recent evidence indicates that destruction of target cells by non-phagocytic mechanisms may be the important phenomenon related to activated or specifically sensitized cells of the macrophage-histiocyte compartment. Granger and Weiser (8) demonstrated *in vitro* that homograft target cell destruction can be produced by immune peritoneal macrophages and that the cell destruction apparently results from a non-phagocytic mechanism involving cell contact. Hibbs *et al.* (6) also found that macrophages from mice chronically infected with Toxoplasma have the capacity to nonspecifically destroy target cells *in vitro* by a non-phagocytic mechanism. Hibbs (9) further showed that mouse peritoneal macrophages activated *in vivo* by chronic infection with BCG are cytotoxic against tumor cells *in vitro* and that the cytotoxicity is mediated by lysosomal enzymes of macrophage origin. Lysosomes of activated macrophages are secreted directly into the cytoplasm of susceptible target cells, presumably at regions of cell contact. These results suggest a local membrane fusion or "destabilization" that occurs during direct contact of neoplastic target cells and activated macrophages. In fact, the underlying basis of activated macrophage-mediated destruction of tumor cells, whether specific or nonspecific, may be found in a cell membrane property of the effector and/or target cell. The molecular aspects of this phenomenon could be of extreme importance to tumor immunology.

It is important to acquire further morphological and functional data on apposed membranes of neoplastic target cells and effector cells of the macrophage-histiocyte compartment in relevant experimental models where activation of macrophages is known to effect immunotherapy. The purpose of this study was to evaluate morphologically and functionally, in strain-2 guinea pigs with transplanted syngeneic tumors, the interaction between cells of the macrophage-histiocyte compartment and tumor cells during the course of BCG-mediated tumor regression. Ultrastructural studies were carried out with tissues collected at the tumor transplantation site and in draining lymph nodes at various intervals after intralesional injection of BCG. In addition, the interaction of neoplastic cells with host immune cells was studied *in vitro*. In these studies, cultured line-10 tumor cells were overlayed with adherent cells from lymph nodes of animals treated with BCG. These studies included Nomarski time-lapse cinematography coordinated with electron microscopy.

METHODS AND RESULTS

Inbred strain-2 guinea pigs and the transplantable syngeneic line-10 hepatocarcinoma were used in these studies. The antigenic and biologic properties of the transplantable tumors developed from the primary cellular hepatocarcinoma originally induced with the water soluble carcinogen, diethylnitrosamine, have been described previously (10). In this experimental model, guinea pigs are injected intradermally with 1×10^6 line-10 hepatocarcinoma cells. Under these conditions, tumors grow progressively and metastasize to regional lymph nodes. Untreated guinea pigs die as a consequence of metastases 60-90 days after tumor injection. The regression of transplanted syngeneic hepatocarcinoma established in the skin of strain-2 guinea pigs and the elimination of regional lymph node metastases can be achieved in the majority of guinea pigs by an intratumoral injection of viable BCG (11,12). Initial studies with this model established several facts: 1) The efficacy of a single intratumoral BCG injection is limited by tumor size and when metastasis is confined to the first regional lymph node (12,13); 2) there is a requirement for early host reactivity to BCG antigens, which is mediated by sensitized lymphocytes (13,14); 3) histologic and ultrastructural studies of BCG-treated regressing tumors and metastases in regional lymph nodes suggest that cells of the macrophage-histiocyte compartment are most essential to the destruction of tumor cells *in vivo* (1,3); and 4) during and following BCG-mediated tumor regression in the skin or elimination of regional lymph node metastases, there is development of systemic humoral and cell-mediated tumor immunity (4,13).

Interaction in vivo of cells of the macrophage-histiocyte compartment with tumor cells during BCG-mediated tumor regression. The histologic and ultrastructural description of major changes that occur in draining lymph nodes and the cutaneous tumor site at various intervals after intralesional injection of BCG has been described elsewhere (1-3). This report will concentrate on the morphologic aspects of tumor cell cytotoxicity by effector cells of the macrophage-histiocyte compartment. It is important at this point to define the nomenclature used with these descriptions, primarily because of the difficulty of interpreting the extensive literature on classic tuberculin granulomatous disease.

The general term "histiocyte" refers to a cell type distinguishable from conventional circulating macrophages and phagocytic mononuclear cells and consistent with the characteristics of the "epithelioid cells" associated with the granulomatous reactions. Granted, there may be different morphologic

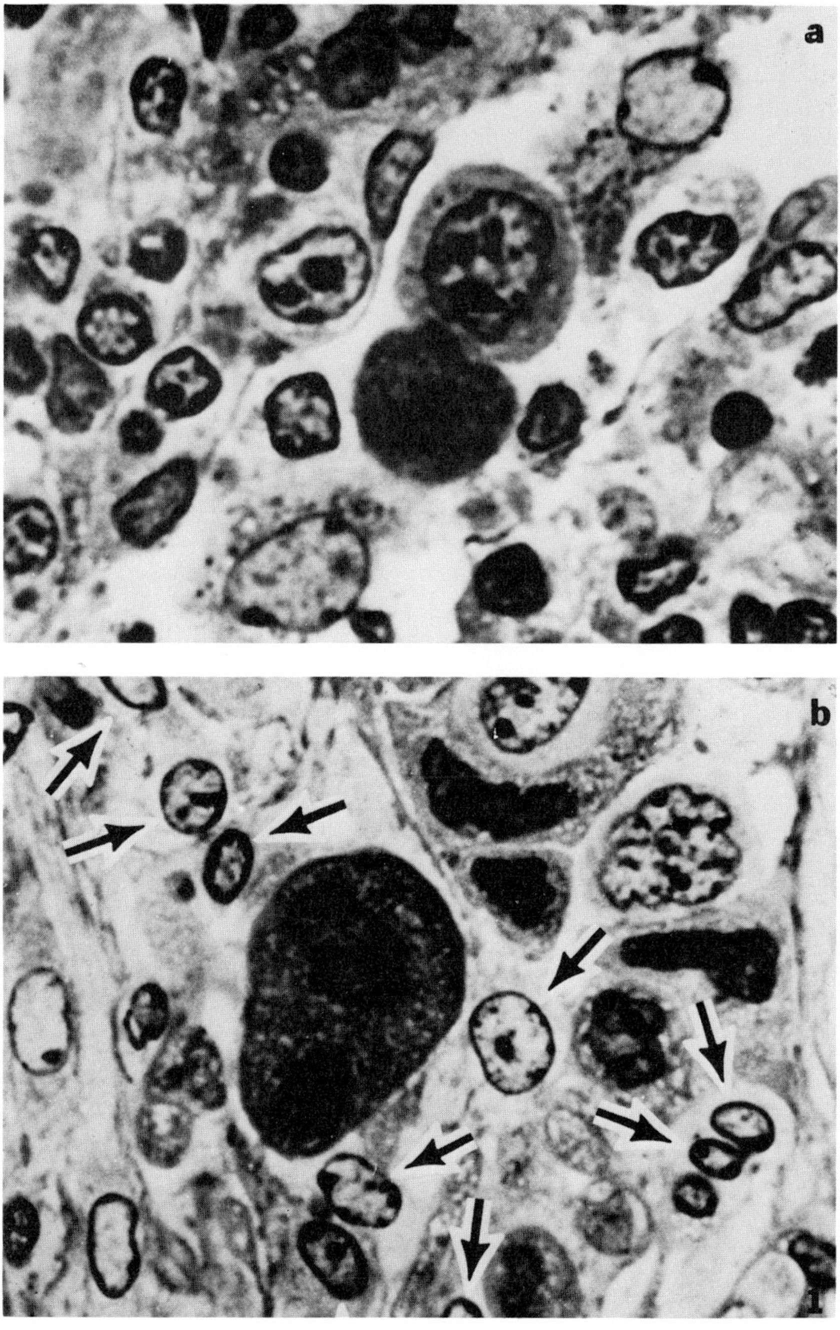
a
b
1

appearances of the same cell type commonly grouped into the general macrophage-histiocyte compartment. Also, it is recognized that in the early host response, phagocytosis of a limited number of bacilli by macrophages initially activates this cell compartment. However, the general absence of active phagocytosis and a representative number of cell inclusion bodies in the enlarged, activated compartment of effector cells tends to argue against phagocytosis as a primary function. We reject the commonly used terms "epithelioid" and "epithelial-like cell" because they are based on resemblance and are misleading with respect to origin and function of the active cytotoxic cell.

Morphologically, the histiocytes observed in medullary sinuses of the lymph nodes responding to BCG treatment are large and irregular. The abundant cytoplasm is quite eosinophilic. The large ovoid nucleus contains finely clumped chromatin and one or two large nucleoli. When they are organized as granulomas or tubercles in the cortex and paracortex of lymph nodes, these cells have indistinct cytoplasmic margins that appear to merge or form a syncytium with neighboring histiocytes.

Between 4 and 16 days after intralesional injection of BCG, numerous examples of interaction between activated histiocytes and tumor cells were observed at the tumor site, as well as in various regions of the draining lymph nodes. In many cases we observed degeneration of tumor cells associated with or surrounded by histiocytes. The association of tumor cells and histiocytes in the subcapsular marginal sinus of the regional lymph nodes, as observed from 1 μ sections, is shown in Figure 1a. Several histiocytes are associated with the surface of the tumor cells and the latter are dark and pycnotic, indicative of cell degeneration. Such "rosette" formations of tumor cells surrounded by histiocytes and occasional lymphocytes (Fig. 1b) were commonly observed in lymph nodes and in the skin tumor during the course of BCG-mediated tumor regression. The plasmalemmae of the line-10 tumor cell and the histiocyte are generally very closely apposed; and the distortion of the cytoplasm of histiocytes, in an attempt to make contact with the tumor cells, indicates that this is an active rather than a passive function of the histiocyte (Fig. 1a). Numerous electron-dense, round bodies and intracellular tubules containing electron-dense material could be observed in the histiocyte cytoplasm. Often these are polarized in the region of cell surface contact.

The interaction of histiocytes and line-10 tumor cells in the regional lymph node of BCG-treated guinea pigs is shown on the ultrastructural level in Fig. 2. The subsequent effect of interaction between histiocytes and tumor cells was degeneration of the hepatocarcinoma cells. The cytoplasma of the

Fig. 1a. *(Shown at left) Histiocytes in contact with 2 metastatic tumor cells 8 days after treatment.* × *950.* **Fig. 1b.** *Histiocytes (arrows) among hepatocarcinoma cells 8 days after treatment. Both mitotic and degenerate tumor cells are present.* × *950.*

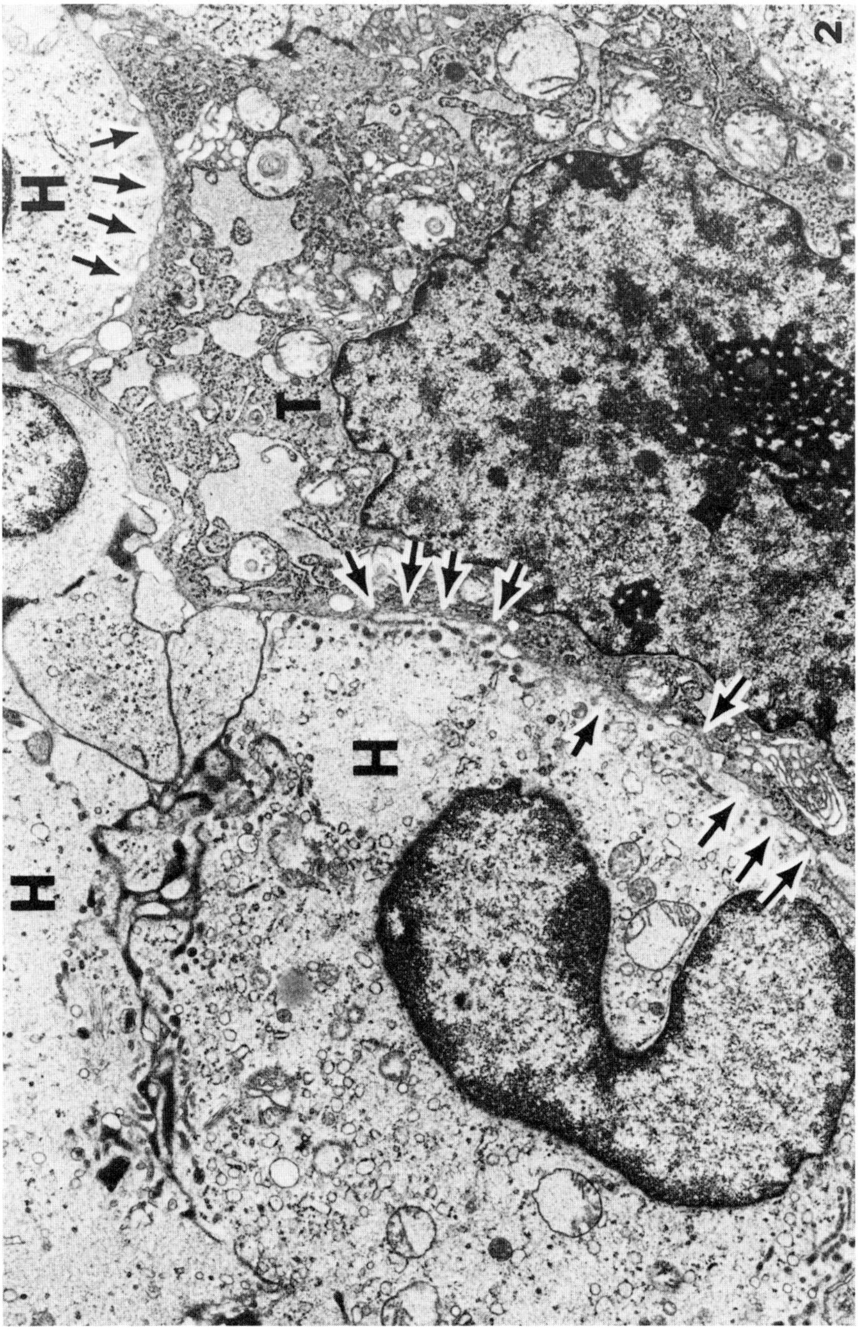
2
H
T
H
H

tumor cell shown in Fig. 2 is dark (electron-dense) and contains numerous irregular vesicles and ribosomes which appear to have lost their normal polysomal organization. The mitochondria are severely disrupted and the pleomorphic, pycnotic nucleus contains several nucleoli.

The cytoplasm of the histiocyte contains a well developed Golgi apparatus, large and small vesicles of rough endoplasmic reticulum, and numerous lysosomes. Because of their large nucleoli and prominent nuclei these cells have been called epithelioid cells by other investigators. Although kinetic evidence concerning the specific origins of these cells is not yet available, their morphological characteristics suggest a mesenchymal origin from stromal or primitive reticular cells.

Interaction between histiocytes and hepatocarcinoma cells is frequently seen both in the tumor site and the regional lymph nodes. The destruction of tumor cells by cells resembling activated histiocytes is a common feature of BCG-induced regressing tumors and reactive lymph nodes. Although morphology alone cannot ascertain the functional mechanism of cell interaction, the ultrastructure shown in Fig. 2 suggests areas of apparent intercellular bridges between the membranes of histiocytes and tumor cells. These areas are observed with regularity in tissue samples obtained from the regional lymph nodes and the skin tumor sites, and seem to be an integral part of the mechanism by which BCG-activated histiocytes destroy the tumor cells. As seen in Fig. 2, adjacent to these apposed cell surface regions, the histiocytes have numerous intracytoplasmic channels containing electron-dense material which is also found extracellularly. Higher magnification of the intercellular bridges between histiocytes and tumor cells are shown in Fig. 3. Morphologically, these cell networks are distinct from the common, electron-dense "tight junctions" which can be observed within homogenous cell populations.

Interaction in vitro of line-10 cells and cells of the macrophage-histiocyte compartment from regional lymph nodes of BCG-tumor-cured guinea pigs. Line-10 hepatocarcinoma cells adapted to growth *in vitro* were grown on 25 mm coverslips and overlayed with lymphoid cells harvested from the lymph node regional to a BCG-treated skin tumor. The nodes were surgically excised from guinea pigs 6 weeks after intralesional BCG treatment, when skin tumor had completely regressed. The tumor cell preparations were incubated with lymph node cells for 1.5 hours at 37°C, then washed 2 times with CMEM tissue culture media. Thus, only adherent lymphoid cells which had attached to tumor cells or to glass remained on the coverslip which was placed into a tissue chamber (Nicholson Precision Instruments, Bethesda, Maryland) and

Fig. 2. *(Shown at left) Areas of apparent fusion (arrows) of the plasmalemmae of histiocytes (H) and an electron dense hepatocarcinoma cell (T) 8 days after treatment. Note that the histiocytes have numerous intracytoplasmic channels containing electron-dense material, which is also found extracellularly around these cells.* × *11,000.*

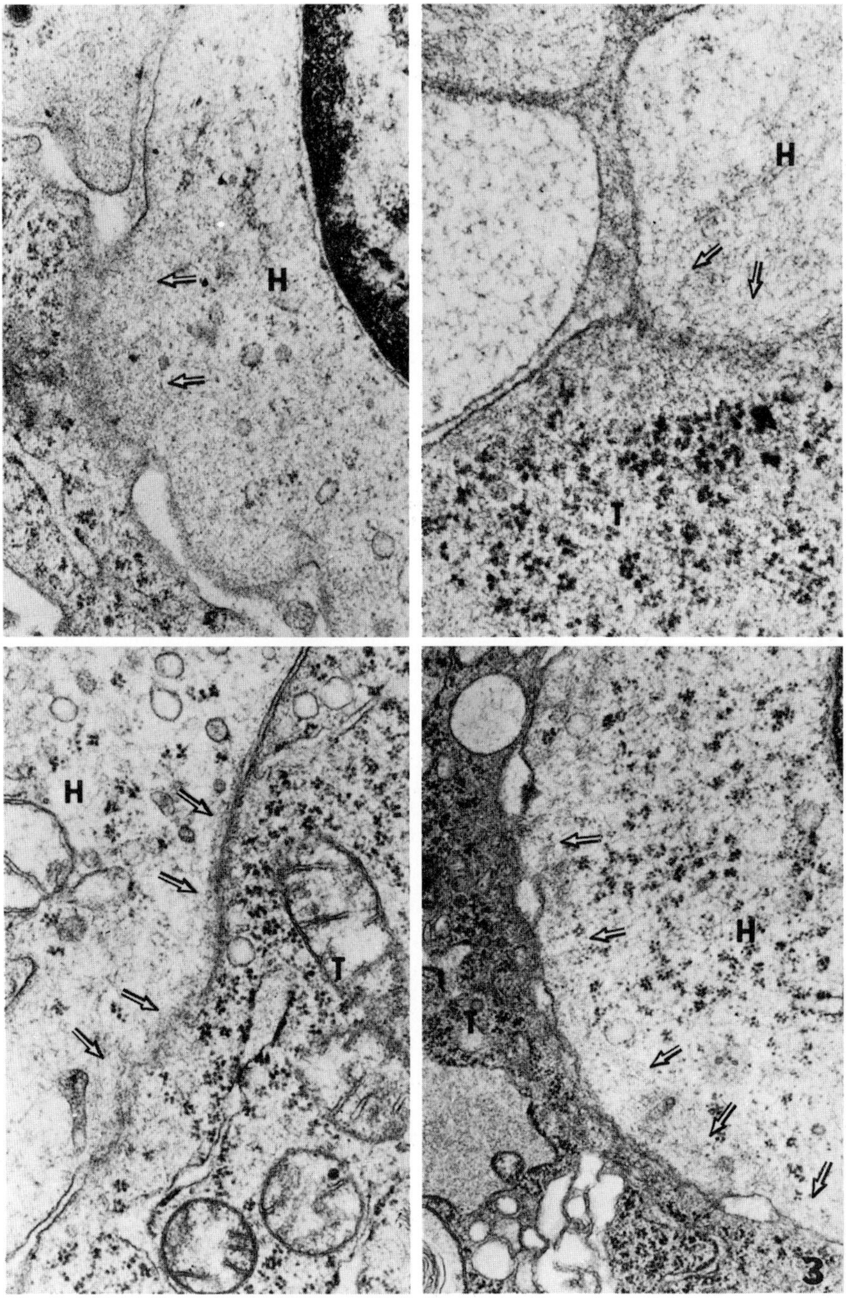
H
H
T
H
T
T
H
3

examined in a Zeiss photo microscope III. The temperature of the chamber was kept at 37°C by means of an air stream incubator (Nicholson Precision Instruments, Bethesda, Maryland). Specific areas showing histiocyte-tumor contact were selected, photographed on a GAF 500 color film, and the sequence of events in the histiocyte-tumor interaction was recorded for 2 hours with a time-lapse Bolex camera. Coverslips with line-10 cells and adherent lymph node cells were removed at 1.5 hours, 72 hours, and 5 days. Also additional coverslips were fixed in methanol and stained with Giemsa stain. Light microscopic evaluation of these preparations showed adherent lymph node cells attached to line-10 tumor cells (Fig. 4). The cells which adhered to tumor cells were both mature lymphocytes and large mononuclear cells morphologically resembling tissue macrophages or histiocytes.

Interference microscopy. The cine-photomicrographs obtained after 1.5 hours of incubation of adherent lymph node and tumor cells indicate that initial contact of adherent lymph node cells to tumor cells occurs rapidly. Figures 5 and 6 are a direct visualization of the lymphoid cell-tumor interaction. Figure 5 shows blebbing of cytoplasmic pseudopodia of large mononuclear cells on tumor cells. A pulsation at the tumor cell-adherent cell junction can be detected in the set of frames of Fig. 5. The recurring protuberances of the adherent cell cytoplasm between frames a through e took approximately 1 min 40 sec. The persistence of this adherent cell activity between frame e through f is shown over an elapsed time of 3 min 20 sec. The entire surface activity in Fig. 6 is over a 7 min 20 sec sequence. Thus, an active undulation of the adherent cell membrane can be demonstrated at the line-10 tumor cell surface. A number of adherent cells were observed to attach to various regions of the tumor cell. It was not unusual to find a cluster of cells along the thin cytoplasmic projection of the tumor cell as well as around the vicinity of the nucleus of the tumor cell.

Time-lapse photomicrographs of 72 hour samples generally showed clusters of adherent cells on the surface of tumor cells. At the end of 5 days incubation, very few adherent lymph node cells were detected and the remaining tumor cells were normal in appearance.

Transmission electron microscopy (TEM). Samples of the above preparation were fixed at 1.5 hours, 36 hours and 5 days incubation. The samples were fixed in 2.5% cacodylate buffered glutaraldehyde followed by 1% cacodylate buffered osmiumtetroxide, dehydrated in a graded series of ethanol and embedded as a monolayer in Epon-Araldite mixture. Specific areas in the

Fig. 3. *(Shown at left) Areas of apparent adhesion (arrows) between the plasmalemmae of histiocytes (H) and hepatocarcinoma cells (T). Upper left-upper right—Subcapsular sinus of the SDA lymph node 8 days after BCG treatment.* × *25,000 and 40,000 respectively. Lower left-lower right—The s.c. tumor transplantation site 8 and 16 days after BCG treatment.* × *30,000 and 35,000 respectively.*

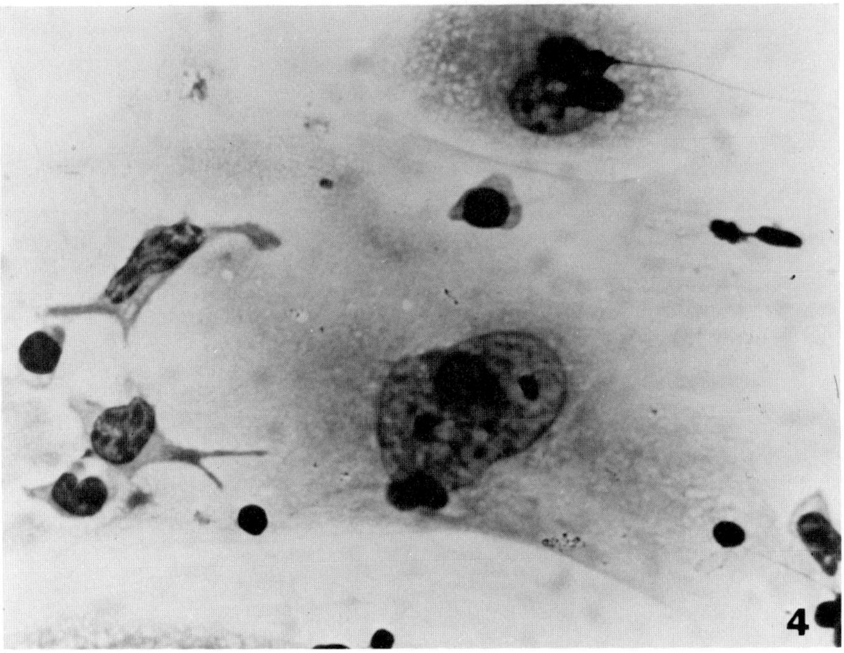

Fig. 4. *Photomicrograph of line-10 cells with adherent lymph node cells attaching to the tumor cell surface.* × *800.*

monolayer containing tumor cells with attached adherent lymph node cells were chosen. Serial sections of the monolayers were cut perpendicular to the long axis of the growing cells to determine the orientation of the lymph node cells to the tumor cells. Monolayers of samples obtained after 72 hours and 5 days incubation were cut in a similar manner, and also cut along the longitudinal axis of the tumor cells to determine the extent of adherent cell-tumor interaction as well as the distribution of lysosomes and residual bodies that were first observed in 36 hour samples. The sections were cut with a diamond knife on a LKB Ultratome III. Because of the flexibility of the orientation head of this microtome we were able to cut thin sections of the same cell from two different planes perpendicular to each other. Thin sections were picked up on Formvar coated one-hole grids or coated 150 mesh copper grids, stained with uranyl acetate and lead citrate, and examined in an Hitachi 12-A electron microscope.

Fig. 5. *(Shown at right) Nomarski cinematography 1.5 hours after culture in vitro of line-10 cells and adherent lymph node cells.* × *400.*

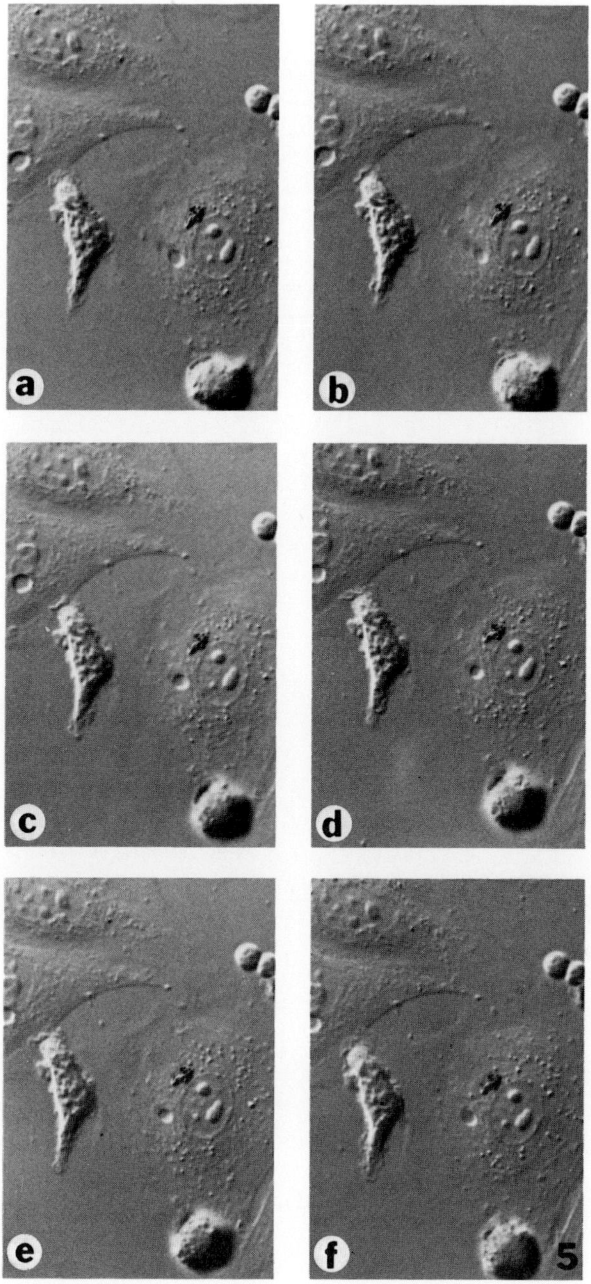
a
b
c
d
e
f
5

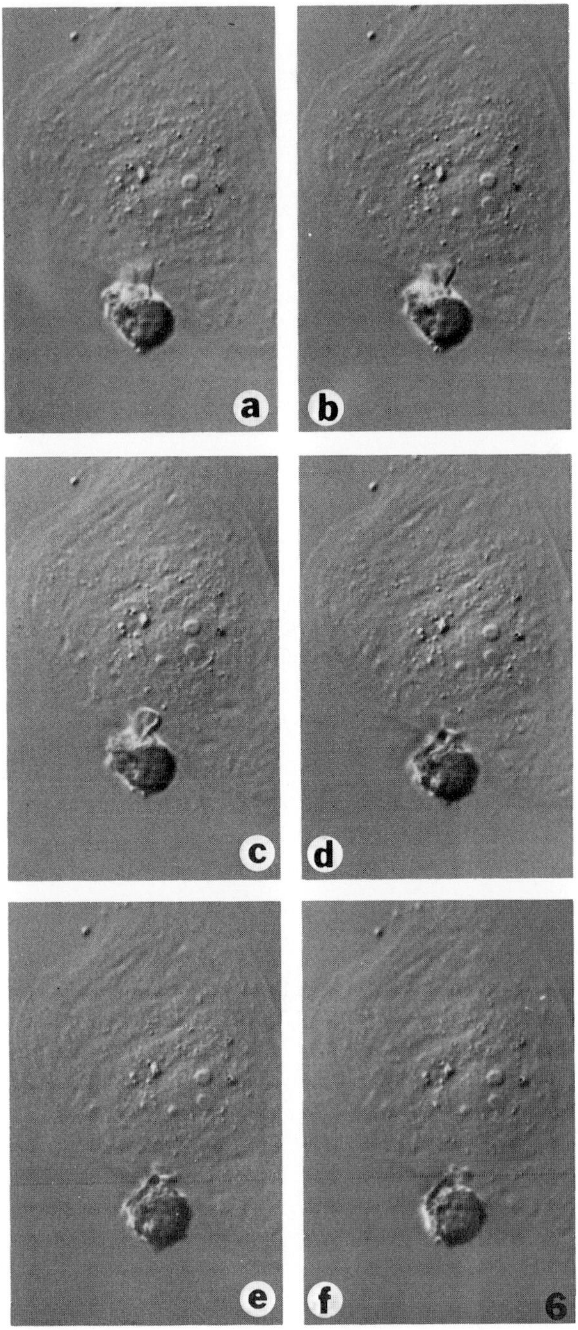

a
b
c
d
e
f
6

Samples taken after 1.5 hours of incubation showed adherent lymph node cells on the surface of line-10 tumor cells. Morphologically, these cells were classified as histiocytes, as described above. Figure 7 shows a histiocyte attached by a cytoplasmic extension to a tumor cell. The latter has large vesiculated areas and swollen rough endoplasmic reticulum. The histiocyte shows numerous microtubules radiating from the region of the centriole and dilated Golgi bodies. A number of "primary" lysosomes, as well as phagosomes, "secondary lysosomes," were also observed. There is an apparent discontinuity of the tumor cell membrane at the point of contact with the histiocyte cytoplasmic extension.

A similar association of histiocytes with tumor cell surfaces can be seen in Figure 8a. This photograph also shows where microvilli of the tumor cell, with a low radius of curvature, have attached to the histiocyte. Apparent discontinuity of histiocyte-tumor cell surface is shown in Figure 8b.

By day 3, electron microscopy of tumor cell-histiocyte interactions showed marked identation of the tumor cell. These indentations were always opposite cytoplasmic extensions of the histiocyte (Fig. 9a). Wide areas of contact between histiocytes and tumor cells showed regions of membrane destabilization. This could not be a sectioning artifact because serial sections of these regions showed no continuous limiting membrane of the histiocyte or tumor cell. Furthermore, serial sections cut perpendicular to this plane also support the observation of membrane destabilization. High magnification of the histiocyte cytoplasmic extensions suggest microtubular formation of histiocyte origin penetrating to tumor cell junction (Fig. 9b). In addition, our electron microscopic observation at the tumor cell-histiocyte interaction sites indicates that some of the cytoplasmic extensions of the histiocyte may penetrate for quite a distance into the cytoplasm of the tumor cell. Support for this observation is not only obtained from static sections, but also from serial sectioning so that cytoplasmic extensions can be traced back to their histiocyte origin (Fig. 9b).

Another type of association of histiocyte with tumor cell is seen in Figure 10. The histiocyte appears to be partially enveloped by the tumor cell. Areas of membrane destabilization between the two cells can also be observed (Fig. 10b). Numerous microfilaments, dilated rough-surfaced endoplasmic reticulum, and primary and secondary lysosomes can be observed in tumor cells. Many tangential sections of microtubules of histiocyte origin are observed aligned perpendicular to the region of membrane destabilization (Fig. 10a). The most prominent feature of tumor cells at this time is the presence of large residual bodies containing partially digested mitochondria and membranes, and dilated rough surface endoplasmic reticulum with granular contents in the cisternae.

Fig. 6. *(Shown at left) Nomarski cinematography 1.5 hours after culture in vitro of line-10 cells and adherent lymph node cells.* × *400.*

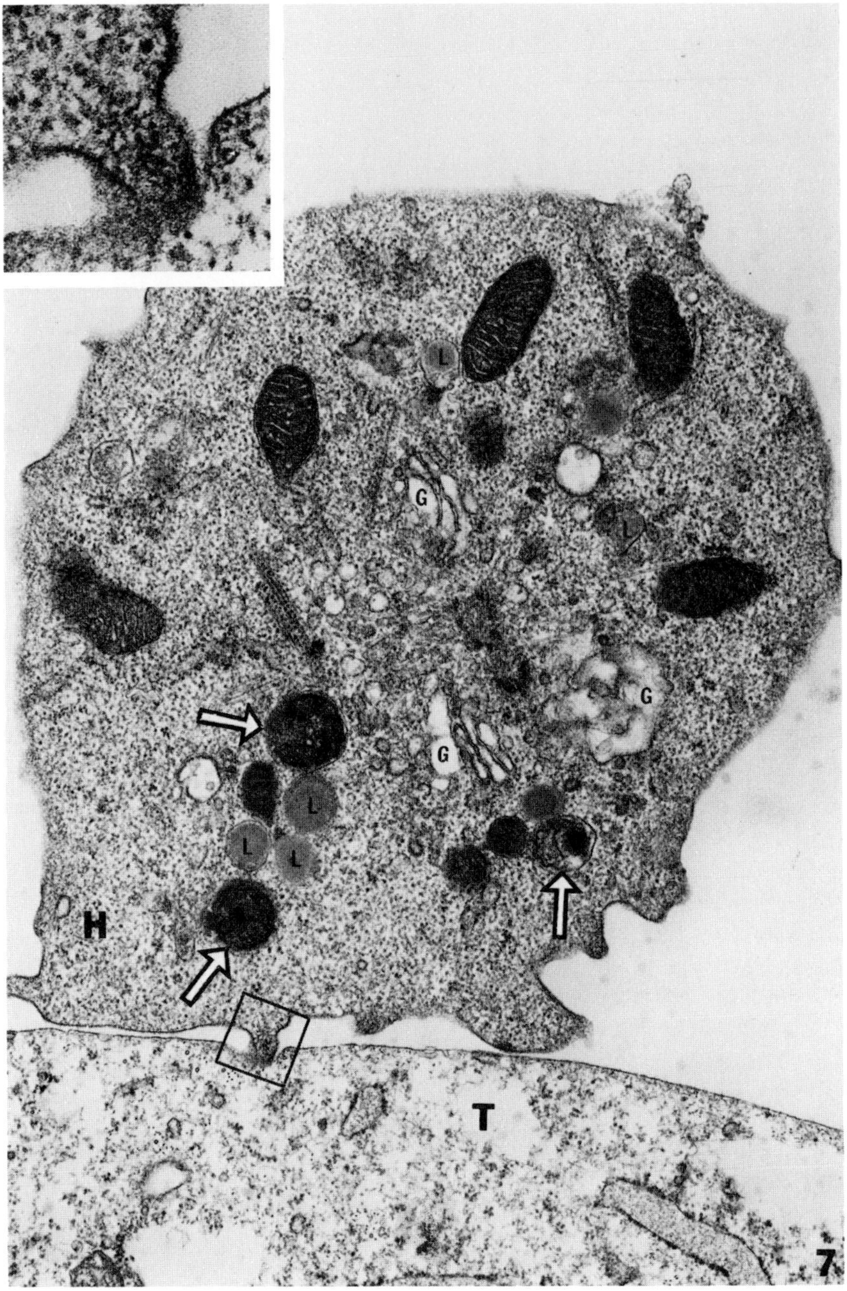

L
G
L
G
G
L
L
L
H
T
7

Numerous dense osmiophilic bodies of various sizes, which resemble lysosomes, were also observed in tumor cell cytoplasma after 3 days of incubation. These osmiophilic bodies were very closely associated with dilated endoplasmic reticulum and were detected in the majority of tumor cells at the 72 hour intervals (Fig. 10c).

CONCLUSION

Macrophage-mediated destruction of tumor cells has been demonstrated *in vitro* and *in vivo* in a variety of syngeneic, allogeneic and xenogeneic experimental systems. Cytotoxic macrophages have been isolated from specifically immune animals, as well as from animals stimulated nonspecifically with various agents. The general consensus is that the destruction of tumor cells by macrophages requires cell surface contact but is accomplished by a nonphagocytic process. The possibility of transfer of lysosomes or lysosomal products of macrophage origin to tumor cells, resulting in heterocytolysis, has been proposed by Hibbs (9).

In the present study we tested adherent cells isolated from lymph nodes in which elimination of metastases had been accomplished subsequent to BCG-intratumoral injection of a regional skin tumor. Thus, it was known at the outset of the experiment that functional BCG-activation of mononuclear cells had occurred. Also, the guinea pigs from which these regional lymph nodes were isolated were specifically immune to the syngeneic tumor and could reject a subsequent tumor challenge.

The adherent lymph node cells which participated in cytotoxicity *in vitro* of the line-10 tumor cells were morphologically classified as cells belonging to the macrophage-histiocyte compartment. They had the appearance of "activated" mononuclear cells characteristic of the tuberculous response and were observed *in vivo* to be associated with BCG-mediated tumor regression. Histochemical studies of these cells during the tuberculous reaction by Dannenberg (14) demonstrated that these cells have high levels of β-galactosidase, acid phosphatase, β-glucuronidase, cytochrome oxidase, and succinic dehydrogenase. Morphologically, this would be characterized by an increased number of primary lysosomes in the cells. Since, during the course of our study, there was no evidence of phagocytosis of tumor cells by these BCG-activated cells, we prefer to classify them not as activated macrophages but as histiocytes, which denotes a tissue cell of the macrophage-histiocyte series which is not primarily phagocytic.

With respect to the process of tumor cell cytotoxicity as mediated by these histiocytes, our morphological data prompt us to speculate that initial

Fig. 7. *(Shown at left) Electron micrograph showing interaction of histiocyte (H) and line-10 tumor cell (T) after 1.5 hours of incubation in vitro. The histiocyte-tumor cell contact (inset) when viewed at higher magnification showed tumor cell membrane discontinuity.* × *37,000. Inset* × *130,000.*

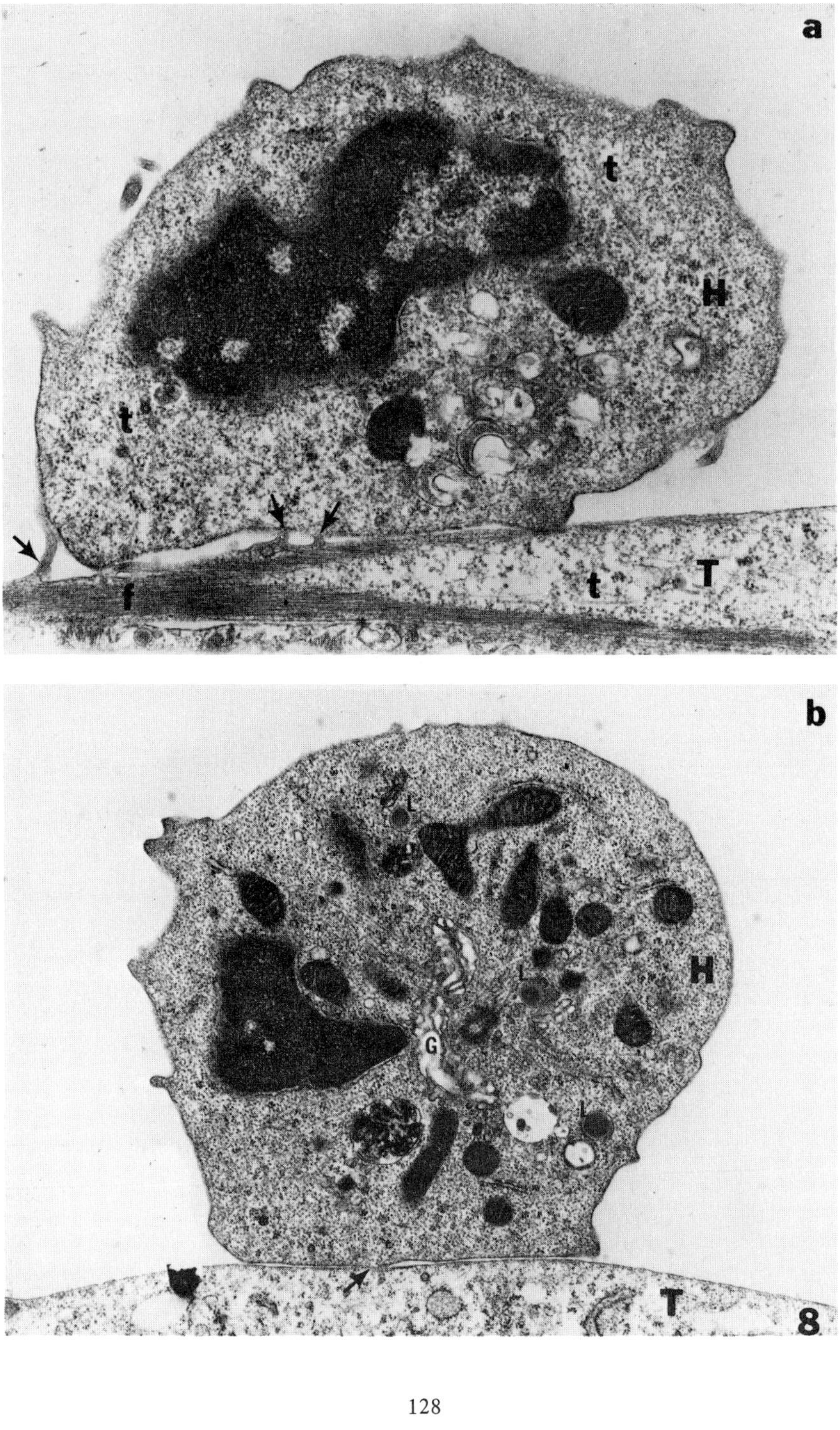
a
t
H
t
f
t
T
b
L
H
G
L
L
T
8

contact involves a "grappling" of the tumor cell by cytoplasmic extensions of the histiocyte. The cytoplasmic extensions protrude into the tumor cell cytoplasm predominantly by invagination of the tumor cell. Distinct microtubules can be seen throughout the length of these cytoplasmic extensions. The cytoplasmic extensions of the histiocytes appear to circumscribe a broader region of cell surface contact where membrane destabilization is observed. Morphologically, this region of membrane destabilization suggests the possibility of an intercellular bridge which provides transport through cell membranes. Tangential to the region of membrane destabilization, classic microtubules of histiocyte origin can be observed. These microtubular structures have been shown to be involved in the transport of intracellular products as well as in alteration of cell shape (15). During the time course of the present study, primary lysosomes initially detected only in histiocytes were later observed also in neoplastic target cells. Indeed, if these lysosomes were of histiocyte origin, the mechanism of exocytosis from histiocytes, either through the region of membrane destabilization and/or through the cytoplasmic extensions via transport along microtubules, may have been involved in the histiocyte-mediated tumor cell cytolysis.

REFERENCES

1. Hanna, M. G., Jr., B. Zbar and H. J. Rapp (1972). Histopathology of tumor regression after intralesional injection of *Mycobacterium bovis*. I. Tumor growth and metastasis. *J. Natl. Cancer Inst. 48*:1441-1455.

2. Hanna, M. G., Jr., B. Zbar and H. J. Rapp (1972). Histopathology of tumor regression after intralesional injection of *Mycobacterium bovis*. II. Comparative effects of vaccinia virus, oxazolone, and turpentine. *J. Natl. Cancer Inst. 48*:1697-1707.

3. Snodgrass, M. J. and M. G. Hanna, Jr. (1973). Ultrastructural studies of histiocyte-tumor cell interactions during tumor regression mediated by intralesional injection of *Mycobacterium bovis*. *Cancer Res. 33*:701-716.

4. Hanna, M. G., Jr., M. J. Snodgrass, B. Zbar and H. J. Rapp (1973). Histopathology of tumor regression after intralesional injection of *Mycobacterium bovis*. IV. Development of immunity to tumor cells and BCG. *J. Natl. Cancer Inst. 51*:1897-1908.

5. Alexander, P. and R. Evans (1971). Endotoxin and double stranded RNA render macrophages cytotoxic. *Nature New Biol. 232*:76-78.

Fig. 8a. *(Shown at left) Histiocyte (H) and line-10 tumor cell (T) interaction after 1.5 hours of incubation in vitro. Both cells have prominent microtubules (t) but the tumor cell also contains abundant microfilaments (f). Cytoplasmic extensions or folds (arrows) of the tumor cell are in contact with histiocyte. × 31,000.* **Fig. 8b.** *A cross section of histiocyte in contact with a tumor cell after 1.5 hours of incubation in vitro. Microtubules are seen radiating from the region of the centriole and Golgi bodies (G). Lysosomes (L) and phagosomes are also observed. The region of contact between histiocyte and tumor cells (arrow) suggests membrane destabilization. × 22,000.*

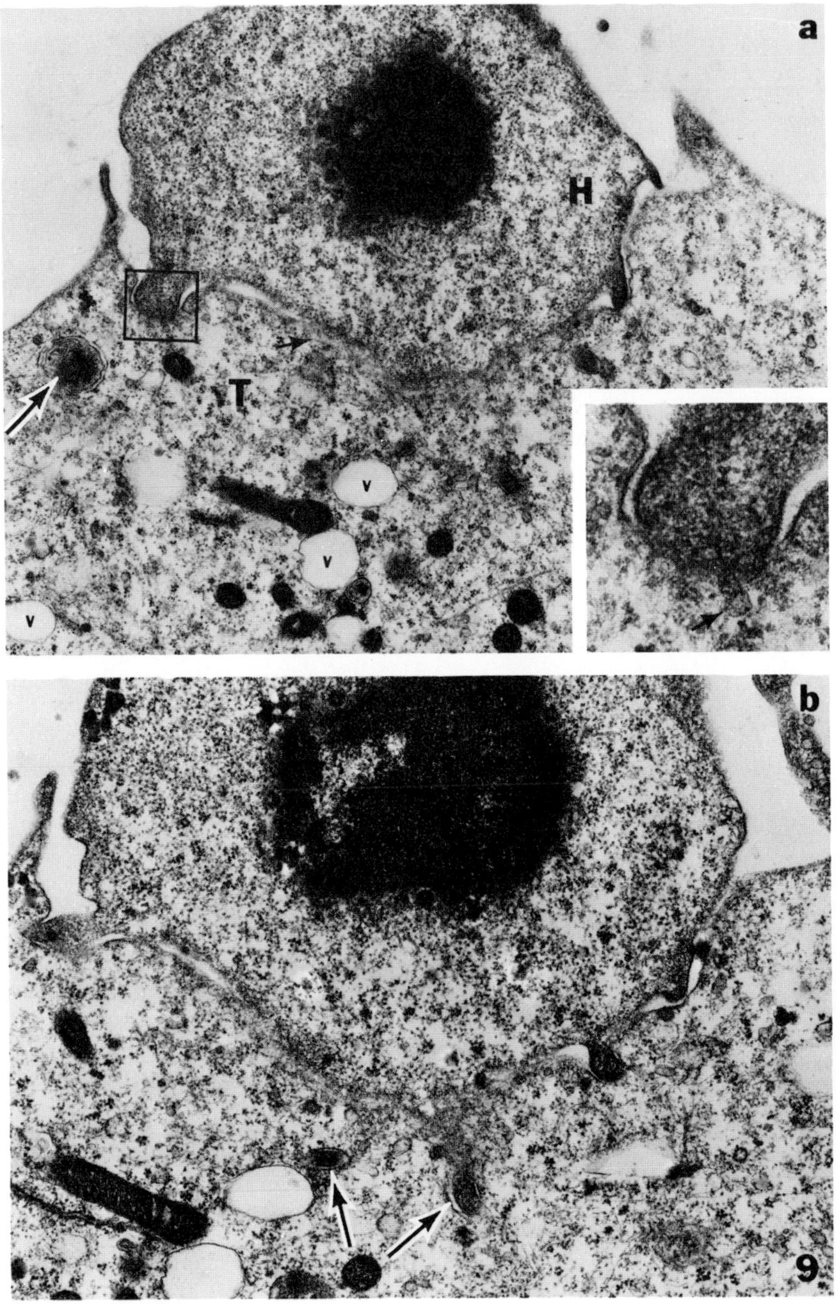
a
H
T
v
v
v
b
9

6. Hibbs, J. B., Jr., L. H. Lambert, Jr. and J. S. Remington (1972). Possible role of macrophage mediated nonspecific autotoxicity in tumor resistance. *Nature New Biol. 235*:48-50.

7. Chambers, V. C. and R. S. Weiser (1969). The ultrastructure of target cells and immune macrophages during their interaction *in vitro*. *Cancer Res. 29*:301-317.

8. Granger, G. A. and R. S. Weiser (1964). Homograft target cells: Specific destruction *in vitro* by contact interaction with immune macrophages. *Science 145*:1427-1429.

9. Hibbs, J. B., Jr. (1974). Heterocytolysis by macrophages activated by Bacillus Calmette-Guérin: Lysosome exocytosis into tumor cells. *Science 184*:468-471.

10. Zbar, B., H. T. Wepsic, H. J. Rapp, T. Borsos, B. S. Kronman and W. H. Churchill, Jr. (1969). Antigenic specificity of hepatomas induced in strain-2 guinea pigs by diethylnitrosamine. *J. Natl. Cancer Inst. 43*:833-841.

11. Zbar, B. and T. Tanaka (1971). Immunotherapy of cancer: Regression of tumors after intralesional injection of *Mycobacterium bovis. Science 172*:271-273.

12. Zbar, B., I. D. Bernstein, G. L. Bartlett, M. G. Hanna, Jr. and H. J. Rapp (1972). Immunotherapy of cancer: Regression of intradermal tumors and prevention of growth of lymph node metastases after intralesional injection of living *Mycobacterium bovis* (Bacillus Calmette-Guérin). *J. Natl. Cancer Inst. 49*:119-130.

13. Zbar, B., H. T. Wepsic, T. Borsos and H. J. Rapp (1970). Tumor-graft rejection in syngeneic guinea pigs: Evidence for a two-step mechanism. *J. Natl. Cancer Inst. 44*:475-481.

14. Dannenberg, A. M., Jr. (1968). Cellular hypersensitivity and cellular immunity in the pathogenesis of tuberculosis: Specifically, systemic and local nature, and associated macrophage enzymes. *Bacteriological Rev. 32*:85-102.

15. Fawcett, D. W. (1966). *An Atlas of Fine Structure. The Cell - Its Organelles and Inclusions* (ed. D. W. Fawcett). W. B. Saunders Company, Philadelphia, p. 219.

Fig. 9a. *(Shown at left) Electron micrograph of histiocyte (H) and line-10 tumor cell (T) after 72 hours incubation in vitro. There is marked indentation of the tumor cell at the site of histiocyte attachment and pronounced invagination opposite the cytoplasmic extension of the histiocyte (inset). A wide area of contact between histiocyte and tumor cell show regions of membrane destabilization and is confirmed by serial sections. Inset also shows a microcytoplasmic fold of the histiocyte projecting into the tumor cell (arrow).* × *25,000. Inset* × *70,000.* **Fig. 9b.** *Serial section of region shown in 9a. Note cytoplasmic extensions (arrows) of the histiocyte that appears to penetrate the tumor cell.* × *31,200.*

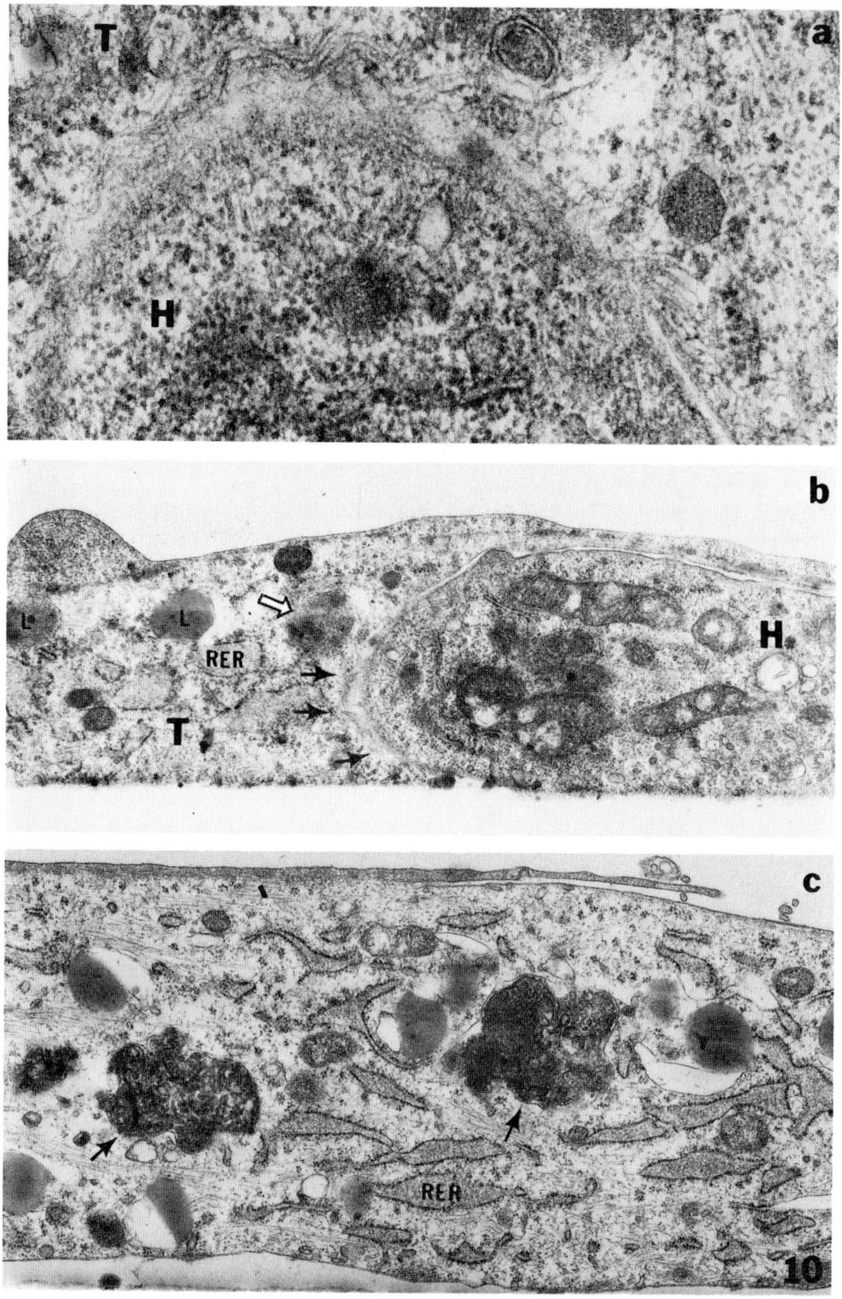

T
a
H
b
L
L
RER
T
H
c
RER
10

Fig. 10a. *(Shown at left) Micrograph of the histiocyte (H) – tumor (T) cell contact showing areas of membrane destabilization. Arrows indicate limiting membrane fragments of both cells at the areas of contact. Numerous tangential sections of microtubules and microfilaments are observed in both cells. Microtubules of the histiocyte appear to be aligned perpendicular to the area of membrane destabilization.* × *68,000.* **Fig. 10b.** *Histiocyte (H) and line-10 tumor (T) interaction after 72 hours of incubation in vitro. The histiocyte appears to be partially enveloped by the tumor cell, although areas of membrane destabilization between the two cells are observed (arrows). The tumor cell contains dilated rough endoplasmic reticulum RER, vacuoles (V), lysosomes (L), and phagosome (white arrow). Mitochondria of the histiocyte are clustered in close proximity to the area of membrane destabilization.* × *18,400.* **Fig. 10c.** *Line-10 tumor cell after 72 hours of incubation in vitro with histiocytes. The most prominent feature of the tumor cell is the presence of large electron-dense residual bodies (arrows) containing partially digested mitochndira and membranes. Note also the dilated rough endoplasmic reticulum with very granular material in the cisternae. Dense osmiophilic bodies that are closely associated with the dilated rough endoplasmic reticulum are frequently observed.* × *16,800.*

MECHANISMS OF TARGET CELL DESTRUCTION BY ALLOIMMUNE PERITONEAL MACROPHAGES[1]

Keith L. McIvor, Charles E. Piper[2], and Robert B. Bell[3]

Department of Bacteriology and Public Health
Washington State University
Pullman, Washington 99163

Cell mediated immunity, involving both lymphocytes and macrophages, is considered of primary importance in allograft as well as tumor rejection. Many years ago, Gorer (1) was the first to suggest that the macrophage may be involved in the rejection of certain types of tumors, mainly the ascites form. Since that time the specific contact destruction of allogenic target cells by alloimmune macrophages has been well documented both *in vivo* and *in vitro* (2,3,4,5,6).

Tumor cell destruction by macrophages can occur by any of several mechanisms. Bennett, Old and Boyse (7) described phagocytosis and the destruction of tumor cells by peritoneal macrophages from mice in the presence of isoantibody. Target cell destruction by a non-phagocytic mechanism following contact of target cells by macrophages has been described. Cytotoxicity or cytoinhibition of target cells may be immunologically specific ("armed" macrophages) (4,5,8,9,10), nonspecific for any adjacent cell ("activated" macrophages) (11) or nonspecific and kill cells with transformed membranes ("angry" macrophages) (8,12,13,14)

We have been particularly interested in determining the mechanism of killing of tumor cells by alloimmune macrophages during the rejection of an ascites tumor allograft in mice. In our studies we have employed the SaI tumor which is a dibenzanthracene induced tumor that was initiated in the A/JAX mouse in 1948. SaI is maintained by weekly serial intraperitoneal

[1] This study was supported in part by Grant CA12162 from the National Cancer Institute, National Institutes of Health, Bethesda, Maryland.

[2] Present Address: School of Veterinary Medicine, University of Pennsylvania, New Bolton Center, Kennett Square, Pennsylvania 19348.

[3] Present Address: The Johns Hopkins University, School of Medicine, Department of Laboratory Animal Medicine, Baltimore, Maryland 21205.

injections of 0.2 ml containing approximately 25 million SaI tumor cells. This dose is uniformly lethal to the A/JAX mouse in 8-10 days. When a similar intraperitoneal dose of SaI tumor cells is given to the C57BL/6 mouse, the tumor will be rejected in approximately 10-12 days. At the time of rejection, the peritoneal cavity will contain a cell population consisting of predominantly macrophages and in large numbers, up to 10^8. This alloimmune peritoneal macrophage population can be collected, washed, and used for *in vivo* and *in vitro* tests. Even though a macrophage rich population can easily be obtained, some caution should be exercised when the collection of peritoneal cells is based on the number of days after the injection of tumor cells. There is tremendous variation from animal to animal with respect to the percentage of macrophages and tumor cells present on any one day following injection. On day 10, the percentage of macrophages can vary from a low of 4% to 94%. Other characteristics of this tumor system are that the ascites form of SaI is more effective for inducing a macrophage response than normal allogeneic or xenogeneic tissue and SaI induced macrophages are more effective at destroying specific target cells than allogeneic tissue induced macrophages.

During the past decade, considerable information has accumulated concerning the Sarcoma I tumor system. It seems certain that phagocytosis is not the mechanism of killing(15). Although SaI alloimmune macrophages can phagocytize tumor cells, this event is rare. The first step in the sequence of events leading to the destruction of target cells is specific recognition mediated by a cytophilic factor, presumably antibody. Granger and Weiser (5) reported the very rapid and specific adherence of macrophages to target cells. This adherence occurred within 3-4 minutes and was very firm. In contrast, alloimmune macrophages or "normal" macrophages will stick to glass as well as "non-specific" target cells, however, the adherence is weaker, takes longer (30-60 minutes) and does not result in cell death. That specific recognition is mediated by a cytophilic antibody is supported by the report that a specific hemagglutinin can be eluted by heat from SaI alloimmune macrophages (16). In addition, adherence and killing is abolished by trypsinization (16).

That the killing events are both specific and begin early have been established by a variety of *in vitro* and *in vivo* studies. There is morphological evidence of cell damage in 3-4 hours (5) and killing could not be reversed following 1 hr of contact of immune cells with target cells (17).

Metabolic activity is required on the part of the macrophage. Pretreatment of the macrophage with the metabolic inhibitors, actinomycin-D, or chloramphenicol prevented the formation of plaques on monolayers of target cells (18). In contrast the same treatment of target cells had no effect on plaquing.

Actual death of the cell may be due to a heat-labile cytotoxin that we have designated specific macrophage cytotoxin (SMC) (9). Whether SMC is solely responsible for the death of target cells is not certain as there may be several soluble factors released from macrophages following contact with the target cells (19,20,21). Some of the properties of these soluble toxins have recently been compared (21). It is very possible that the macrophage may release one or more of these materials depending on the stimulus, environmental conditions, and incubation time. Release of particulate particles, such as lysosomes, is also a likely possibility (22).

The procedure for obtaining SMC is essentially the same as previously described (9). Alloimmune macrophages are obtained from the C57BL/6 following rejection of the ascites form of SaI. Twenty million well washed peritoneal cells (approximately 90-95% macrophages) are incubated for 2 hours with 10 million L-cells. The culture supernatant is removed, centrifuged to remove cellular debris, and assayed for cytotoxic activity. Specific contact, mediated through a cytophilic receptor, is essential for the release of SMC (9). Trypsinization of the alloimmune macrophage population prior to contact with the target cells, blocks the release of SMC. This suggests that a cytophilic protein receptor is required for activity. When alloimmune macrophages are incubated by themselves or when they are incubated with cells other than that used to sensitize the animal, there are minimal amounts of cytotoxin present in the culture supernatant. Further, the 2 hr culture supernatant of stimulated macrophage incubated with target cells is not cytotoxic.

The characteristics of SMC show it to be unique from other reported mouse *in vitro* cytotoxins (23). Specific macrophage cytotoxin is detected in the culture supernatant after 2 hours of incubation. The cytotoxicity of SMC affects only specific allogeneic cells and it is not mediated through heat labile serum components. SMC is inactivated by heating at 56°C for 30 minutes and it is trypsin sensitive. The molecular weight has been estimated to be 150-200,000.

Although a considerable amount of information on lymphotoxin has been done with mitogen induced material, it is apparent that lymphotoxin is also released by the specific interaction of immune lymphocytes and specific target cells. An important consideration is the potential role that lymphocytes might play in our system for it has been well established that immune lymphocytes of spleen or lymph node origin can cause the *in vitro* destruction of specific target cells. Even nonimmune lymphocytes when treated with PHA will inhibit the growth of target cells or cause plaques in monolayers of target cells.

Since 20 million peritoneal cells are allowed to interact with target cells, there may have been as many as 1.0×10^6 lymphocytes present. It is possible that this number of lymphocytes could have been the source of the cytotoxin released into the supernatant. In order to determine whether or not lymphocytes participated in release of cytotoxin, the following experiment was done. Immune peritoneal cells were collected, washed in the usual manner and 20 million were allowed to fix on glass at 37°C for 1 hour. The resulting monolayer of alloimmune peritoneal macrophages was washed 5 times with tissue culture medium. The lymphocytes present should have been largely removed by these washings since they have little tendency to adhere to glass. To the washed monolayer, 10 million L-cells were added. The immune cell-target cell interaction was allowed to proceed for 2 hours at 37°C and the supernatant was tested for the presence of SMC on L-cells.

In addition to the macrophage population, a lymphocyte-rich preparation (95% lymphocytes) was made and studied. The lymphocyte preparation was made from the mesenteric lymph nodes from the same mice from which the immune peritoneal macrophages had been collected. They were washed, resuspended in medium and 20 million lymphocytes were added to a monolayer of 10 million L-cells. The mixture was incubated for 2 hours at 37°C and the supernatant was tested for the presence of cytotoxin. The number of lymphocytes in the mixture was at least 10 times the number of contaminating lymphocytes present in the peritoneal macrophage preparation. Control supernatants included SMC prepared in the usual manner from alloimmune macrophages and "used medium" from a 2-hour culture of L-cells.

The results presented in Fig. 1 show that SMC resulted from the interaction of macrophages and L-cells, regardless of whether the macrophages were first placed on glass or were added directly to the L-cells. In contrast, the suspension of immune lymphocytes on L-cells did not produce any detectable cytotoxic substance in the 2 hours of incubation. After 48 hours of

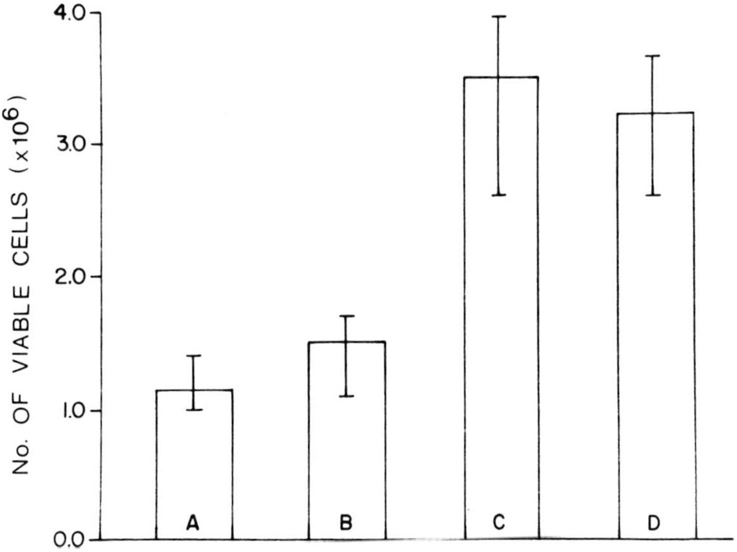

Fig. 1. *The effect of supernatants from a lymphocyte-rich or "pure" alloimmune macrophage interaction with L-cells on growth of L-cells: A. Treated with SMC from macrophages on L-cells; B. Treated with SMC from macrophages seeded on glass for one hour, washed, and L-cells added; C. Treated with supernatant from a two-hour interaction of a lymphocyte-rich preparation and L-cells: D. Treated with "used" medium.*

incubation, the culture supernatant of either alloimmune macrophages or lymphocytes and L-cells is cytotoxic for L-cells (9). This late macrophage toxin has been characterized and named macrophage toxic factor by Kramer and Granger (20) and found to be very similar to lymphotoxin. It seems certain that the macrophage is responsible for the release of SMC.

As there are reports of the release of both early (19,21) and late (20) macrophage toxins, we were interested in determining the optimal incubation period for maximum production of SMC. Twenty million alloimmune macrophages were incubated on L-cells at 37°C for varying time intervals. The culture supernatant from different reaction bottles which had been continually incubated for intervals of 1-10 hours were assayed for cytotoxicity. Figure 2 shows that SMC production reached detectable levels between 1 and 2 hours, stayed at a constant level for 2-6 hours, and then began to decline at 8-10 hours. Additional experiments were conducted to determine if SMC was released over the entire 6-hour incubation period. In these experiments the supernatant from the same reaction bottle was decanted at 2-hour intervals and replaced with new 199. When each of these supernatants was assayed,

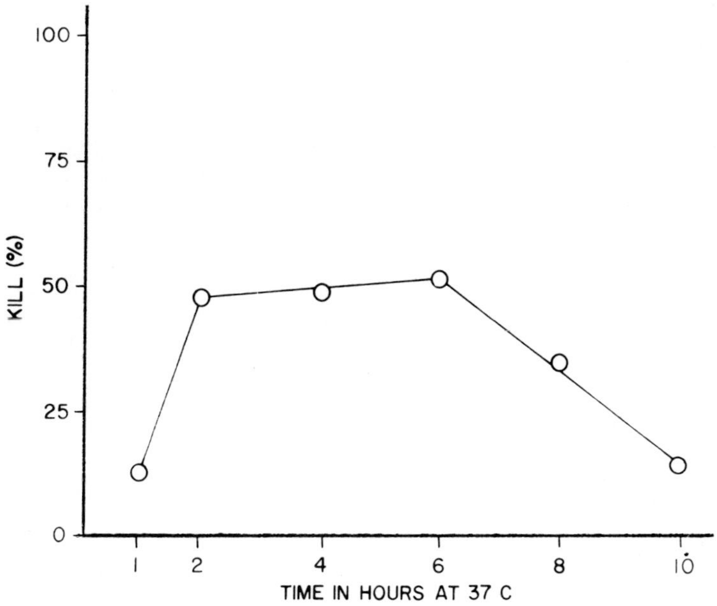

Fig. 2. *Effect of incubation time on production of SMC. Each point is the mean of triplicate cultures. Percent kill was determined by the following:*

$$\% \text{ Kill} = 100 - \frac{\text{No. of Viable Test Cells} \times 100}{\text{No. of Viable Control Cells}}$$

toxicity was obtained throughout the 6 hours of incubation. These experiments show that SMC is released during the first few hours of the interaction.

As SMC is stable at 37°C for at least 72 hours (23), the fact that SMC appears to decline in the culture supernatant after 6 hours may be due to adsorption to specific target cells. Approximately 50% of the toxicity of SMC was removed by a 2-hour adsorption of 37°C on three different monolayers of specific target L-cells, whereas it is not adsorbed with Hela cells (23).

We were interested in determining if additional adsorption would remove more cytotoxicity. Five milliliter aliquots of SMC were adsorbed for 1 hr at 37°C on 1.0×10^7 L-cells or Hela cells. At the end of one hour, the adsorbed material was removed and placed on another monolayer of L-cells or Hela cells. This procedure was repeated two additional times resulting in a total adsorption of 4 hours on 4 separate monolayers. SMC that had been adsorbed for 4 hours on four separate monolayers of Hela cells showed slight decrease in cytotoxicity, but the cytotoxicity of SMC was reduced from 80% to 15% when adsorption was on L-cells (Table 1). In another experiment, aliquots of SMC were adsorbed for 1 hour on 1.0×10^7 L-cells. At the end of one hour, an aliquot was removed, filtered, and tested for cytotoxic activity. The remaining aliquots were transferred to new monolayers of 1.0×10^7 L-cells. The above procedure was repeated each hour until one aliquot had been adsorbed on 4 separate monolayers for a total of 4 hours. The reduction of cytotoxicity of SMC is shown in Table 2. Unadsorbed SMC killed 63% of the treated L-cells, whereas SMC that had been adsorbed for 4 hours on L-cells kill 21% of the cells. There was a gradual reduction in cytotoxicity over the 4-hour period. These experiments support the concept that SMC specifically binds to target cells.

The specificity of SMC was originally explored using L-cells and primary cultures of allogeneic, syngeneic and xenogeneic fibroblasts (9). In these experiments no significant killing of syngeneic or xenogeneic fibroblasts

TABLE I

The Effect of Specific Macrophage Cytotoxin on L-cells Following Adsorption on L-cells or Hela Cells

Treatment	Adsorption (Hour)	Viable Cells/ Field[a]	Growth Inhibition (%)
Medium 199 alone	–	116	–
Medium 199 on L-cells	4	100	14
SMC alone	–	23	80
SMC on L-cells	4	98	15
SMC on Hela cells	4	39	66

[a]Average number of viable cells remaining after 48 hrs. Assays were performed in Lab-tex culture dishes in duplicate. Ten high-power fields were counted and the range of viable cells was less than ±20%.

TABLE 2
The Effect of Specific Macrophage Cytotoxin on L-Cells Following Adsorption for Various Lengths of Time

Treatment	Adsorption (Hour)	Viable Cells/ Field[a]	Growth Inhibition (%)
Medium 199 alone	–	187	–
SMC alone	–	58	63
SMC on L-cells	1	77	58
SMC on L-cells	2	92	51
SMC on L-cells	3	130	30
SMC on L-cells	4	162	13
SMC on L-cells[b]	4	146	21

[a]Average number of viable cells remaining after 48 hrs. Assays were performed on Lab-tex culture dishes in duplicate. Ten high-power fields were counted and the range of viable cells was less than ±20%.

[b]Adsorbed on one monolayer of 1.0×10^7 cells for 4 hours.

occurred. The results showed that SMC displayed the cytotoxicity expected of a specific cytotoxin; namely, its cytotoxicity was related to the target antigens present in test cells. When SMC was tested on several xenogeneic cell lines (Hep cells, Vero cells, Hela cells and embryonic ferret skin) there was approximately the same number of viable cells remaining after 24 hours of incubation with SMC as there were in controls (23). However, it is known that lymphotoxin is dose specific and not species specific, but a 4x dose of SMC had no effect on these xenogeneic cell lines (unpublished observations). The possibility that higher doses may show some effect is speculative.

The specificity of action is compatible with the previous findings that subsequent to specific recognition and adherence, presumably by antibody, there is a second specific step in the killing of target cells (16) and partial plaques are formed when mixed monolayers of specific target cells and control Hela cells are treated with alloimmune macrophages. The degree of clearing correlates with the percentage of L-cells present (24). Additional support for the specificity of SMC is supplied by its specific adsorption, and that its cytotoxicity can be inhibited by pretreatment of target cells by specific hyperimmune serum (23). The latter also suggests that SMC may bind to target cell membrane through transplantation antigens or a very closely related site.

It has been shown that purified human lymphotoxin causes an early decrease in the number of polysomes and an increase in the rate of RNA synthesis (25). We were interested in determining the effect of SMC on target cells. DNA and RNA metabolism was monitored by exposing 2×10^5 L-cells to SMC for 12 hours. SMC treated and control cultures were pulse labeled for one hour with either ^{3}H-thymidine or ^{3}H-uridine following 3, 7, and 11 hours of exposure. Table 3 shows the results of such an experiment. The uptake and incorporation of ^{3}H-thymidine is rapidly reduced by SMC and by 12 hours ^{3}H-thymidine levels are approximately one-half of controls. In contrast, the uptake and incorporation of ^{3}H-uridine are initially stimulated, however, by 12 hours they become reduced to less than control values.

In comparing target cell alterations induced by SMC with those reported for human lymphotoxin, two similarities are apparent. Both SMC and human lymphotoxin cause increases in the accumulation and incorporation of ^{3}H-uridine into RNA. Rosenau, *et al.* (25) have also reported that the cytotoxic effect of human lymphotoxin is potentiated and accelerated by actinomycin D. This feature is also common to SMC. SMC plus actinomycin D (0.5 μg/ml) showed a synergistic effect when tested on L-cells, whereas, the effect of hydroxyurea (0.1 μ mole/ml) or cycloheximide (0.1 μg/ml) with SMC was only additive. Human lymphotoxin and SMC have considerable differences with respect to molecular weight, heat lability, source and method of production and specificity. However, both may react with the cell membrane and trigger similar intracellular events. If SMC does exert its toxic effect on target cell membranes, it is conceivable that membrane alteration might result in observable changes in macromolecular synthesis. PHA stimulation of resting lymphocytes results in part in the activation of nuclear DNA dependent RNA polymerase (26). Further, tumor cell lines exposed to immunoglubulin specific for cell surface antigens develop increased levels of DNA synthesis (27).

If the affect of SMC is to inhibit DNA synthesis, cell death may not occur until the cell needs to divide. Generally, it is acknowledged that the growth of cells in tissue culture is enhanced by increases in serum concentrations. In fact Rubin and Koide (28) have reported that the rate of DNA synthesis in cultures of animal cells is directly proportional to the serum concentration. We have observed that without fetal calf serum in the culture medium, L-cells maintain themselves but minimal division occurs. In order to determine the effect of serum concentration on the toxicity of SMC, 2×10^5 L-cells were exposed to either SMC or control medium to which various concentrations of calf serum had been added. The results, Figure 3, show that the toxicity is substantially reduced when no calf serum was present in the

TABLE 3
The Effect of SMC on RNA and DNA Metabolism of L-cells[a]

Time (Hours)	^{3}H-Uridine Pools	^{3}H-Uridine Incorporation	^{3}H-Thymidine Pools	^{3}H-Thymidine Incorporation
4	1.22	1.15	0.73	0.78
8	1.14	1.06	0.64	0.71
12	0.92	0.83	0.52	0.62

[a]Results expressed as ratio of SMC treated cells (cpm per μg)/control cells (cpm per μg)

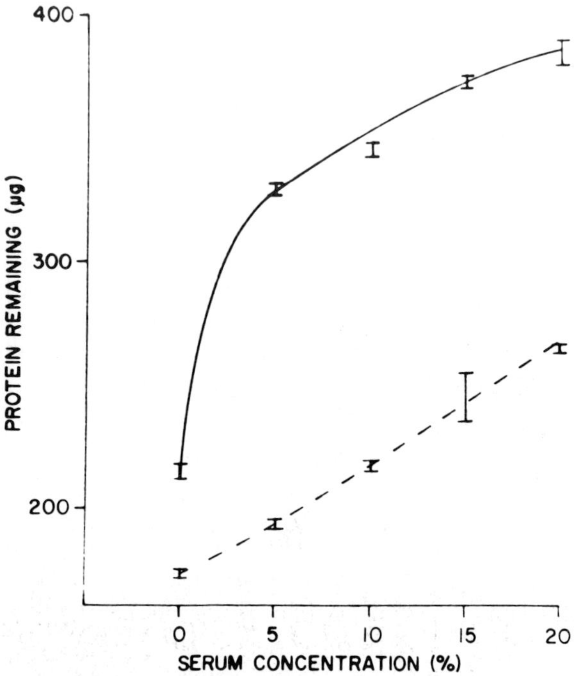

Fig. 3. *Effects of serum concentration on the toxicity of SMC. Control (—); SMC 0.5 cytotoxic units per ml (----).*

medium and suggests that the non-dividing cell is not as sensitive to SMC killing as the dividing cell. There have been several reports about the selective effect of the macrophage on neoplastic cells as compared to non-neoplastic cells (12,13,29). It is possible that if the effect of the macrophage is on DNA synthesis, the neoplastic cell may be more severely affected as it is not regulated by contact inhibition as is the non-neoplastic cell.

Recently, we have investigated the effect of SMC on the uptake of tritiated thymidine by Con A stimulated A/JAX or C57BL/6 spleen cells. Spleen cells from both species will be stimulated and take up increased amounts of tritiated thymidine when exposed to Con A. If the effect of SMC is to inhibit DNA synthesis, Con A stimulation should be blocked. Further, if SMC is specific for A/JAX spleen cells, only Con A stimulation of A/JAX spleen cells should be blocked. The results of such an experiment are shown in Fig. 4. The uptake of tritiated thymidine by Con A stimulated A/JAX spleen is essentially blocked when SMC is present, whereas C57BL/6 spleen cells are only partially suppressed. Presumably the A/JAX spleen cells do not respond because of specific killing. Nelson (30) has demonstrated the presence of factors in macrophage culture supernatants that will depress lymphocyte

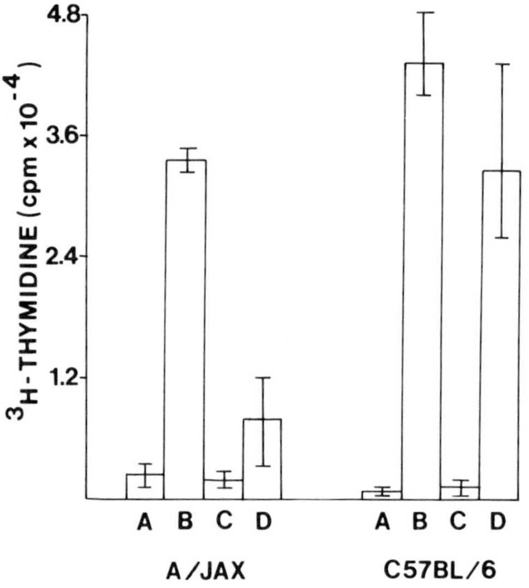

Fig. 4. *Effects of SMC on the concanavalin A response of syngeneic and allogeneic spleen cell cultures. MEM (A); MEM and 2 μg/ml Con A (B); SMC, 0.5 cytotoxic units per ml (C); SMC, 0.5 cytotoxic units per ml and 2 μg/ml Con A (D).*

transformation. The nonspecific partial suppression of C57BL spleen cells may be the result of such factors. It seems unlikely that the essentially 100% blockage of A/JAX spleen cells would be due entirely to suppressive factors. Whether or not the suppression of C57BL/6 spleen cells represents any regulatory effect remains to be elucidated but it is consistent with the hypothesis that the macrophage may be the source of an immunoregulatory α-globulin (31).

To date, SMC as well as lymphotoxin and other soluble cytotoxins have been obtained and investigated *in vitro*. It is assumed that these toxins exist *in vivo* and should be present during the rejection of tumor. Their true biological significance is dependent upon their presence *in vivo*. Preliminary evidence suggesting the presence of SMC *in vivo* during the rejection of Sarcoma I tumor has been obtained (McIvor and Moore, unpublished data). Table 4 shows the toxicity of ascites and culture supernatants of peritoneal exudate cells during various stages of rejection. Cytotoxicity to L-cells of 10% ascites fluid was minimal at the beginning and end of the rejection process and maximal when the tumor macrophage ratio reached approximately 1. Three-hour culture supernatants of peritoneal exudate cells from the various stages of rejection were similarly cytotoxic to L-cells. Cytotoxicity was heat labile and specific, suggesting SMC. These data not only suggest that SMC may be present *in vivo* during the rejection of tumor, they support the concept that

TABLE 4
Inhibition of Growth of L-cells by 10% Ascites Fluid and Peritoneal Cell Incubation Supernatants from C57BL/6 Mice at Various Stages of Rejection

Rejection Stage	Tumor Cells Remaining (%)	Growth Inhibition (%±SD)[a] 10% Ascites	PEC Culture Supernatant
A	>80	14±20 (3)	4.6±6 (5)
B	60-80	25±20 (7)	19±17 (19)
C	30-60	44±16 (6)	46±11 (5)
D	10-30	34±13 (3)	32±17 (5)
E	<10	3±5 (11)	15±17 (7)

[a]Number in parenthesis indicates number of experiments. Assays were performed in triplicate in Lab-tex culture dishes and growth inhibition was determined after 48 hours by the following formula:

$$100 - \frac{\text{No. of viable test cells} \times 100}{\text{No. of viable control cells}}$$

specific contact is necessary for the release of SMC. Prior to the presence of sufficient macrophages in the peritoneal cavity there are minimal amounts of cytotoxin release. When sufficient tumor cells are no longer present to interact with macrophages and trigger the release of SMC, toxicity in the ascites decreases. However, the macrophage population at the end of the rejection process is capable of releasing SMC, providing it is triggered with specific target cells. In fact it is with this population of cells that SMC is routinely made *in vitro*.

The concept that SMC is responsible for target cell death is attractive and is compatible with the observation of Granger (24) that advanced degenerative changes occur within target cells within 3 to 4 hours after contact with alloimmune macrophages.

The fact that plaques are formed in monolayers of target cells by alloimmune macrophages does not appear to be consistent with the release of a soluble toxin. In other laboratories the formation of plaques on tumor cells by macrophages from Toxoplasma infected mice (32) and BCG stimulated macrophages (11) has been interpreted as evidence against a soluble toxin. A relatively small number of macrophages ($1 \times 10^6 - 2 \times 10^6$) are used in most plaquing experiments. The apparent lack of toxicity in these culture supernatants may be due to the small number of macrophages available to release cytotoxin. Most likely the cytotoxin in the culture supernatant is "excess" material, as some may be passed directly into or onto target cells. We have observed that when larger numbers (4.0×10^6) of alloimmune macrophages are placed at 2 loci on a monolayer of target cells (approximately 1.0×10^6 covering approximately 10^2 cm) that the monolayer in the plaquing bottle is essentially destroyed. Further, specific macrophage cytotoxin may not act at any appreciable distance beyond the area of cell overlay because of its utilization by target cells, dilution effect, adsorption, or destruction by enzymes released by injured cells.

The failure of others to detect a soluble toxin in the culture supernatant may be due to different experimental systems that have been employed. In our system peritoneal macrophages are obtained 10-12 days following a single intraperitoneal injection of 25-30 million tumor cells. Other investigations have used macrophages activated with BCG (11) or taken from chronically infected mice (32) or mice that had received three injections of tumor cells (33). The length of time macrophages are cultured on glass or plastic may be important. When cultured on glass, SaI alloimmune macrophages rapidly lose their ability to form plaques (16) presumably due to membrane turnover and loss of specific recognition. In addition, the release of a soluble toxin from normal rat peritoneal cells is substantially less after 24 hours (21). Further, the time that the culture supernatant is examined for cytotoxic factors may be critical. The time of release of SMC as well as other soluble toxins is apparently restricted to the first few hours of interaction between immune cells and target cells.

To summarize, the killing of target cells by alloimmune peritoneal macrophages may take place in the following manner: (1) initial specific recognition and cell adherence occurs due to the interaction of cell-bound antibody with target cell antigen; (2) intimate membrane contact stimulates membrane phagocytosis and "triggers" the release of SMC; (3) SMC acts directly on the target cell membrane; (4) killing is initiated by a blockage of DNA synthesis, followed by inhibition of RNA, protein synthesis and lysis of the cell. The killing mechanism *in vivo* may be similar and heat labile serum components do not appear to be involved. Although the specificity suggests an antibody, attempts to demonstrate the presence of antibody in SMC have failed. The possibility that SMC is an enzyme should be considered. Amos (34) proposed that immune cells may release adaptive enzymes which are directed at substrates on specific target cells and which might act preferentially at sites of damage on target cells.

ACKNOWLEDGEMENTS

We wish to thank Ann Moore and Laurel Druffel for their expert technical assistance.

REFERENCES

1. Gorer, P. A. (1956). Some recent work on tumor immunity. *Adv. Cancer Res. 4*:149-186.

2. Old, L. J., E. A. Boyse, B. Bennett and F. Lilly (1963). Peritoneal cells as an immune population in transplantation studies. *Cell-bound Antibodies.* B. Amos and H. Koprowski, Eds. Wistar Institute Press, Philadelphia.

3. Bennet, B. (1965). Specific suppression of tumor growth by isolated peritoneal macrophages from immunized mice. *J. Immunol. 95*:656-664.

4. Tsoi, Mang-So and R. S. Weiser (1968). Mechanisms of immunity to Sarcoma I allografts in the C57BL/Ks mouse. I. Passive transfer studies with immune peritoneal macrophages in X-irradiated hosts. *J. Nat. Cancer Inst. 40*:23-30.

5. Granger, G. A. and R. S. Weiser (1964). Homograft target cells: Specific destruction *in vitro* by contact interaction with immune macrophages. *Sci. 145*:1427-1429.

6. Pearsall, N. N. and R. S. Weiser (1968). The macrophage in allograft immunity. I. Effects of silica as a specific macrophage toxin. *J. Reticuloendothelial Soc. 5*:107-120.

7. Bennett, B., L. J. Old and E. A. Boyse (1964). The phagocytosis of tumor cells *in vitro. Transplantation 2*:183-202.

8. Krahenbuhl, J. L. and J. S. Remington (1974). The role of activated macrophages in specific and nonspecific cytostasis of tumor cells. *J. of Immunol. 113*:507-516.

9. McIvor, K. L. and R. S. Weiser (1971). Mechanisms of target cell destruction by alloimmune peritoneal macrophages. II. Release of a specific cytotoxin from interacting cells. *Immunology 20*:315-322.

10. den Otter, W., R. Evans and P. Alexander (1972). Cytotoxicity of murine peritoneal macrophages in tumor allograft immunity. *Transplantation 14*:220-226.

11. Germain, R. N., R. M. Williams and B. Benacerraf (1975). Specific and nonspecific antitumor immunity. II. Macrophage-mediated nonspecific effector activity induced by BCG and similar agents. *J. Nat. Cancer Inst. 54*:709-718.

12. Hibbs, J. B., Jr., L. H. Lambert, Jr. and J. S. Remington (1972). Control of carcinogenesis: A possible role for the activated macrophage. *Sci. 177*:998-1000.

13. Hibbs, J. B., Jr. (1973). Macrophage nonimmunologic recognition: Target cell factors related to contact inhibition. *Sci. 180*:868-870.

14. Keller, R. and V. E. Jones (1971). Role of activated macrophages and antibody in inhibition and enhancement of tumor growth in rats. *Lancet 2*:847-849.

15. Baker, P., R. S. Weiser, J. Jutila, C. Evans and R. Blandau (1962). Mechanism of tumor homograft rejection: The behavior of Sarcoma I ascites tumor in the A/JAX and C57BL/Ks mouse. *Ann. N.Y. Acad. Sci. 101*:46-63.

16. Weiser, R. S., E. Heise, K. McIvor, S. Han and G. Granger (1969). *In vitro* activities of immune macrophages. *Cellular Recognition* R. T. Smith and R. A. Good, Eds. Appleton-Century-Crofts, New York.

17. McIvor, K. L. and R. S. Weiser (1971). Mechanisms of target cell destruction by alloimmune peritoneal macrophages. I. The effect of treatment with sodium fluoride. *Immunology 20*:307-313.

18. Granger, G. A. and R. S. Weiser (1966). Homograft target cells: Contact destruction *in vitro* by immune macrophages. *Sci. 151*:97-99.

19. Sintek, D. E. and W. B. Pincus (1970). Cytotoxic factor from peritoneal cells: Purification and characteristics. *J. Reticuloendothel. Soc. 8*:508-521.

20. Kramer, J. J. and G. A. Granger (1972). The *in vitro* induction and release of a cell toxin by immune C57BL/6 mouse peritoneal macrophages. *Cell. Immunol. 3*:88-100.

21. Reed, William P. and Zolton J. Lucas (1975). Cytotoxic activity of lymphocytes. V. Role of soluble toxin in macrophage inhibited cultures of tumor cells. *J. of Immunol. 115*:395-404.

22. Hibbs, J. B., Jr. (1974). Heterolysis by macrophages activated by bacillus Calmette-Guerin: Lysosome exocytosis into tumor cells. *Science 184*:468-471.

23. Piper, C. E. and K. L. McIvor (1975). Alloimmune peritoneal macrophages as specific effector cells: Characterization of specific macrophage cytotoxin. *Cell. Immunol. 17*:423-430.

24. Granger, G. A. (1965). Studies on *in vitro* homograft rejection in mice. Doctoral thesis, University of Washington, Seattle, Washington.

25. Rosenau, W., M. L. Goldberg and G. C. Burke (1973). Early biochemical alterations induced by lymphotoxin in target cells. *J. of Immunol. 111*:1128-1135.

26. Pogo, B. (1972). Early events in lymphocyte transformation by phytohemagglutinin I. DNA-dependent RNA polymerase activities in isolated lymphocyte nuclei. *J. Cell. Biol. 53*:635-641.

27. Shearer, W. T., G. W. Philpott and C. W. Parker (1973). Stimulation of cells by antibody. *Science 182*:1357-1359.

28. Rubin, H. and T. Koide (1973). Inhibition of DNA synthesis in chick embryo cultures by deprivation of either serum or zinc. *J. Cell. Biol. 56*:777-786.

29. Meltzer, M. S., R. W. Tucker, K. K. Sanford and E. J. Leonard (1975). Interaction of BCG-activated macrophages with neoplastic and nonneoplastic cell lines *in vitro*: Quantitation of the cytotoxic reaction by release of tritiated thymidine from prelabeled target cells. *J. Nat. Cancer Inst. 54*:1177-1184.

30. Nelson, D. S. (1973). Production by stimulated macrophages of factors depressing lymphocyte transformation. *Nature 246*:306-307.

31. Copperband, S. R., A. M. Badger, R. C. Davis, K. Schmid and J. A. Mannick (1972). The effect of immunoregulatory α-globulin (IRA) upon lymphocytes *in vitro. J. of Immunol. 109*:154-163.

32. Hibbs, John B., Jr., Lewis H. Lambert and Jack S. Remington (1972). Possible role of macrophage mediated nonspecific cytotoxicity in tumor resistance. *Nature (New Biol.) 235*:48-50.

33. Evans, R. and P. Alexander (1972). Role of macrophages in tumor immunity. II. Involvement of a macrophage cytophilic factor during syngeneic tumor growth inhibition. *Immunology 23*:627-636.

34. Amos, D. B. (1962). The use of simplified systems as an aid to the interpretations of mechanisms of graft rejection. *Prog. in Allergy 6*:468-538.

CYTOSTATIC AND CYTOCIDAL EFFECTS OF ACTIVATED NONIMMUNE MACROPHAGES

R. Keller

Immunobiology Research Group
University of Zurich
Schönleinstrasse 22
CH-8032 Zurich/Switzerland

INTRODUCTION

It is now rather widely appreciated that macrophages, apart from their well established important role in pathological processes such as inflammation and resistance to microorganisms, and in immunity, could represent major effectors in the destruction of tumor cells (1-3). *In vitro* studies in the early 1970's performed independently by several groups (4-6) have reanimated and substantiated such a concept. In subsequent work it was brought out that macrophages have the capacity to interact with eukaryotic targets in a variety of ways. Such studies have been of particular importance showing that the macrophage effects on tumor cells can be either immunologically specific (2,3,7,8) or nonspecific (4-6,9). In the latter category, macrophages from animals infected with nematode (4) or protozoan parasites (6,10,11), bacteria such as BCG (12) and *Listeria monocytogenes* (6,11), or pretreated with a large array of stimulants such as peptone (4,13), Freund's complete adjuvant (14,15), endotoxin (5), double-stranded RNA (5) or killed *Corynebacterium parvum* (16,17) have in each instance acquired rather similar capacities of interacting with a variety of tumor targets *in vitro*. This communication seeks to summarize and evaluate the accumulated data on *in vitro* interaction of nonimmune, activated macrophages (AM) with target cells, considers the technical difficulties peculiar to this area and identifies new directions for exploration.

IN VITRO EFFECTS ON TARGET CELL PROLIFERATION

Two main consequences of the *in vitro* interaction of AM with targets have thus far been detected and analysed to some degree. The first expressions of the interaction are on target cell proliferation. Then, under certain defined conditions, destructive capacities of AM leading to cytocidal and/or cytolytic target cell damage are expressed.

It seems now probable that proliferation of target cells can be either inhibited or enhanced, depending on the kind and/or degree of macrophage activation, the actual ratio of macrophages to targets, and the susceptibility of the target cell.

1. Cytostatic capacities of AM

There is now considerable evidence attesting to the cytostatic potential of AM (13,15-24).

1.1. *Methodological aspects*

As a method of assessing residual target cell proliferation, the incorporation of a pulse label of tritiated thymidine has provided reproducible data. Since macrophages in culture remain in the G_1 or G_0 phase of the cell cycle, incorporation of methyl-[^{3}H]-thymidine ([^{3}H]-TdR) into DNA in this system reflects solely proliferation of target cells. It could be argued that the AM effect is merely on thymidine incorporation. In fact, macrophages lack thymidine kinase activity, and thus contain a sizable thymidine pool which might compete with the label (25). However, various observations strongly suggest that the macrophage effects on target cell proliferation by far exceed such a trivial action. Experiments with a variety of spontaneously replicating targets including lymphoblastoid lines have indicated that macrophage-mediated inhibition of thymidine incorporation is paralleled or followed by a decrease in uridine incorporation, by a standstill or a decrease in the number of targets, a decrease in the number of mitoses and by marked decrease in the number of targets with high nuclear DNA content (13,20,21; Keller unpublished; Keller, R., Bregnard, A., Gehring, W. J., and Schroeder H. E., in preparation). It remains to be determined, however, how far the later consequences of the interaction are mediated by cytostatic and/or cytolytic principles. Other important objections against such observations are based on the fact that, especially in experiments extended over several days, changes in cell density and related nutrient depletion might decisively affect proliferation. Although dependence on the fluctuation of such factors within a realistic range cannot be fully excluded, the observations that the presence of a similar number of nonstimulated peritoneal cells or of the nonadherent portion of peptone-induced cells, or a much higher number of tumor cells alone diminished proliferation only slightly or not at all, provide strong evidence against a major role for such changes (13,18,20,21,23,24,26). Moreover, medium removed from 2 to 4 day tumor cell cultures fully supported further growth of targets (Keller unpublished). Altogether, these observations indicate that determination of residual target cell proliferation by a pulse of tritiated thymidine truly reflects changes occurring in targets. Assessment of residual target cell proliferation by pulse labeling with ^{125}I-iododeoxyuridine has led to similar results. It seems advantageous, however, to confirm such findings by parallel enumeration of targets remaining after various intervals.

1.2. *Evidence that activated mononuclear phagocytes are the effector cells which mediate cytostasis.*

In the author's lab, peritoneal cells were obtained either from untreated donor DA rats (170-200 g), or 3 days after intraperitoneal injection of 10 ml 10% proteose peptone (13). Cultures were prepared by seeding approximately 2×10^6 macrophages into 35×10 mm plastic Petri dishes. Effector cells were allowed to adhere for 60 min at 37°C. The non-adhering cells were then removed by intensive washing. When peptone-induced peritoneal cells had been seeded, at least 96% of the cells remaining on the dishes after this procedure showed the characteristics of mononuclear phagocytes (morphology, adherence, phagocytosis, resistance to X-irradiation; 13,18, Keller, Bregnard, Gehring and Schroeder, in preparation). Moreover, no cytostatic activity evolved when interaction took place in the presence of silica, an agent selectively toxic for mononuclear phagocytes (13). To monolayers consisting of 2×10^6 macrophages, usually 2×10^5 target cells were added. Since approximately 3.5×10^6 macrophages constitute a confluent monolayer, these represent half to two third coverage of the surface.

Unfortunately, results obtained with effectors from normal, nonstimulated rats (NM) are not readily comparable to those obtained with AM. First, peptone stimulation, probably by inducing migration of blood monocytes, leads to a 2 to 5 fold increase in the number of peritoneal mononuclear phagocytes which show, moreover, morphological signs of activation such as spreading and ruffled membrane movements. In contrast, among adherent peritoneal cells from normal, untreated rats, only about 70% show the characteristics of mononuclear phagocytes. Furthermore, the assessment of the degree of macrophage activation is rendered difficult, as this function is not static but usually increases in the course of early *in vitro* culture and then decreases again (15,19). Despite these considerable difficulties, the reported differences between NM and AM of the rat in the morphological appearance of their interaction with targets (13,27), in the degree and continuance of cytostasis (15,19), and in the production of a soluble cytostatic factor (20,28; see paragraph 1.5), all point to macrophage activation as the critical process. Similar differences in the cytostatic capacities of AM have been reported to occur in mice (11,22). However, the metabolic and functional requirements involved in increased cytostatic capacity remain quite unknown (19,24).

1.3. *Non-specificity of macrophage-mediated cytostasis*

As the main interests were directed onto possible effects of AM on tumor targets, most earlier studies have been restricted to transformed cell lines (11,13,15-17,22). In the meantime it has been shown, however, that cytostasis mediated by nonspecifically activated macrophages transcends histoincompatibility within (12,24,26) and beyond species (18,21,24,26), cell type (epithelial or lymphoid; 20,21,24,30), growth characteristics (monolayer or suspension; 18,21,24) and was in fact exerted on all rapidly replicating cell lines whether derived from normal or from transformed tissues (18,20,21,24,26). Thus far, prolonged interaction with a majority of 10 macrophages per target led to a distinct inhibition of target cell proliferation in every rapidly proliferating cell line examined (18,21,24). However, the degree and kinetics of macrophage-mediated cytostasis differed markedly from one cell line to another (18,21,24). When a large array of cell lines are ranked according to their susceptibility to cytostasis mediated by DA rat AM, normal replicating lymphoid cells (20), various virus-transformed lines (18,21), P-815 mastocytoma cells (21), and some cell lines derived from human malignant tumors (18,21) are seen to be especially sensitive. Derivatives of the mouse L fibroblast, although consistently blocked after prolonged interaction with macrophages, showed large differences in their initial sensitivity, not corresponding with their degree of malignancy (21); other lines, such as 3T3, CHO, LOPEZ, DMBA- and MCA-induced rat tumor cells, lymphoblastoid cell lines, and also recently explanted fibroblasts derived from normal adult or embryonic rat tissues, were rather resistant to macrophage-mediated cytostasis (18,20,21,24,26). It seems thus highly probable that in rapidly replicating cell lines, factors other than capacity for *in vivo* malignancy or *in vitro* transformation determine susceptibility to macrophage-mediated cytostasis.

1.4. *Kinetics of the cytostatic process*

In the presence of an effector to target cell ratio of 10:1, proliferation of a large number of rapidly replicating cell lines is depressed to approximately 25% of the control within the first 4 h, is reduced to background levels within 12 h and then mostly remained at this base line for several days (13,15,18,21). Other cell lines, particularly lymphoblastoid cell lines (20,21,24), carcinogen-induced syngeneic rat tumor cells (21) and several cell lines originally derived from normal tissues (18,21), were rather resistant to macrophage-mediated cytostasis, and often retain considerable residual proliferation despite the continuing presence of AM.

Macrophage-mediated cytostasis has been shown to be largely dependent on the actual effector to target cell ratio (13,20). Depending on the susceptibility of the target, an effector to target cell ratio of 1:1 either still markedly reduced proliferation (normal lymphocytes, susceptible tumor cell lines), or was without significant effects (lymphoblastoid cell lines, syngeneic carcinogen-induced tumor cell lines, recent explants of syngeneic normal adult or embryonic fibroblasts). When target cells were in majority, the presence of macrophages often resulted in a clear enhancement of target cell proliferation (13,20; see paragraph 2.).

1.5. *Mechanisms by which AM-mediated cytostasis is achieved*

Numerous findings such as the strong parallelism in the appearance of effector/tumor cell aggregates and inhibition of tumor cell proliferation, and the failure of 4 to 8 h macrophage culture supernatants and of macrophage lysates to inhibit tumor cell replication, all pointed towards *cell-to-cell contact* phenomena between functional effectors and targets as important for attaining cytostasis (13,16,22). However, some situations were encountered in which cytostasis was effective despite greatly reduced opportunity of cell-to-cell contact. For example, the interaction between AM and many targets derived from normal tissues did not disclose such close contact despite effective cytostasis (18,20,21,24).

Meanwhile, evidence is rapidly accumulating that cytostasis is mediated by a *soluble factor* secreted by macrophages (20,24,28-32). These data indicate that following appropriate activation, macrophages cultured at optimal densities release a low molecular, heat-stable cytostatic factor which was shown to inhibit the incorporation of $[^3H]$-thymidine and ^{125}I-deoxyuridine into various cells as well as the proliferation and protein synthesis of various cells (20,30-32, Keller unpublished). Optimal conditions for the synthesis, secretion, and catabolism of the soluble mediators and the mechanism by which cytostasis is achieved, have to be determined before its possible *in vivo* significance can reliably be assessed. Present knowledge suggests that a markedly enhanced production of the cytostatic macrophage factor and a high ratio of AM to targets (for example 1:1) is a necessary precondition for its *in vivo* efficacy. As the cytostatic macrophage factor is a small molecule, its efficacy is probably localized to restricted areas. The work of Nelson (28) which shows the presence of such activity in the serum of mice with a graft vs host reaction indicates, however, that in such special situations even a systemic effect of this low molecular factor might be conceivable.

In contrast to the astonishing reproducibility with which cytostasis by activated mononuclear phagocytic cells is mediated, results with their soluble supernatants are not as easily reproduced. This may be due to the variability in the degree and/or kind of macrophage activation, decay or consumption of cytostatic activity, and also depend on the actual concentration of factors inhibiting or enhancing cell proliferation. Observations indicating that cytostasis mediated by macrophage culture supernatants was often distinctly less pronounced than that mediated by the same macrophage monolayer may be interpreted to mean that cytostasis mediated during close contact is more effective than that mediated by the soluble factor (Keller unpublished).

In view of the major role now accorded macrophages in the so-called cooperative effects during the immune response, it is conceivable that enhancement and/or suppression of lymphocyte proliferation by the macrophage and its soluble products could be decisive with respect to the duration and magnitude of that reaction. Although there are indications that the presence of T cells is not required to achieve macrophage-mediated cytostasis (15), it should be emphasized that supernates from antigen- or mitogen-stimulated lymphocytes effectively enhance macrophage cytostatic potential (24,33). The possibility must be envisaged that the MIF-mediated migration and activation of mononuclear phagocytes induced following interaction of lymphocytes with the specific antigen provides the preconditions for inhibition of lymphocyte proliferation, and might thus represent a potent feedback mechanism (20).

2. Macrophage-mediated stimulation of cell proliferation

It has long since been suggested that mononuclear phagocytes capable of multiple functions, might interfere with other cells and thus play a regulatory role on a large array of parameters. However, even the knowledge of their well documented manifold role at various stages of the immune response is far from suggesting an exact concept of their mode of action. Various earlier experiments might be relevant in this context. For example, viability of lymphocytes in culture is increased by the presence of macrophages (34), and macrophage culture supernatants have been found to enhance or support lymphocyte function (35-40), and such capacities seemed to depend upon macrophage stimulation (35,36). We have shown that where macrophages are numerically in the minority there occurs enhanced proliferation of tumor targets (13), of normal lymphocytes (20) and especially marked, of slowly replicating recent explants of fibroblasts (Keller unpublished). Such enhancement of target cell proliferation could reflect some sort of trophic influence of macrophages. Earlier reports indicated that mercaptoethanol somehow substituted for this function of macrophages (34). Using tumor cells and recent syngeneic explants of rat fibroblasts as targets, no evidence for a substitution of the macrophage-mediated enhancement of proliferation by mercaptoethanol could be found (Keller unpublished).

2.1. *Evidence that simulation of cell proliferation is mediated by a soluble factor secreted by macrophages.*

Recent studies have shown that macrophage culture supernatants exhibited both proliferation inhibitory and enhancing capacities probably mediated by different activities (20,29-32) and all evidence points to the macrophage as the source of both materials. According to the work of Unanue and collaborators (32), the stimulatory molecule did not contain H-2 antigen, was resistant to diisopropylfluoro-phosphate treatment, eluted from Sephadex with a size ranging from 15,000 to 21,000 daltons, and was sensitive to chymotrypsin and pepsin.

The relationship between the state of maturation and/or the degree of activation and the formation of the stimulatory molecule remains to be clarified. All available evidence suggests that apart from the macrophage functional activities and the actual ratio of enhancing and inhibitory factors, conditions such as the number of macrophages, the nature and/or susceptibility and number of targets, and the anatomical relationship between effectors and targets may also determine whether stimulatory or cytostatic effects become dominant. The easiness with which the two macrophage factors can now be separated will certainly facilitate the resolution of these questions.

Analysis by impulse cytophotometry of the effects of macrophage culture supernatants exhibiting predominantly stimulatory activity on the proliferation of various syngeneic and xenogeneic tumor targets and recent explants from normal syngeneic tissue has shown that the number of cells being in the S and G_2 phase of the cell cycle were distinctly increased in such populations (Keller and Gehring, unpublished). This indicates that, similar to the cytostatic principle, the stimulation of cell proliferation induced by this factor is real, and that its effect is exerted on a variety of targets from different origin and exhibiting different growth characteristics.

IN VITRO EFFECTS ON TARGET CELL VIABILITY

As outlined in the previous chapter (p. 3), the first expressions of AM were always on target cell proliferation. However, the earliest *in vitro* observations on the consequences of the interaction of target cells with AM have shown that tumor cells undergo conspicuous morphologic changes whereas no such changes were seen with normal cells (4-6,13,27).

In the meantime the methods have been refined, increased in number, and a large array of targets has been examined. On the basis of these data, the present knowledge of the macrophage effects on target cell viability is briefly discussed.

1. Morphological consequences of the interaction of AM with targets

The early studies of the interaction of nonimmune AM with tumor targets were based mainly on morphological criteria (4-6,8,9,13,26,27). These observations indicated that AM, similar to immune macrophages from tumor-immunized animals (2,3,7,41), have the capacity to kill tumor cells and that this destruction is probably mediated during close contact with targets. In sharp contrast, interaction of AM with targets derived from normal tissues was not followed by such conspicuous changes. Further studies have essentially confirmed and extended such observations (18,24,42,43, Keller, Brègnard, Gehring and Schroeder, in preparation).

The analysis of the morphological consequences of the interaction of AM with tumor cells has shown that addition of tumor cells to a monolayer of AM is often followed by an early directed movement of neighboring macrophages onto nearby targets (24). This early phase of the interaction is frequently characterized by an accumulation of AM around targets and the formation of effector/target cell aggregates (5,13,27). Already within the first 12 h of interaction, it is frequently evident that the number of targets is distinctly lower in these cultures than in cultures consisting of target cells alone. As interaction proceeds, the number of target cells progressively further decreases whereas macrophages remain essentially intact (Keller, Bregnard *et al.*). As a consequence, the macrophage/tumor cell ratio may considerably increase. The disappearance of tumor targets with a conspicuous absence of cell debris during their interaction with AM is a rather uniform, consistent occurrence but the underlying basis for this phenomenon is not understood.

EM analysis of the consequences of the AM interaction with tumor cells helped determine, that despite close proximity between effectors and targets, there was no morphological evidence for joint junctions or intrusion of effector cell villi into target cells. As interaction proceeded, disintegrated tumor cells surrounded by macrophages, and macrophages containing phagocytized tumor cell residues within vacuoles were often encountered (Keller and Bächi, unpublished, 24, Keller, Bregnard *et al.*).

Thus, interaction of AM with tumor targets is frequently characterized by the formation of effector/target cell aggregates which favor close cell-to-cell contact. During such close contact, targets are damaged and are then addicted to decay. In other words, killing is effected during close contact; phagocytosis of target cell residues is a secondary event having scavenger rather than killer function. Such close contact is absent when AM are interacted with targets derived from normal tissues.

2. Cytocidal and/or cytolytic activities of AM

The morphological observations showing that interaction of AM with tumor cells is consistently accompanied by a decrease in the number of tumor cells (4,5,9,18,27) and that in cultures containing a central monolayer of AM, tumor cells grow unchecked in the periphery but were fully eliminated in the region of the macrophage monolayer (6,14,42-44), all strongly suggested a cytocidal or cytolytic effect of AM. On the other hand, indicators of immune cytotoxicity such as employed in lymphocyte target studies, release of ^{51}Cr or uptake of trypan blue, remained unaffected during interaction with AM (13,18).

2.1. *Methodological aspects*

Various methodological approaches were made to substantiate the concept that the progressive disappearance of tumor targets during their interaction with AM was due to some unknown cytocidal process.

In a series of experiments, the residual capacity of targets to reestablish growth was assessed. In showing that after interaction with AM for 72 h, syngeneic, allogeneic or xenogeneic cell lines derived from tranformed tissue were often no longer able to reestablish growth, these data attested to the effective killing of tumor targets during their *in vitro* interaction with AM (18). However, both the enumeration of target cells remaining and the assessment of residual *cloning efficiency* were subject to considerable errors.

In the search for more objective methods, various approaches using prelabeled targets have been made. ^{125}*I-iododeoxyuridine* (IUdR) has come into increasing use as a label of target cells for the detection of lymphocyte- (45-49) and macrophage- (17,21) mediated cytotoxicity. These experiments have convincingly shown that stimulated mononuclear phagocytes were extremely effective in lysing tumor targets *in vitro*. Although this method has proved useful, its disadvantages such as toxicity of IUdR and of FUdR often rendered interpretation of results difficult. As an alternative, we have recently passed over to target cell prelabeling with ^{14}C- or [^{3}H]-TdR as indicators of macrophage-mediated lytic activity. As reutilization of the label by macrophages is low and toxicity contributed by the labeling procedures can be neglected when the concentration of the isotope is kept low, the assessment of the release of ^{14}C- or [^{3}H]-TdR from prelabeled targets seems to reliably reflect macrophage-mediated cytolytic potential. It is thus possible to measure cytostatic (residual target cell proliferation) and cytocidal capacities (release of isotope from prelabeled targets) with the same nontoxic isotope. Very recently, an even more sensitive assay has been introduced to detect macrophage-mediated cytocidal or cytolytic capacity (50).

3. Evidence that AM are the effector cells which mediate target cell lysis

The accurate measurement of viability in a variety of targets, and its application to macrophage-mediated effects was essential for furthering the understanding of the processes involved in the interaction between macrophages and other eukaryote cells. Using such objective quantitative methods, it has recently been demonstrated that cells exhibiting the characteristics of mononuclear phagocytes (see paragraph B 1.2.) were effective in killing tumor cells (17,18,21); more recent experiments have shown that the nonadherent portion of peptone-induced peritoneal cells is quite unable to mediate such cytostatic and cytolytic effects (Keller, unpublished). The earlier observations indicating that normal, resting macrophages have no or only moderate anti-tumor effect (5,6,13) have also been confirmed (17). Thus, the few available data may be taken to indicate that the presence of the macrophage is indispensable for, and that macrophage activation is the critical process in attaining increased cytolytic capacities; but as in cytostasis, the metabolic and functional requirements involved remain unknown.

4. Are the cytocidal macrophage effects tumor-specific?

On the basis of morphological grading of macrophage-mediated target cell cytotoxicity, it was concluded that neoplastic cells are uniquely susceptible as contrasted to their normal counterparts (6,13,27,43, Keller, Bregnard *et al.*). This seems to apply to targets of syngeneic, allogeneic or xenogeneic origin. The observation that the viability of certain long established cell lines originally derived from normal tissues was considerably reduced following interaction with AM was interpreted as an expression of their transformation (18). However, other findings suggest that the situation is not as simple as previously supposed and that there are quantitative rather than qualitative differences in susceptibility of normal and tranformed targets to macrophage-mediated cytolysis (21,42,44,51). In particular, the findings showing that transformed cells are affected equally whether grown at permissive or non-permissive temperatures or when they differ considerably in their *in vivo* malignant potential strongly suggest that their susceptibility to the cytocidal macrophage effect is quite independent of the *degree* of malignancy (21).

5. Postulated mechanisms for macrophage-mediated target cell damage

The aforementioned data reliably attest to the macrophage cytocidal and/or cytolytic capacities towards a large array of targets, especially transformed cells. It is evident, however, that the susceptibility to these macrophage effects differs considerably from one target cell to another and does in no way parallel its degree of transformation or *in vivo* malignancy (21). This indicates that the target cell surface structures determining susceptibility to macrophage-mediated cytocidal effects are not invariably correlated with the malignant attributes of the target.

Perusal of the available material makes clear that early and extensive formation of effector/target cell aggregates and effective target cell killing are closely associated. In other words, close contact seems to favour the macrophage cytolytic potential. In showing that macrophage-mediated cytolysis can be inhibited by agents which prevent the exocytosis of macrophage lysosomes such as hydrocortisone or which interfere with the action of lysosomal enzymes such as trypan blue, Hibbs (43) has provided support for the concept that this capacity is mediated by lysosomal enzymes of AM. The results further suggest that lysosomes of AM are secreted directly into the cytoplasm of susceptible target cells which subsequently undergo lysis. Indeed, such a concept fits in with several facts now available.

When it is accepted that close contact between effectors and targets represents an important precondition for the mediation of the macrophage cytolytic effect, several other conceptual views arise. The large differences among a variety of tumor cells in their susceptibility to the macrophage-mediated cytolytic effect are probably due to various properties. Among the various possibilities, differences in membrane fluidity and emission of macrophage chemotactic signals assuring close effector/target cell contact can be envisaged as likely candidates in determining target cell susceptibility and may also contribute to the relative tumor specificity of the cytolytic effect.

Another possibility to be envisaged is that the cytolytic activity is mediated by a soluble toxin secreted by AM. Indeed, immunologically specific (52) and nonspecific (50,52-56) cytotoxic activities have been found in the supernatants of immune and nonimmune AM, respectively. It may thus be postulated that such nonspecific lytic principles released by AM may damage susceptible types of cells without requiring direct macrophage-target cell contact. It is conceivable that these two cytolytic mechanisms, close cell-to-cell contact and mediation by a soluble toxin, may both contribute to the macrophage effects.

GENERAL DISCUSSION AND OUTLOOK

The aforementioned studies have demonstrated that under *in vitro* conditions, macrophages and/or their soluble factors have the potential of affecting the proliferation and/or the viability of a large array of target cells. These astonishingly potent *in vitro* effects are mediated at effector to target cell ratios which seem physiologically plausible and could be attained *in vivo*. How is it then that cancer is not a rarity, i.e, that these effects are not the rule under *in vivo* conditions? In this respect, a variety of issues emerge and some are briefly discussed.

There is evidence to suggest that the macrophage potential contributing to natural tumor resistance is especially critical in the very earliest phases of tumor development, i.e. tumor nidation, and that it is not likely to contribute greatly to resistance against tumors already established (Keller unpublished). The *in vitro* data indicate that macrophages should be able to kill a small number of more or less isolated accessible tumor cells if an appropriate ratio of activated mononuclear phagocytes is locally available. However, already under *in vitro* conditions, the question whether macrophage activation is required is not a consensus (50), although there is considerable evidence to suggest that appropriately activated macrophages have greatly increased cytostatic and cytolytic potential. The limited knowledge of the biochemical background underlying these macrophage functions makes it difficult to assess the role of macrophage "activation" *in vivo*. It may moreover be argued that many of the experimental procedures utilized to mobilize large numbers of peritoneal macrophages and/or their functional activity, such as intraperitoneal injection of peptone, etc. are quite artificial and bear no relationship to normal conditions. In this respect, attempts to duplicate *in vitro* what is believed to happen *in vivo*, i.e., stimulation of lymphocytes by neoantigens with ensuing elaboration of lymphokines, which in term enhance macrophage functional activity, merit special attention.

Another relevant aspect concerns the effector cell population. Peritoneal macrophages have mainly been used in these studies as a very practical convenience. It has been a major assumption, however, that this population is functionally uniform and truly representative of mononuclear phagocytes from different anatomical sites. However, there is growing evidence for macrophage functional heterogeneity, not only between different but also within distinct anatomical sites (57-59). Moreover, expression of macrophage functions may also depend on the degree of its maturation. For example, blood monocytes obtained from healthy individuals show rather weak cytostatic activity and under present conditions were incapable of killing a variety of tumor targets (Keller and Sauter, unpublished). Thus, apart from species differences, many of the macrophage parameters relevant with respect to their cytostatic and cytocidal capacities are still poorly understood.

It is even more difficult to assess the consequences of the *in vivo* interaction of macrophages and targets and a presumed array of factors that interfer with it. It seems now established that tumors contain a characteristic percentage of mononuclear phagocytes, and this percentage varies considerably from one type of tumor to another (60). Moreover, intratumoral injection of immunostimulants such as *Corynebacteria*, BCG or *Listeria monocytogenes* in many instances induces regression of tumor growth. However, the important issue is whether such regression is mediated initially by lymphocytes or directly by macrophages or by cooperation of both. There too it is essential to establish whether there is any relationship between the percentage of macrophages in a tumor and its susceptibility to such infectious agents. Systematic studies of such relationships are likely to provide useful information.

Another urgent issue is the possible effects of tumor growth on macrophage functions. Regarding the subtlety with which the macrophage processes mediating inhibition or promotion of growth are governed, factors such as the emission of chemotactic signals assuring close contact between effectors and tumor targets or the release of macrophage-inactivating material may be decisive in determining tumor growth. During the early phases of tumor growth, there is no clear evidence for macrophage deficiency of the tumor-bearing host or for any discernible anti-macrophage activity by the most part normal functional activity *in vitro*. However, it cannot be excluded that factors affecting the effector/target cell interaction *in vivo* are removed by the isolation procedure.

The *in vitro* findings have shown that some of the macrophage effects are on every eukaryote target whereas others are more or less selective for tumors. The understanding of the underlying processes and of the causes for the differences in susceptibility between normal and transformed cells seems of central importance. Moreover, the issue whether the basic role of macrophages is in the control of normal cell proliferation also deserves more attention.

The aforegoing are but a few of the concerns that have arisen that attest to the complexity of the relevant *in vivo* processes and the continuing limitations in our knowledge. What remains clear, however, is that, under defined conditions, macrophages have the potential for an important role in growth processes and especially so in tumor growth. What is now needed is an improved insight into the subtle conditions which determine the outcome of these interactions whether growth is to be blocked or enhanced.

I thank Dr. Maurice Landy, Schweizerisches Forschungs-institut, Davos, for helpful criticism. The author's work has been supported by the Swiss National Science Foundation (grants 3.516.71 and 3.234.74).

REFERENCES

1. Gorer, P. A. (1956). Some recent work on tumour immunity. *Adv. Cancer Res. 4*:149-186.

2. Granger, G. A. and R. S. Weiser (1964). Homograft target cells: specific destruction *in vitro* by contact interaction with immune macrophages. *Science 145*:1427-1429.

3. Granger, G. A. and R. S. Weiser (1966). Homograft target cells: contact destruction *in vitro* by immune macrophages. *Science 151*:97-99.

4. Keller, R. and V. E. Jones (1971). Role of activated macrophages and antibody in inhibition and enhancement of tumour growth in rats. *Lancet II*:847-849.

5. Alexander, P. and R. Evans (1971). Endotoxin and double-stranded RNA render macrophages cytotoxic. *Nature New Biol. 232*:76-78.

6. Hibbs, J. B., L. H. Lambert and J. S. Remington (1972). Macrophage mediated non-specific cytotoxicity – possible role in tumour resistance. *Nature New Biol. 235*:48-50.

7. Evans, R. and P. Alexander (1972). Mechanism of immunologically specific killing of tumour cells by macrophages. *Nature 236*:168-170.

8. Lohmann-Matthes, M.-L., H. Schipper and H. Fischer (1972). Macrophage-mediated cytotoxicity against allogeneic target cells *in vitro. Europ. J. Immunol. 2*:45-49.

9. Keller, R. (1972). Beziehungen zwischen Tumorwachstum und Immunität. *Schweiz. Med. Wschr. 102*:1149-1151.

10. Hibbs, J. B. (1972). Control of carcinogenesis. A possible role for the activated macrophage. *Science 177*:998-1000.

11. Krahenbuhl, J. and J. S. Remington (1974). The role of activated macrophages in specific and nonspecific cytostasis of tumor cells. *J. Immunol. 113*:507-516.

12. Alexander, P., R. Evans and C. K. Grant (1972). The interplay of lymphoid cells and macrophages in tumour immunity *Ann. Inst. Pasteur 122*:645-658.

13. Keller, R. (1973). Cytostatic elimination of syngeneic rat tumor cells *in vitro* by nonspecifically activated macrophages. *J. Exp. Med. 138*:625-644.

14. Hibbs, J. B., L. H. Lambert and J. S. Remington (1972). *In vitro* non-immunologic destruction of cells with abnormal growth characteristics by adjuvant activated macrophages. *Proc. Soc. Exp. Biol. Med. 139*:1049-1052.

15. Keller, R. (1974). Mechanism by which activated normal macrophages destroy syngeneic rat tumour cells *in vitro*. Cytokinetics, non-involvement of T lymphocytes, and effect of metabolic inhibitors. *Immunology 27*:285-298.

16. Olivotto, M. and R. Bomford (1974). *In vitro* inhibition of tumour cell growth and DNA synthesis by peritoneal and lung macrophages from mice injected with *Corynebacterium parvum. Int. J. Cancer 13*:478-488.

17. Ghaffar, A., R. T. Cullen, N. Dunbar and M. F. A. Woodruff (1974). Anti-tumour effect *in vitro* of lymphocytes and macrophages from mice treated with *Corynebacterium parvum. Brit. J. Cancer 29*:199-205.

18. Keller, R. (1974). Modulation of cell proliferation by macrophages: a possible function apart from cytotoxic tumour rejection. *Brit. J. Cancer 30*:401-415.

19. Keller, R., R. Keist and R. J. Ivatt (1974). Functional and biochemical parameters of activation related to macrophage cytostatic effects on tumor cells. *Int. J. Cancer 14*:675-683.

20. Keller, R. (1975). Major changes in lymphocyte proliferation evoked by activated macrophages. *Cellular Immunol. 17*:542-551.

21. Keller, R. Susceptibility of normal and transformed target cell lines to cytostatic and cytocidal effects exerted by macrophages. *J. Nat. Cancer Inst.*, in press.

22. Krahenbuhl, J. L. and L. H. Lambert (1975). Cytokinetic studies of the effects of activated macrophages on tumor target cells. *J. Nat. Cancer Inst. 54*:1433-1437.

23. Keller, R. (1975). Cytostatic killing of syngeneic tumour cells by activated non-immune macrophages. *Mononuclear Phagocytes in Immunity, Infection and Pathology* (R. van Furth, ed.) Blackwell, Oxford.

24. Keller, R. (1976). Cytostatic and cytocidal effects of activated macrophages. *Immunobiology of the Macrophage*. (D. S. Nelson, ed.) Academic Press, New York.

25. Opitz, H. G., D. Niethammer, H. Lemke, H. D. Flad and R. Huget (1975). Inhibition of ^{3}H-thymidine incorporation of lymphocytes by a soluble factor from macrophages. *Cellular Immunol. 16*:379-388.

26. Keller, R. (1975). *Immunobiology of the Tumor-Host Relationship.* (R. I. Smith and M. Landy, Eds.) Academic Press, New York.

27. Holtermann, O. A., E. Klein and G. P. Casale (1973). Selective cytotoxicity of peritoneal leucocytes for neoplastic cells. *Cellular Immunol. 9*:339-352.

28. Nelson, D. S. (1973). Production by stimulated macrophages of factors depressing lymphocyte transformation. *Nature 246*:306-307.

29. Waldman, S. R. and A. A. Gottlieb (1973). Macrophage regulation of DNA synthesis in lymphoid cells: Effects of a soluble factor from macrophages. *Cellular Immunol. 9*:142-156.

30. Calderon, J., R. T. Williams and E. R. Unanue (1974). An inhibitor of cell proliferation released by cultures of macrophages. *Proc. Nat. Acad. Sci. N. Y. 71*:4273-4277.

31. Calderon, J. and E. R. Unanue (1975). Two biological activities regulating cell proliferation found in cultures of peritoneal exudate cells. *Nature 253*:359-361.

32. Calderon, J., J.-M. Kiely, J. L. Lefko and E. R. Unanue (1975). The modulation of lymphocyte functions by molecules secreted by macrophages. I. Description and partial biochemical analysis. *J. Exp. Med. 142*:151-164.

33. Nathan, C. F., M. L. Karnovsky and J. R. David (1971). Alterations of macrophage functions by mediators from lymphocytes. *J. Exp. Med. 133*:1356-1376.

34. Chen, C. and J. G. Hirsch (1972). The effects of mercaptoethanol and of peritoneal macrophages on the antibody-forming capacity of nonadherent mouse spleen cells *in vitro. J. Exp. Med. 136*:604-617.

35. Gery, K., R. K. Gershon and B. H. Waksman (1972). Potentiation of the T-lymphocyte response to mitogens. I. The responding cell. *J. Exp. Med. 136*:128-142.

36. Gery, K. and B. H. Waksman (1972). Potentiation of the T-lymphocyte response to mitogens. II. The cellular source of potentiating mediator(s). *J. Exp. Med. 136*:143-155.

37. Hoffman, M. and R. W. Dutton (1971). Immune response restoration with macrophage culture supernatants. *Science 172*:1047-1048.

38. Bach, F. H., B. J. Alter, S. Solliday, D. C. Zoschke and M. Janis (1970). Lymphocyte reactivity *in vitro*. II. Soluble reconstituting factor permitting response to purified lymphocytes. *Cellular Immunol. 1*:219-227.

39. Schrader, J. W., (1973). Mechanism of activation of bone marrow-derived lymphocyte. III. A distinction between a macrophage-produced triggering signal and the amplifying effect on triggered B lymphocytes of allogeneic interactions. *J. Exp. Med. 138*:1466-1480.

40. Wood, D. D. and S. L. Gaul (1974). Enhancement of the humoral response of T cell-depleted murine spleens by a factor derived from human monocytes *in vitro*. *J. Immunol. 113*:925-933.

41. Bennett, B., L. J. Old and E. A. Boyse (1964). Retention Funct. Differentiation Cult. Cells, Symposium 1964, *Wistar Inst. Monogr.* No. 1, p. 87-98.

42. Cleveland, R. P., M. S. Meltzer and B. Zbar (1974). Tumor cytotoxicity *in vitro* by macrophages from mice infected with *Mycobacterium bovis* strain BCG. *J. Nat. Cancer Inst. 52*:1887-1895.

43. Hibbs, J. B. (1974). Heterocytolysis by macrophages activated by Bacillus Calmette-Guérin: Lysosome exocytosis into tumor cells. *Science 184*:468-471.

44. Kaplan, A. M., P. S. Morahan and W. Regelson (1974). Induction of macrophage-mediated tumor-cell cytotoxicity by pyran copolymer. *J. Nat. Cancer. Inst. 52*:1919-1923.

45. Cohen, A. M., J. F. Burdick and A. S. Ketcham (1971). Cell-mediated cytotoxicity: an assay using ^{125}I-iododeoxyuridine-labeled target cells. *J. Immunol. 107*:895-898.

46. Seeger, R. C. and J. J. T. Owen (1973). Measurement of tumor immunity *in vitro* with ^{125}I-iododeoxyuridine-labeled target cells. *Transplantation 15*:404-408.

47. Seeger, R. C., S. A. Rayner and J. J. T. Owen (1974). An analysis of variables affecting the measurement of tumor immunity *in vitro* with ^{125}I-iododeoxyuridine-labeled target cells. Studies of immunity to primary Moloney sarcoma. *Int. J. Cancer 13*:697-713.

48. LeMevel, B. P. and S. A. Wells (1973). A microassay for the quantitation of cytotoxic antitumor antibody: use of ^{125}I-iododeoxyuridine as a tumor cell label. *J. Nat. Cancer Inst. 50*:803-806.

49. Oldham, R. K. and R. B. Herberman (1973). Evaluation of cell-mediated cytotoxic reactivity against tumor associated antigens with ^{125}I-iododeoxyuridine-labeled target cells. *J. Immunol. 111*:1862-1871.

50. Reed, W. P. and Z. J. Lucas (1975). Cytotoxic activity of lymphocytes. V. Role of soluble toxin in macrophage-inhibited cultures of tumor cells. *J. Immunol. 115*:395-404.

51. McLaughlin, J. F., N. H. Ruddle and B. H. Waksman (1972). Relationship between activation of peritoneal cells and their cytopathogenicity. *J. RESoc. 12*:293-304.

52. McIvor, K. L. and R. S. Weiser (1971). Mechanisms of target cell destruction by alloimmune peritoneal macrophages. II. Release of a specific cytotoxin from interacting cells. *Immunology 20*:315-322.

53. Sintek, D. E. and W. B. Pincus (1970). Cytotoxic factor from peritoneal cells: purification and characteristics. *J. RESoc. 8*:508-521.

54. Kramer, J. J. and G. A. Granger (1972). The *in vitro* induction and release of a cell toxin by immune C57Bl/b mouse peritoneal macrophages. *Cellular Immunol. 3*:88-100.

55. Heise, E. R. and R. S. Weiser (1969). Factors in delayed sensitivity: lymphocyte and macrophage cytotoxins in the tuberculin reaction. *J. Immunol. 103*:570-576.

56. Melsom, H., G. Kearny, S. Gruca and R. Seljelid. (1974). Evidence for a cytolytic factor released by macrophages. *J. Exp. Med. 140*:1085-1096.

57. Daems W. Th. and P. Brederoo (1973). Electron microscopical studies on the structure, phagocytic properties, and peroxidatic activity of resident and exudate peritoneal macrophages in the guinea pig. *Z. Zellforsch. 144*:247-297.

58. Rice, S. G. and M. Fishman (1974). Functional and morphological heterogeneity among rabbit peritoneal macrophages. *Cellular Immunol. 11*:130-145.

59. Walker, W. S. (1976). *Immunobiology of the Macrophage* (D. S. Nelson, ed.) Academic Press, New York, in press.

60. Evans, R. (1972). Macrophages in syngeneic animal tumours. *Transplantation 14*:468-473.

DISCUSSION

D. Bernard Amos, Chairman

The various papers presented in this session stand by themselves and need no further emphasis from the chairman. Instead, I should like to touch upon some aspects of the microcosm that constitutes a progressing tumor.

The meeting in general has served to show how large a component of host cells there may be in a tumor. Some of this migration into the tumor may be directed by the host, but some is almost certainly directed by the tumor. The discussion by Dr. Snyderman in another section of these proceedings is relevant to this point. Factors which alter the flow of macrophages and lymphocytes through the tumor or which cause them to remain in the tumor are very relevant to the mediation of immunity *in vivo*.

We cannot assume that all of the host cells accumulating in a tumor are tumoricidal. Indeed many of the cells may be neutral bystanders trapped in the tumor by chemotactic and other factors. From Dr. Hibbs' presentation we know that normal macrophages can even potentiate tumor cell growth. It has long been known that normal lymphocytes can also have feeder or growth potentiating effects as well as cytotoxic activities.

An overall impression which has been strengthened during this meeting is the requirement for constant cooperation between cells. Thus, macrophages held in culture for more than 2 days begin to lose their reactivity but can regain it after exposure to immune lymphocytes and antigen. This suggests that for any continuing activity of macrophages *in vivo*, the presence of activated lymphocytes is also necessary. Dr. Hanna showed the complex interactions that can be visualized between the macrophage and the tumor cell. Killing by macrophages appears to follow a different pathway from that used by cytotoxic lymphocytes and both could presumably cooperate in being cytotoxic. Lysosomal activation seems to be a necessary prerequisite for macrophages but the cytotoxic lymphocyte, whether acting passively and through antibody, or whether actively immune, is often a small lymphocyte with little evidence of lysosomal proliferation.

A constant concern is that reactions measured *in vitro* do not reflect events occurring *in vivo*. At least three sources of error may be introduced. Reactions may occur *in vitro* that are not paralleled by events *in vivo*. Of primary concern in this regard is lymphocyte dependent antibody mediated cytotoxicity which is a highly potent cytotoxic process *in vitro* but is thought to be of doubtful significance *in vivo* since passively transferred antibody does not lead to immediate cytolysis of the tumor. This may not be a valid argument, however, since in the absence of an active inflammatory reaction the necessary Fc receptor cells and the antibody may not gain access to the tissue cells. Reactions that occur *in vivo* may not be demonstrable *in vitro*. Mouse complement is nonlytic for mouse tumor cells sensitized by allo-antibody *in vitro*. Guinea pig complement may be active in this system. *In vivo*, mouse complement is as potent as guinea pig complement when the target cells are retained in diffusion chambers. Further, short range forces such as local antibody production by B lymphocytes is difficult to evaluate *in vitro* and although lytic plaques can be demonstrated with nucleated targets, very little emphasis has been placed on B cell activity *in vivo*. Finally, the definition of cells involved in certain immune reactions may be erroneous. Two examples may be cited. 1) It is assumed that cytotoxic lymphocytes are T cells because effector cell populations treated with anti-Thy 1 sera lose their potency. However, reciprocal experiments with anti-B cell sera are rarely carried out and there is evidence (a) that the Thy 1 antigen can be present on cells that are not typical T cells and (b) that B cell as well as T cell markers may be present on some subclasses of lymphocytes. 2) Experiments involving cytotoxic lymphocytes or tumoricidal macrophages are almost invariably carried out using mixed populations of cells. It is difficult to obtain a population of either cell type that is completely free from the other. This is of some concern to this meeting where many cell preparations are made from peritoneal exudate cells. A contamination of 5-10% lymphocytes may seem trivial, but these cells could be very important through their own activities, or through their cooperation with the macrophages.

It is usually assumed that the host's defenses to autochthonous tumors is a rather weak one. I believe this to be frequently erroneous. The Rous sarcoma virus in mice produces tumors which are highly lethal in newborns, the tumor derived in newborns and lethal to newborns is immediately rejected by adults. Mammary tumor induced tumors are lethal to strains that carry the virus but are strongly resisted by similar mice not preconditioned by the virus. Carcinogen induced tumors which are lethal to the original host may yet immunize strongly following removal or when transferred to syngeneic hosts. Consequently it is easy to believe that the tumor host carries a highly potent immune defense system, but this is blunted by the normal regulatory mechanisms that control all immunologic reactions.

A study of mechanisms would require at least two components additional to those reported at this meeting. One is a reversion to direct methods of examination such as those conducted by Algire and his colleagues (1,2). These investigators developed highly sophisticated chambers that permitted direct visualization of the tumor and its blood supply. The procedures developed could now be modified to permit the introduction of specific classes of effector cells or of cell free factors. Another need is to intensify our efforts to understand normal regulatory mechanisms. This is a necessary prerequisite to the development of procedures which will allow us to selectively, but transiently, ablate control. This would be hazardous. Loss of regulation might permit the induction of autoimmunity to tissues other than the tumor. However, it would potentially allow the unleashing of primed immune effectors against the tumor. The model for study of such control processes need not be a tumor and a simpler symbiont such as monilia or even a hapten-carrier model would provide the basic data. Although there is a tendency to decry immunologic processes in tumor surveillance, I believe that this is a passing phase and that eventually tumor immunity will be found to be as potent as transplantation immunity is at present. The papers presented in this session are helping us build toward that knowledge.

REFERENCES

1. Algire, G. H. and F. Y. Legallais (1949). Recent developments in the transparent chamber technique as adapted to the mouse. *J. Nat. Cancer Inst. 10*:225-253.

2. Algire, G. H. and R. M. Merwin (1955). Vascular patterns in tissues in grafts within transparent chambers in mice. *Angiology 6*:311-318.

SESSION IV

Functional Expression of Macrophages and Neoplasia

Chairman: Osias Stutman

HUMAN PULMONARY MACROPHAGES IN DISEASE AND NEOPLASIA

David W. Golde, M. D.

Division of Hematology-Oncology
Department of Medicine
UCLA School of Medicine
Los Angeles, California

Grant Support: California Lung Association, USPHS grant CA 15688, and a grant from Brown and Williamson Tobacco Corp., Philip Morris Inc., R. J. Reynolds Tobacco Co., United States Tobacco Co., and Tobacco Associates, Inc.

INTRODUCTION

The alveolar macrophage is a crucial element in the pulmonary ecology and a major factor in the defense of the lung against environmental hazards (1,2). Relatively little is known about the activities of the human alveolar macrophage because it has been difficult in the past to obtain this cell in man. Our knowledge of macrophage function therefore derived largely from studies of monocytes cultivated *in vitro* (monocyte-derived macrophages). The development of a catheter technique for bronchopulmonary lavage and the widespread application of fiberoptic bronchoscopy have enabled investigators to recover human pulmonary macrophages for study (3-5). In this paper, some of our recent work with the human lung macrophage will be summarized.

MATERIALS AND METHODS

Pulmonary macrophages were obtained by bronchopulmonary lavage from normal smokers and nonsmokers and patients with acute leukemia, pulmonary infiltrates, and pulmonary alveolar proteinosis. Bronchopulmonary lavage was performed by the method of Finley (3,6). A number 16 or 19 Metras catheter is passed into a lower-lobe bronchus under local anesthesia and fluoroscopic control. Normal saline is introduced in 100-ml aliquots (total 300 ml/lavage) and the fluid withdrawn. The lavage effluent is mixed with equal volumes of Hank's balanced salt solution containing 20% fetal calf serum and antibiotics (7). The cells are then recovered by centrifugation at 150 G for 10 minutes, washed twice, and suspended in McCoy's 5A medium with 20% fetal calf serum and antibiotics.

Viable cell counts are performed and cytocentrifuge preparations made for morphological and histochemical studies (7,8). A portion of the cells are fixed in buffered glutaraldehyde and processed by routine methods for electron microscopy (9). DNA synthetic activity is assessed by radioautographic analysis after pulse labeling with ^{3}H-thymidine (7,8). The cells are cultured in Leighton tubes (5,10) or in Marbrook chambers as described for human hematopoietic cells (11). Tests of functional capacity include adherence to glass (5), phagocytosis of yeast and bacteria, and tests for the presence of cell surface receptors for immunoglobulin (8). Microbicidal function was determined by the specific staining assay of Lehrer using *Candida pseudotropicalis* (12). Chemotaxis was measured with a modified Boyden chamber technique using a 8-μ-pore size nucleopore filter (13). Production of colony-stimulating activity (CSA) is determined by assaying conditioned medium from macrophage cultures on normal human bone marrow using the agar plate method (14,15).

RESULTS

The pulmonary macrophages have characteristic ultrastructural features and, in cigarette smokers, "smoker inclusions" are clearly visible at the light and electron microscopic level (Fig. 1 & 2) (4,9,16). The smoker inclusions contain granular and amorphous material, lipid and rod-like crystalline structures believed to be kaolinite (Fig. 3) (16). The macrophages stain positively with PAS after diastase digestion (indicative of glycolipid), methyl green

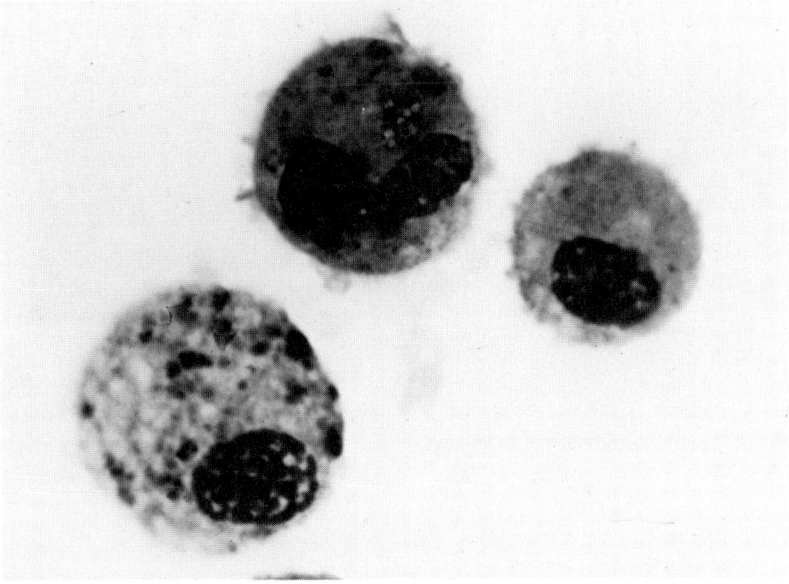

Fig. 1. *Pulmonary macrophages obtained by lavage from a normal cigarette smoker. Note the dark "smoker inclusions." (Giemsa stain).*

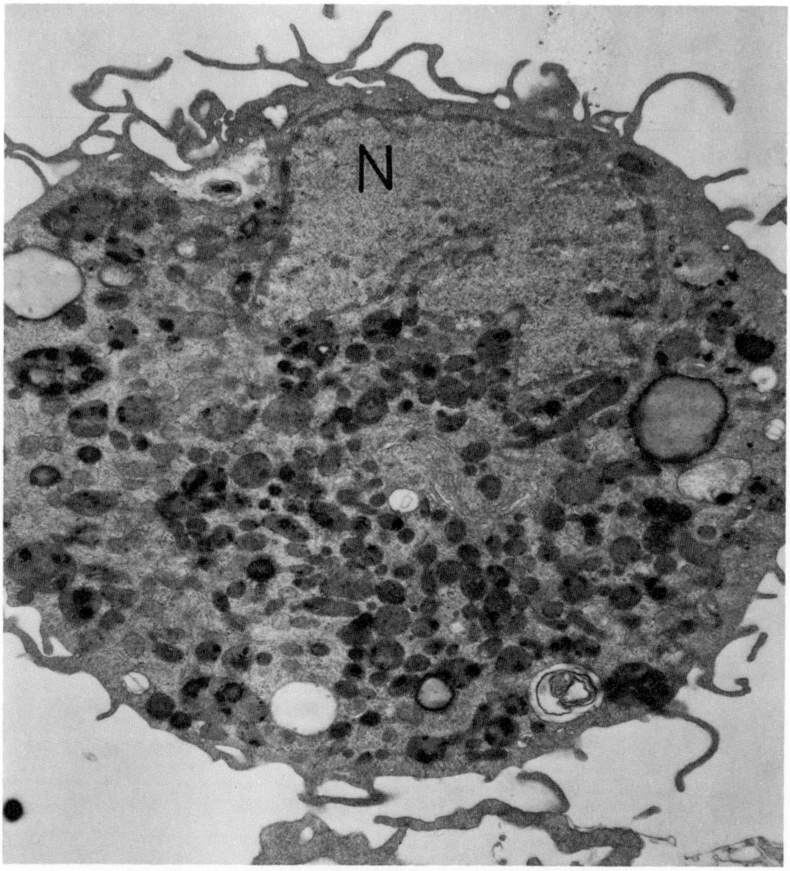

Fig. 2. *Electron micrograph of an alveolar macrophage from a smoker. N – nucleus.*

pyronine (indicative of RNA), and with fat stains such as oil red O and Sudan black. Alveolar macrophages stain intensely for α-naphthyl butyrase, a histochemical marker for cells of the mononuclear phagocyte series. Macrophages from normal individuals usually do not stain heavily for hemosiderin (17). In certain anticoagulated patients and patients with leukemia who have "occult" pulmonary hemorrhage, the alveolar macrophages contain large quantities of hemosiderin and hemoglobin (17,18). The pulmonary macrophages have receptors for IgG as determined by rosette formation with anti-D coated erythrocytes (Fig. 4) (8).

Radioautographic studies show that normally 0.35-1.25% of the macrophages will take up ^{3}H-thymidine after pulse labeling (7). The cells incorporating the tracer can be clearly identified as macrophages (Fig. 5) and blocking studies with appropriate concentrations of hydroxyurea or cytosine arabino-

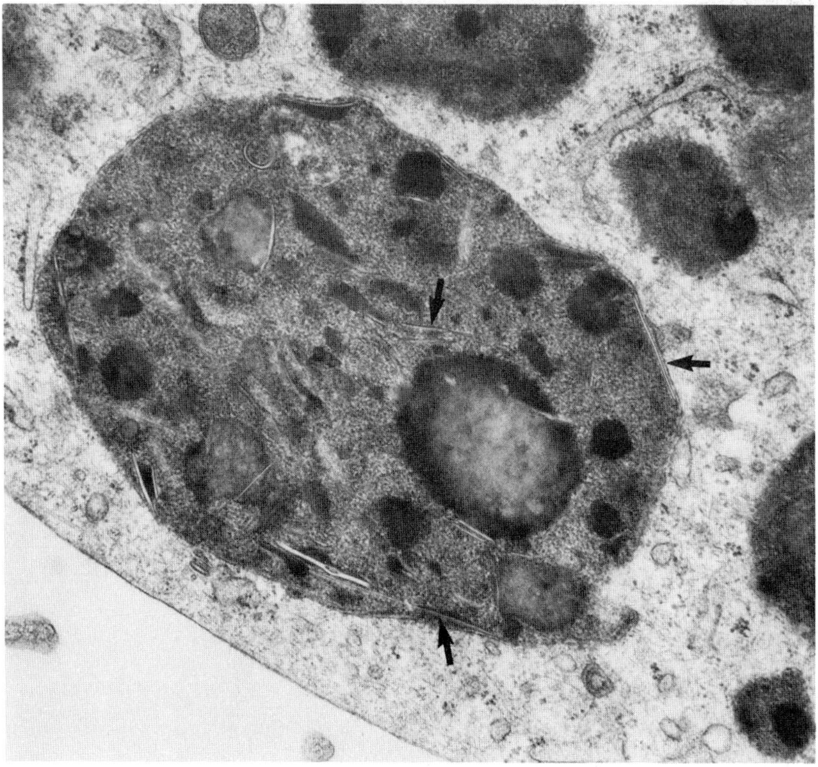

Fig. 3. *High power view of a smoker inclusion at the periphery of the cell. Inclusion contains lipid and rod-like structures believed to be kaolinite (arrows).*

side suggest that the ^{3}H-thymidine uptake represents prereplicative DNA synthesis (7,8). Macrophages obtained from patients with acute leukemia remain morphologically and functionally intact and are capable of scheduled DNA synthesis (8). The macrophage population in these patients appears to sustain itself through long periods of monocytopenia.

Confirmation that the human alveolar macrophage population is at least in part sustained by an influx of bone marrow-derived monocytes was obtained in studies of a patient who underwent bone marrow transplantation. This female patient had aplastic anemia and was transplanted with histocompatible male bone marrow cells. A successful graft was documented clinically and cytogenetically. Several months later the patient underwent bronchopulmonary lavage and macrophages were obtained which were clearly shown to contain the Y chromosome by quinacrine fluorescence. These observations suggest that the human alveolar macrophage population may be

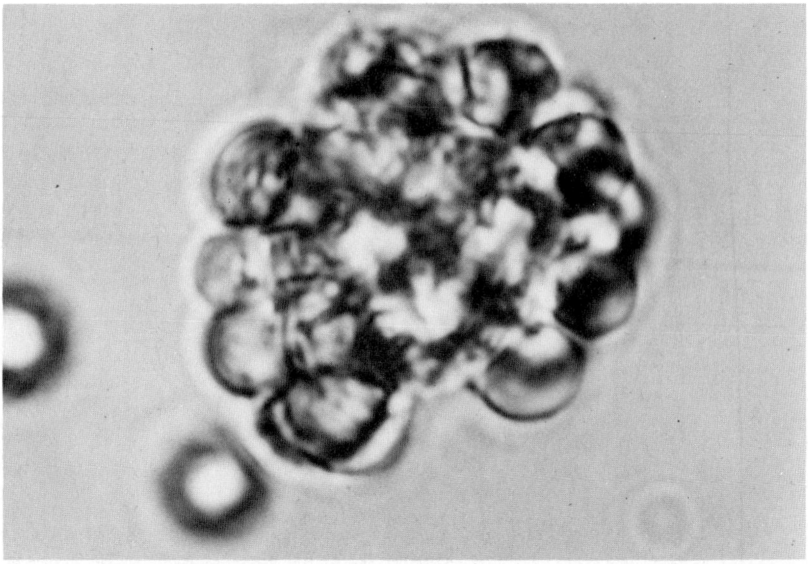

Fig. 4. *Demonstration of IgG receptors on surface of alveolar macrophage by rosette formation with anti-D coated erythrocytes.*

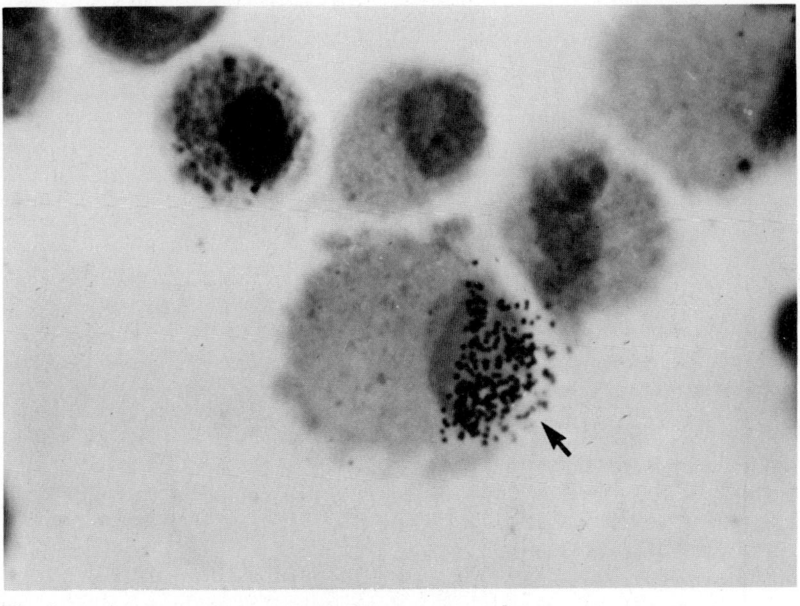

Fig. 5. *Radioautographic preparation demonstrating* ^{3}*H-thymidine uptake (arrow) in alveolar macrophage lavaged from a normal subject.*

maintained by two mechanisms: influx of monocytes from the peripheral blood and by replication of macrophages *in situ*.

When conditioned medium from Leighton tube or suspension cultures of alveolar macrophages was assayed against normal human bone in agar plates, prominent colony-stimulating activity was observed (15). Similarly, alveolar macrophages from patients with acute leukemia were shown to produce substantial quantities of CSA (8). Since many myeloid leukemic cells respond to CSA *in vitro* (19), the production of CSA by lung macrophages may influence the course of leukemia in man (8). The demonstrated production of CSA by human alveolar macrophages suggests that these cells may stimulate granulopoiesis in times of need and recruit more monocytes to maintain the alveolar macrophage population for pulmonary defense.

In Marbrook cultures of cells obtained by bronchopulmonary lavage, lymphocytes were occasionally observed to undergo "spontaneous" blastic transformation. Normally, few lymphocytes are seen in pulmonary washings from individuals who smoke heavily; however, in nonsmokers 5-25% of the cells in the lavage fluid may be lymphoid. In some suspension cultures, phytohemagglutinin (PHA) was added and five days later substantial lymphocyte transformation was observed. The proliferative response of lymphocytes in the pulmonary washings was documented radioautographically by ^{3}H-thymidine incorporation (Fig. 6).

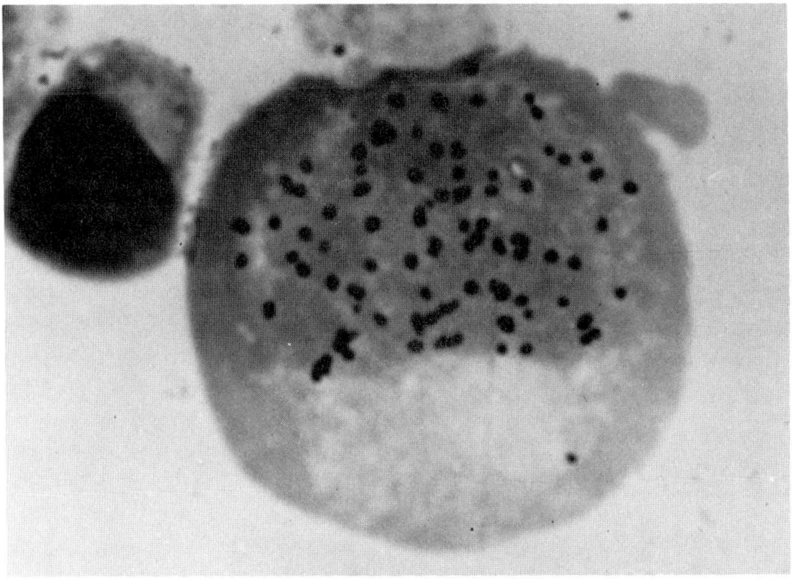

Fig. 6. *Radioautographic preparation demonstrating ^{3}H-thymidine uptake in transformed lymphocyte from PHA-stimulated culture of cells obtained at bronchopulmonary lavage. Note also small unstimulated lymphocyte.*

The lung macrophages in patients with pulmonary alveolar proteinosis are morphologically and functionally defective. These cells have increased amounts of PAS-positive material in their cytoplasm and most show evidence of vacuolization and fat accumulation. Some of the cells resemble the foamy macrophages seen in postobstructive lipoid pneumonia (Fig. 7) (20). By electron microscopy the alveolar proteinosis cells have giant phagosomes, many of which contain lamellated material (Fig. 8). Other cells are diffusely vacuolated. Although these cells phagocytized normally, they were defective in their ability to adhere to glass (< 50% of control) and to chemotax in Boyden chambers. More importantly, these cells manifest a prominent defect in their ability to kill ingested *Candida pseudotropicalis.*

DISCUSSION

The available data on the human alveolar macrophage suggests that these cells originate from bone marrow stem cells and arrive at the lung via the circulating monocyte. In addition, the macrophage has proliferative capacity suggesting that the lung macrophages can replenish their numbers by replication *in situ* and are not wholly dependent on peripheral blood monocytes (7). In patients with acute leukemia the lung macrophage population is maintained through long periods of monocytopenia and cytotoxic chemotherapy (8). Direct evidence for a hematopoietic derivation of the alveolar macrophages in man was obtained by studies on a female patient with a successful bone

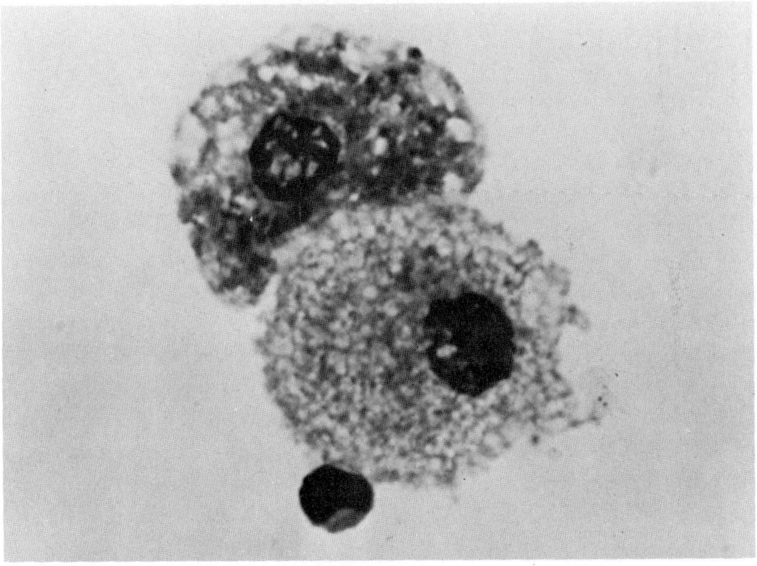

Fig. 7. *Cells lavaged from patient with pulmonary alveolar proteinosis showing macrophages with marked vacuolization and pyknotic nuclei. Lymphocytes were morphologically normal.*

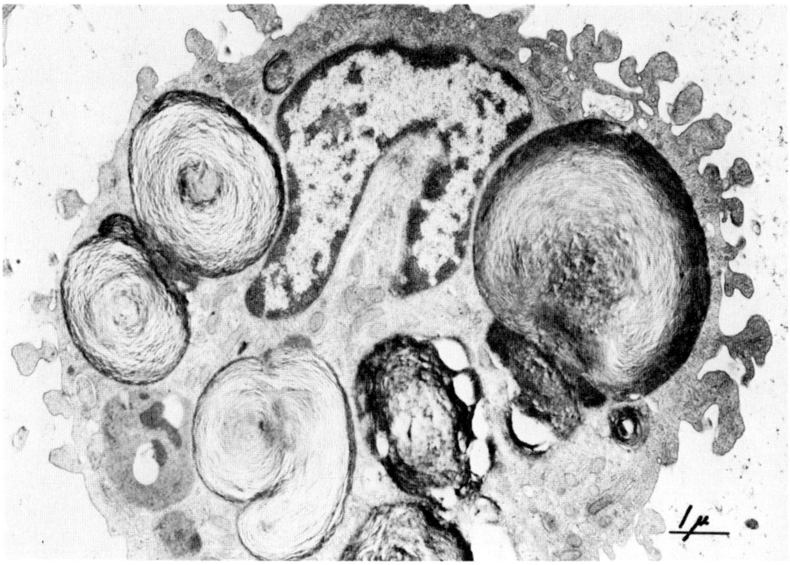

Fig. 8. *Macrophage from patient with alveolar proteinosis with giant phagolysosomes containing concentrically arranged lipid-like material.*

marrow graft from a male donor in whom macrophages containing the Y chromosome were obtained by bronchopulmonary lavage. These data in man are consistent with a large body of information relative to the derivation of alveolar macrophages in animals (21-23).

The alveolar macrophages show many of the functional characteristics of mononuclear phagocytes in other locations. One of these properties is the ability to produce colony-stimulating activity (CSA) (8,14,15). CSA is a glycoprotein believed to be a humoral regulator of granulocytopoiesis and monocytopoiesis (24). The production of CSA by alveolar macrophages suggests a means whereby these cells may regulate their own numbers as well as influence granulopoiesis. Thus, under appropriate circumstances these cells could theroretically increase their elaboration of CSA, thereby causing the production of more monocytes and granulocytes for host defense.

Lymphocytes present in the bronchopulmonary spaces of man were shown to be capable of a proliferative response to PHA. The proximity of immunocompetent lymphoid cells and macrophages in the lung environment suggests that the critical elements for complex immunologic reactions are available (10) and may function importantly in local defense and response to neoplasia (25).

The alveolar macrophage in pulmonary alveolar proteinosis is a defective cell. These cells show morphologic and functional alterations indicative of severe cellular injury. It seems likely that the macrophage abnormality is acquired and is due to ingestion of the PAS-positive proteinaceous material in the alveoli. Thus the macrophage may become defective due to its abnormal environment. Patients with alveolar proteinosis have an extraordinary incidence of exotic pulmonary infections including a variety of fungal diseases and, most prominently, infection with Nocardia (26). It seems reasonable to speculate that the increased incidence of such infections relates to the macrophages with reduced fungicidal capacity. If this is the case, it can provide a rational basis for attempts to remove the proteinaceous material for reasons of pulmonary defense.

With the increased use of bronchopulmonary lavage and fiberoptic bronchoscopy there has been a rapid advance in our knowledge of the human lung macrophage. This area of investigation will likely flourish as the techniques of cell biology are applied to the study of these important cells.

ACKNOWLEDGEMENT

The author thanks Dr. Martin J. Cline, Dr. Theodore N. Finley, Dr. Gordon Johnston, and Dr. Mary Territo for major contributions to these studies.

REFERENCES

1. Cohen, A. B. and W. M. Gold (1975). Defense mechanisms of the lungs. *Ann. Rev. Physiol. 37*:325-350.

2. Goldstein, E., W. Lippert and D. Warshauer (1974). Pulmonary alveolar macrophage. Defender against bacterial infection of the lung. *J. Clin. Invest. 54*:519-528.

3. Finley, T. N., E. W. Swenson, W. S. Curran, G. L. Huber and A. J. Ladman (1967). Bronchopulmonary lavage in normal subjects and patients with obstructive lung disease. *Ann. Intern. Med. 66*:651-658.

4. Harris, J. O., E. W. Swenson and J. E. Johnson, III (1970). Human alveolar macrophages: Comparison of phagocytic ability, glucose utilization, and ultrastructure in smokers and nonsmokers. *J. Clin. Invest. 49*:2086-2096.

5. Cohen, A. B. and M. J. Cline (1971). The human alveolar macrophage: Isolation, cultivation *in vitro*, and studies of morphologic and functional characteristics. *J. Clin. Invest. 50*:1390-1398.

6. Finley, T. N. and A. J. Ladman (1972). Low yield of pulmonary surfactant in cigarette smokers. *N. Engl. J. Med. 286*:223-227.

7. Golde, D. W., L. A. Byers and T. N. Finley (1974). Proliferative capacity of human alveolar macrophage. *Nature 247*:373-375.

8. Golde, D. W., T. N. Finley and M. J. Cline (1974). The pulmonary macrophage in acute leukemia. *N. Engl. J. Med. 290*:875-878.

9. Pratt, S. A., M. H. Smith, A. J. Ladman and T. N. Finley (1971). The ultrastructure of alveolar macrophages from human cigarette smokers and nonsmokers. *Lab. Invest. 24*:331-338.

10. Hanifin, J. M. and M. J. Cline (1970). Human monocytes and macrophages. Interaction with antigen and lymphocytes. *J. Cell Biol. 46*:97-105.

11. Golde, D. W. and M. J. Cline (1973). Growth of human bone marrow in liquid culture. *Blood 41*:45-57.

12. Lehrer, R. I. (1975). The fungicidal mechanisms of human monocytes. I. Evidence for myeloperoxidase-linked and myeloperoxidase-independent candidacidal mechanisms. *J. Clin. Invest. 55*:338-346.

13. Boyden, S. (1962). The chemotactic effect of mixtures of antibody and antigen on polymorphonuclear leucocytes. *J. Exp. Med. 115*:453-466.

14. Golde, D. W. and M. J. Cline (1972). Identification of the colony-stimulating cell in human peripheral blood. *J. Clin. Invest. 51*:2981-2983.

15. Golde, D. W., T. N. Finley and M. J. Cline (1972). Production of colony-stimulating factor by human macrophages. *Lancet 2*:1397-1399.

16. Brody, A. R. and J. E. Craighead (1975). Cytoplasmic inclusions in pulmonary macrophages of cigarette smokers. *Lab. Invest. 32*:125-132.

17. Golde, D. W., W. L. Drew, H. Z. Klein, T. N. Finley and M. J. Cline (1975). Occult pulmonary haemorrhage in leukaemia. *Br. Med. J. 2*:166-168.

18. Finley, T. N., A. Aronow, A. M. Cosentino and D. W. Golde (1975). Occult pulmonary hemorrhage in anticoagulated patients. *Am. Rev. Respir. Dis. 112*:23-29.

19. Metcalf, D., M. A. S. Moore, J. W. Sheridan and G. Spitzer (1974). Responsiveness of human granulocytic leukemic cells to colony-stimulating factor. *Blood 43*:847-859.

20. Cohen, A. B. and M. J. Cline (1972). *In vitro* studies of the foamy macrophage of postobstructive endogenous lipoid pneumonia in man. *Am. Rev. Respir. Dis. 106*:69-78.

21. Soderland, S. C. and Y. Naum (1973). Growth of pulmonary alveolar macrophages *in vitro. Nature 245*:150-152.

22. Godleski, J. J. and J. D. Brain (1972). The origin of alveolar macrophages in mouse radiation chimeras. *J. Exp. Med. 136*:630-643.

23. Bowden, D. H. and I. Y. R. Adamson (1972). The pulmonary interstitial cell as immediate precursor of the alveolar macrophage. *Am. J. Pathol. 68*:521-528.

24. Golde, D. W. and M. J. Cline (1974). Regulation of granulopoiesis. *N. Engl. J. Med. 291*:1388-1395.

25. Kaltreider, H. B. and S. E. Salmon (1973). Immunology of the lower respiratory tract. Functional properties of bronchoalveolar lymphocytes obtained from the normal canine lung. *J. Clin. Invest. 52*:2211-2217.

26. Davidson, J. M. and W. M. Macleod (1969). Pulmonary alveolar proteinosis. *Br. J. Dis. Chest 63*:13-28.

THE EMPLOYMENT OF GLUCAN AND GLUCAN ACTIVATED MACROPHAGES IN THE ENHANCEMENT OF HOST RESISTANCE TO MALIGNANCIES IN EXPERIMENTAL ANIMALS

N. R. Di Luzio, R. McNamee, E. Jones,
J. A. Cook and E. O. Hoffmann

Department of Physiology
Tulane University School of Medicine

Department of Pathology
Louisiana State University Medical Center

New Orleans, Louisiana 70112

In view of the unique role the reticuloendothelial system plays in maintaining the purity of the internal environment, a variety of attempts have been made during the past 20 years to develop pharmacological agents which possess the ability to specifically enhance the functional activity of this unique system. Among one of the first agents employed in an attempt to delineate the physiological and immunological role of the reticuloendothelial system (RES) was zymosan. Zymosan was the name given by Pillemer and Ecker (1) to a yeast cell wall fraction which had the property of inactivating the third component of complement and adsorbing properdin. This cell wall preparation, derived from *Saccharomyces cerevisiae,* was initially demonstrated to be an effective reticuloendothelial (RE) stimulant by Benacerraf and Sebestyen (2). Zymosan is a complex cell wall residue consisting of protein, lipid and complex polysaccharides, namely mannan and glucan (3). Di Carlo and Fiore (4) reported that the composition of the yeast cell wall on a dry weight basis was approximately 58% glucan and 18% mannan. Glucan comprises the inner cell wall with mannan comprising the outer cell wall (5). Since the observations of Benacerraf and Sebestyen (2), zymosan has been uniformly demonstrated to produce marked stimulation of the RES. These events include increased phagocytosis, increased rate of intracellular degradation of phagocytized particulates, increased resistance to certain infections, increased properdin levels, enhanced humoral immunity and inhibition or regression of certain experimental tumors (6,10).

In view of the profound biological activities produced by the administration of zymosan, studies were initiated in our laboratory in the late 1950's to isolate the component of zymosan which possessed the specific ability to initiate activation and proliferation of the RES and thereby increase a variety of host defense mechanisms. In an extensive study of various components present in zymosan, we reported in 1961 that the active RE stimulant in zymosan was glucan (11). Glucan has been characterized as a water insoluble polyglucose or neutral polysaccharide consisting of a chain of gluco-pyranose units united by a β (1→3) glucosidic linkage (12). In addition, a minor β (1→6) glucan component has also been reported (13). The latter component of yeast glucan has recently been found to be inactive relative to macrophage activation (14).

In studies conducted in our laboratory to define the influence of macrophage activation on tumor growth, it was observed that the simultaneous subcutaneous administration of glucan with Shay myelogenous leukemia cells significantly inhibited growth of the tumor (15). In subsequent clinical studies involving three types of metastatic lesions, the intralesional administration of glucan produced, in all cases studied, a prompt and striking reduction in the size of the lesion (16) in 5-10 days. Regression of the glucan injected tumor was associated with necrosis of the malignant cells and a pronounced monocytic infiltrate.

Since glucan appeared to offer distinct advantages (16-18) over other currently employed forms of immunotherapy which make use of viable organisms, such as BCG or *C. parvum,* the present studies were undertaken to extend our initial observations on the utilization of glucan in the prevention and treatment of the Shay myelogenous leukemia tumor. In view of our recent studies which appeared to denote the importance of the number and function of host macrophages in resistance in neoplasia, as well as tumor macrophages number and function in regard to growth and dissemination of the malignant cells (18), additional studies were conducted in which varying concentrations of glucan-activated peritoneal macrophages were added to tumor cells at the time of transplantation. The influence of altered tumor-macrophage cell ratios on growth and dissemination of the tumor was ascertained.

Although intralesional glucan was effective in autochthonous tumors in man and in the rat leukemia model, in view of the allogenic nature of the acute myelogenous leukemia tumor, additional studies were conducted evaluating the tumor inhibitory effect of glucan in two syngenic mouse tumor models. The common ancestry of various rat strains may limit genetic dissimilarity as Palm and Wilson (19) point out that the 52 existing inbred rat strains are virtually all descendants of the original Wistar colonies. Our composite experimental studies denote that glucan activation of macrophages, either pre- or post-tumor cell transplantation, significantly modified the course of the malignancy in both the rat and mouse models. Additionally, the growth as well as dissemination of tumor cells from the primary site appears to be regulated by the number of macrophages which exist within the primary tumor site.

MATERIALS AND METHODS

Long Evans Hooded rats, 3-4 weeks old, were employed as hosts for the Shay chloroleukemia tumor (20). Since the features of the tumor, particularly in respect to its veroperoxidase content, as well as its virulence, have changed since it was first isolated by Shay *et al.* in 1951 (20), the tumor whose current features are listed in Table 1 will be designated in the paper as the Shay myelogenous leukemia rat tumor model rather than chloroleukemia.

The features of tumor model listed in Table 1 are essentially derived from the studies of Lapis and Benedeczky (21) and Handler and Handler (22), as well as our studies.

Two syngenic mouse tumors were also employed, the adenocarcinoma BW10232 and melanoma B16, spontaneous tumors of C57B1/6J mice which were first delineated in 1958 and 1954, respectively (Jackson Laboratory, Bar Harbor, Maine).

Glucan was prepared from Active Dry Yeast (Standard Brands, Inc., New York) by a modification of the method of Hassid *et al.* (23). The yield of glucan approximates 6%. The particulate glucan was suspended in a 5% dextrose and water solution and sterilized for subsequent use.

TABLE 1
Major Features of Shay Myelogenous Leukemia Rat Tumor

1. Induced in Wistar rats by prolonged methylchlanthrene administration (1951).
2. Homogenous polygonal myeloblastic cells – loosely arrayed.
3. No intercellular attachments.
4. Large nuclei-varied shape and size.
5. Little cytoplasm and intracellular material – few mitochondria.
6. Presence of virus-like particles of C type.
7. Few – if any – pigment granules (veroperoxidase).
8. Extremely rapid growth – any site.
9. Rapid dissemination to other organs (bone marrow, spleen, lung, liver, spinal cord, brain, thymus, lymph nodes, muscle).

RESULTS

The Shay myelogenous leukemia tumor was specifically selected as the tumor of choice in view of our previous studies on the role of recognition factors in controlling macrophage surveillance of malignant cells (24-26) and the desire to have the circulating leukemic cells exposed to the fixed macrophage populations which are readily activated by glucan. The rapid dissemination of the tumor cells from the primary site also allows evaluation of the effectiveness of therapy on the secondary as well as the primary lesions. The increased susceptibility of the leukemic rat to bacterial infections also effectively permits an evaluation of macrophage activation on this enhanced bacterial susceptibility, an important facet of human neoplastic disease.

The influence of the simultaneous administration of glucan on growth of 20×10^6 subcutaneously implanted Shay tumor cells is presented in Table 2. In agreement with previous observations (15,18), the administration of glucan significantly decreased tumor growth. Since glucan when injected subcutaneously in rats produced a profound monocytic infiltrate due to its chemotactic nature, the inhibition of tumor growth probably reflects an alteration in tumor macrophage ratio in favor of the latter cell. In preliminary studies undertaken to evaluate this possibility, it was observed that the administration of glucan intralesionally produced a 76% increase in the number of tumor macrophages 12 hours after glucan was administered. At 24 hours the enhancement in tumor macrophage content was no longer present.

In an effort to determine whether glucan may be used as a treatment modality following the administration of leukemic cells, rats were transplanted with 5×10^6 Shay myelogenous leukemic cells intravenously. One to 5 days following transplantation, glucan was administered in 5% glucose intravenously in the amount of 0.2 mg daily. Control animals were injected with isotonic glucose. As can be noted (Figure 1), significant enhancement in survival was observed in the glucan-treated group. Additionally, studies have indicated the

TABLE 2.
Influence of Subcutaneous Implant of Glucan (4 mg) on Growth of Shay Myelogenous Leukemia Cells[+]

Group	No.	Body Weight	Tumor Weight, g
Saline	42	218 ± 2	10.0 ± 1.1
Glucan	42	231 ± 5	4.6 ± 0.9

[+]Tumor weight was determined 10 days post transplantation. Values are expressed as mean ± standard error.

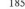

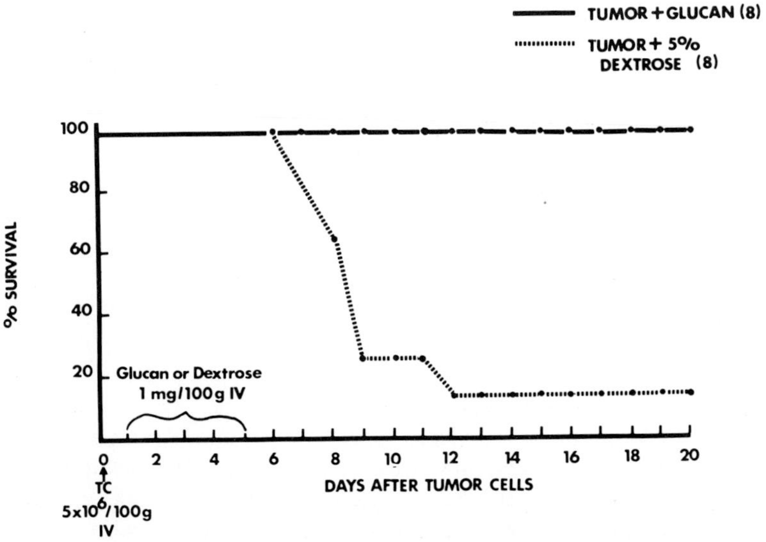

Fig. 1. *Influence of glucan on survival of rats administered 5 × 10^6 Shay myelogenous leukemic cells/100 g intravenously. Glucan (0.2 mg) in dextrose (0.8 mg) or 1 mg of dextrose was given daily on days 1-5.*

development of leukemia at early intervals following leukemic cell transplant was identical in the glucan and the dextrose-treated group. However, leukocyte levels rapidly normalized in the glucan group denoting rejection of the leukemic cell transplant. There were no recurrences of leukemia in any of the survivors in the glucan-treated group.

The influence of glucan administered intravenously on the growth of the adenocarcinoma and melanoma mouse tumors is presented in Tables 3 and 4. Glucan in the amount of 0.2 mg/mouse, or glucose, was administered days 1, 6, 10 and 15 following the subcutaneous injection of 0.5 × 10^6 adenocarcinoma tumor cells. The animals were killed at day 20, tumor weight ascertained. In agreement with the observations in the Shay myelogenous

TABLE 3.
Inhibitory Influence of Glucan on Growth of Adenocarcinoma BW 10232

Group	No.	Wgt., g Body	Wgt., g Tumor
Glucose	8	25	4.21
Glucan	10	20	0.98

0.5 × 10^6 tumor cells injected SQ on Day 0. Glucan (0.2 mgIV)/glucose injections day 1, 6, 10 and 15. Killed on day 20.

TABLE 4.
Inhibitory Influence of Glucan on Growth of Melanoma B16

Group	No.	Wgt., g Body	Tumor
Glucose	7	21	1.26
Glucan	9	20	0.39

1×10^6 tumor cells injected SQ day 0. Glucan (0.2 mg IV) given days 1, 6, 10 and 15. Killed day 21.

leukemia model, the glucan treated mice showed a 76% inhibition of growth in the adenocarcinoma tumor at day 20. Likewise, a rather comparable mean 69% inhibition of tumor growth was observed in the mice injected with 1×10^6 melanoma cells, subcutaneously and treated with glucan in an identical fashion (Table 4).

In an effort to further evaluate the importance of tumor macrophages to the growth of the primary tumor, as well as to its dissemination, the myelogenous leukemic cells were administered to normal rats either alone or in the presence of varying concentrations of glucan activated peritoneal macrophages. As can be noted in Table 5, in two experiments which were

TABLE 5.
Influence of Addition of Glucan Induced Peritoneal Macrophages on Growth of Shay Acute Myelogeneous Leukemia Tumor in Rats

Group	Tumor Cells ($\times 10^6$)	Peritoneal Macrophages Added ($\times 10^6$)	Tumor Weight (g) Exp 1	Exp 2
Control	20	–	5.9 ±0.66	18.8 ±1.73
Control	40	–	–	18.4 ±1.73
Experimental	20	2	2.9 ±0.71$^+$	14.6 ±1.87
Experimental	20	10	2.3 ±0.63$^+$	13.0 ±2.65
Experimental	20	20	2.4 ±1.10$^+$	12.5 ±1.00$^+$

In experiment 1, the groups number 5-7 rats, while 5-6 rats composed each group in experiment 2. An exception to this was the 16 animals which comprised the control group injected with 40×10^6 tumor cells. Tumor weights were ascertained on day 10 in Exp 1 and Day 12 in Exp 2.

Peritoneal macrophages were obtained 4 days following the intraperitoneal administration of 10 ml of a 0.5% suspension of glucan. Tumor cells and glucan activated macrophages were subcutaneously administered.

$^+p<.05$.

conducted in which tumor weights in the control groups varied by a factor of 3, a significant inhibition of tumor weight was observed, particularly when macrophage:tumor cell ratios approximated 1:1. In addition to the inhibition of tumor growth as reflected by the weight of the tumor, distinct histological changes were noted in liver, lung and spleen, as well as in the tumor of the animals bearing tumor implants with varying macrophage populations.

In the control groups which received tumor cells alone, liver showed a heavy infiltrate of tumor cells which compressed and displaced parenchymal cells (Fig. 2). A heavy infiltrate of tumor cells, particularly in the red pulp, was also observed in the spleen (Fig. 3). Megakaryocytes were present in extremely small numbers. In the tumor itself, which was characterized by the presence of myeloblastic cells, limited areas of necrosis and hemorrhage were observed. A relatively small number of mononuclear cells were present.

In the group that received tumor cell:macrophage implants at the ratio of 10:1, the infiltrate of tumor cells in the liver was not as prominent and there appeared to be significant foci of tumor cells undergoing necrosis (Fig. 4). The tumor infiltrate of lung was quite extensive as was that of spleen. The tumor

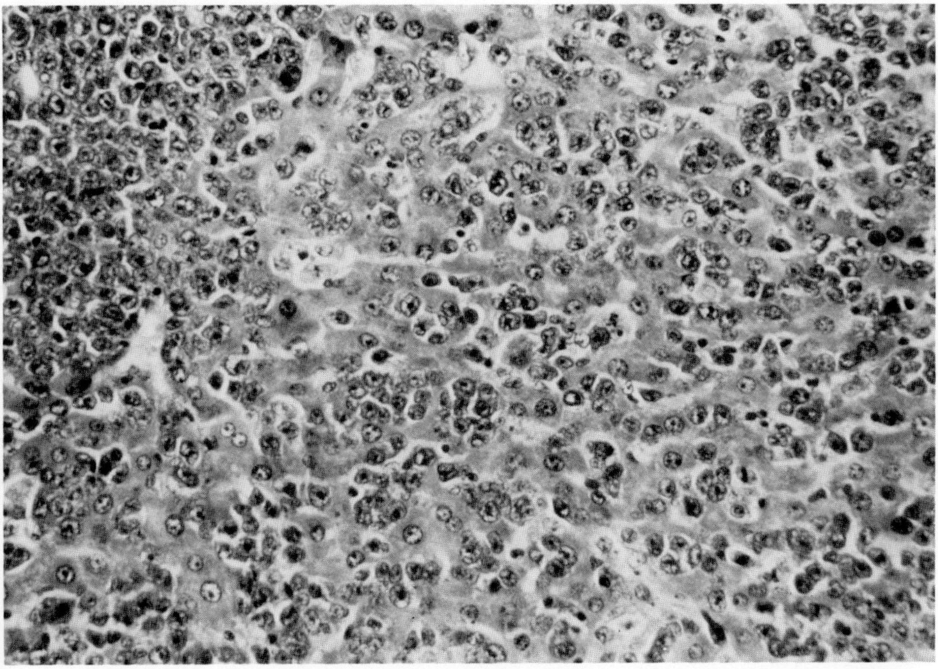

Fig. 2. *Liver from a control rat injected with tumor cells and saline shows a heavy infiltrate of tumor cells on the 12th day. In certain areas hepatocytes have been completely replaced by tumor cells. (H & E 250×).*

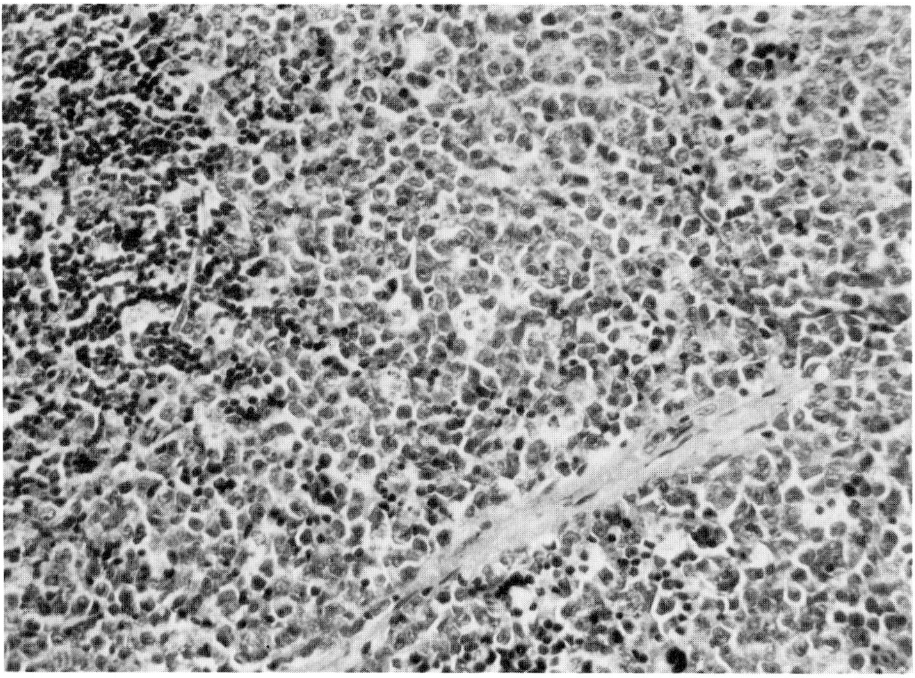

Fig. 3. *Spleen of a control animal injected with tumor cells and saline show tumor infiltrates in the red pulp on day 12. Large aggregates of tumor cells appear to occlude the sinusoids. A small area of normal spleen is observed at the upper left (H & E 250×)*

presented irregularities in necrosis and hemorrhage and a mild infiltrate of vacuolated macrophages.

In the animals which received tumor cells:macrophages in the ratio of 2:1, the liver showed a significant decrease in tumor cell infiltrates and indeed in some livers only a few tumor cells were present. The infiltrate of tumor cells in the lung was characterized as mild to absent. Tumor infiltration of the spleen was significantly reduced compared to the control group (Fig. 5).

The most prominent histiological findings were observed in those animals which received macrophages and tumor cells in the ratio of 1:1. In this group the presence of tumor cells in liver were judged to be slight to absent (Fig. 6). When tumor cells were present they appeared to be undergoing destruction by the mononuclear population. The lung appeared normal and the spleen, relative to degree of tumor infiltrates, was characterized as mild to absent. The tumor presented more extensive areas of necrosis and hemorrhage and had a moderate infiltrate of vacuolated mononuclear cells. These findings denote that by increasing tumor macrophage population and enhancing the

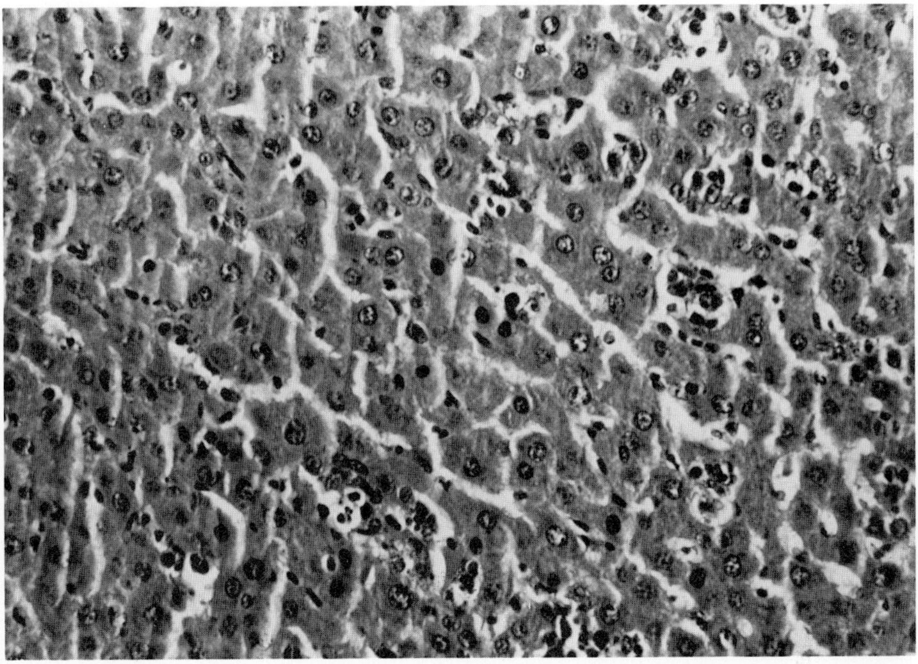

Fig. 4. *Liver of an animal that received tumor cells and glucan stimulated macrophages (10:1 ratio). There is clear evidence of tumor cell infiltration in the sinusoids but many of these tumor cells appear to be undergoing necrosis. Day 12. (H & E 250×).*

ratio of macrophages to tumor cells, a decreased dissemination of malignant cells occurred in association with a more extensive necrosis of the primary lesion.

Studies were also undertaken to provide an evaluation of the comparative effectiveness of BCG and glucan in the myelogenous leukemia rat model. As denoted in Table 6, BCG effectively enhanced 28 day survival. However, the 33% survival was significantly less than the 100% survival noted in the glucan-treated group. Since routes of administration were different and equivalent doses cannot be established, the greater survival of the glucan group over the BCG treated group must be viewed with a certain degree of reservation.

DISCUSSION

It has been amply demonstrated that macrophages, particularly those which are activated either specifically or non-specifically, have the ability to destroy malignant cells by both a phagocytic and an as yet undefined contact

TABLE 6.
Comparative Influence of Pretreatment of Glucan or BCG on Survival of Long-Evans Rats Following the Subcutaneous Administration of Shay Myelogenous Leukemia Cells

Group	No.	28 Day Survival (Percent)
Saline	6	0
BCG	6	33
Glucan	6	100

Agents were administered −7, −5, −3, and on day 0. 0.1 ml of BCG (Glaxo Research Ltd) were given intraperitoneally. Glucan (2 mg) was given intravenously. Tumor cells (20×10^6) were injected subcutaneously on day 0.

lysis mechanism (27,28). Krahenbuhl and Lambert (29) observed that activated macrophages had an enhanced ability to inhibit DNA synthesis in tumor cells. Direct contact between macrophages and target cells was required for cytostasis. The mechanism by which macrophages exert their cytotoxic effect

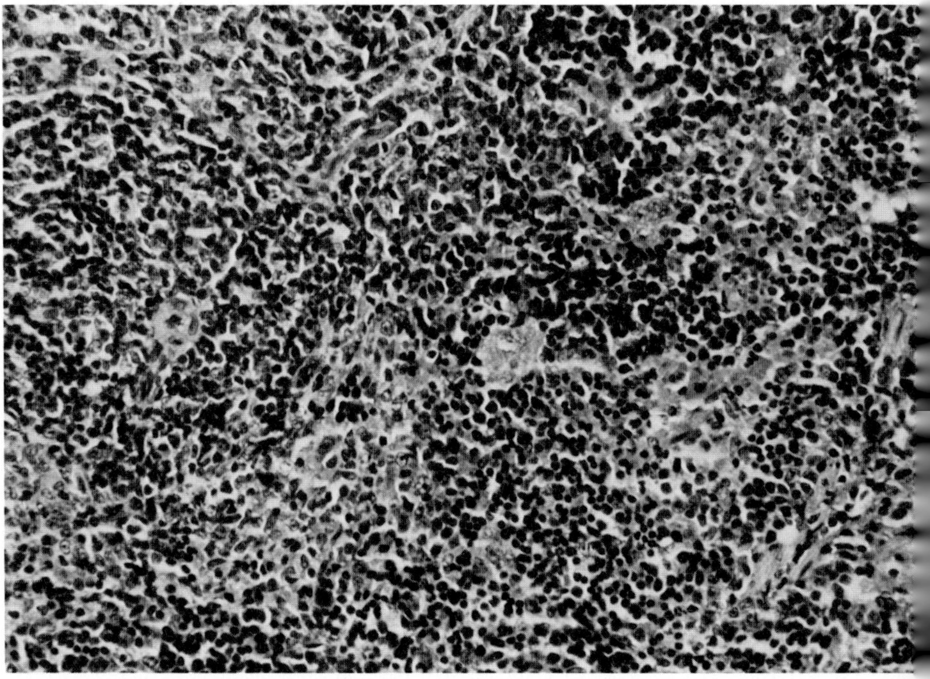

Fig. 5. *Spleen from an animal injected with tumor cells and glucan stimulated macrophages (2:1 ratio), presents few tumor infiltrates in the red pulp but the rest of the tissue is rather normal. Day 12. (H & E 250×).*

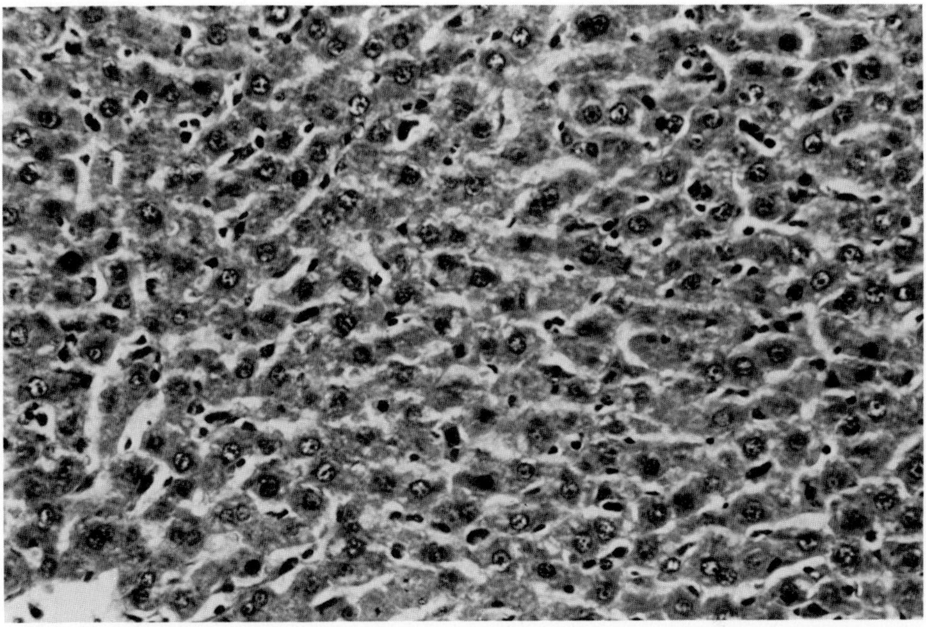

Fig. 6. *Liver of an animal that received tumor cells and glucan stimulated macrophages (1:1 ratio) possesses essentially normal structure denoting an absence of disseminated tumor cells. Day 12. Kupffer cells are prominent. (H & E 250×).*

on tumor cells is not as yet established. One possibility is the anti-microbial myeloperoxidase-hydrogen peroxide-halide system. Employing four different assays of cytotoxicity, a cytotoxic effect of this anti-microbial system was demonstrated by Clark *et al.* (30) on mouse ascites lymphoma cells. The comparative contribution of the lysosomal system and the peroxidase system to the tumor cell killing ability of macrophages is as yet to be defined.

The importance of macrophages to inhibition of tumor growth was recently stressed by Haskill *et al.* (31). Employing velocity sedimentation to fractionate enzymatically or mechanically dispersed tumor cell suspensions, the effector cells within two rat sarcomas were found to be activated macrophages. Haskill *et al.* (31) also reported that the proliferation of macrophages *in vitro* was inhibited by the presence of tumor cells. Whether glucan enhanced activation and proliferation of macrophages may overcome any inhibitory action of the tumor on macrophage effector cells remains to be ascertained.

Our composite studies indicate that tumor macrophage populations play a significant role in determining the degree at which tumor cells disseminate to peripheral sites. This finding is a fundamental confirmation of the observations of Birbeck and Carter (32) who predicated a difference in behavior of a metastatic and non-metastatic lymphoma due to variations in intratumor host macrophage populations. The previous studies of Gershon *et al.* (33) also add to the concept that failure of macrophage mobilization and activation intralesionally contributes significantly to the dissemination of tumor cells. Gershon *et al.* (33) observed that sinus histiocytosis, which resulted in the region of a non-metastasizing lymphoma was absent in lymph nodes draining a metastasizing lymphoma. The clinical importance of such observations may be denoted by the studies of Baum *et al.* (34). These investigators studied macrophage phagocytic activity in patients with breast cancer. Baum *et al.* (34) reported that as long as the macrophage response of the host remained intact, as assayed by phagocytic response, the tumor remained localized to the breast and underlying muscle. In those individuals in whom the tumor disseminated to lymph nodes and beyond, profound impairments were seen in macrophage function. These studies further contribute to an appreciation of the potential importance of macrophages as determinant cells in tumor cell dissemination.

Keller (35) has demonstrated that activated peritoneal macrophages rapidly and effectively eliminate syngenic tumor cells *in vitro*. Keller's studies indicated effector:target cell ratios of 10:1 and 5:1 as well as a pronounced inhibition of thymidine incorporation of tumor cells at macrophage:target cell ratios of 1:1. In the present study, employing an *in vivo* system, we observed that dissemination of leukemic cells from the primary subcutaneous site to liver, lung and spleen was effectively inhibited when macrophages were added to establish tumor cell:macrophage ratios at 2:1 and 1:1 and to a more limited degree at 10:1. Similarly, Eccles and Alexander reported that a high macrophage content of the tumor was associated with decreased metastases while conversely mouse tumors which possess low macrophage content showed increased dissemination (36).

Eccles and Alexander (37) have also indicated the existence of a monocytic defect in tumor induced "anergy." Immunological competence was restored in rats possessing tumor implants by the administration of peritoneal macrophages, but not lymphocytes. Eccles and Alexander (37) suggested that the resulting immunological anergy which develops as the tumor grows is due to the fact that the tumor competes for the available blood monocytes. Eccles and Alexander concluded that the state of anergy in association with tumor development may not be a failure of immunological recognition or reactivity, but may be due to the unavailability of monocytes to fulfill their role as modulators of immunological events. It is therefore possible, by increasing the availability of macrophages through our mechanisms of glucan-induced macrophage proliferation and activation, that immunological competence can be maintained in the presence of tumor development.

It is evident on the basis of our experimental and clinical studies that glucan provides a unique means to initiate an enhancement of host resistance to neoplasia by macrophage activation and proliferation with a resulting significant increase in level of host resistance. It is obvious that the ability to induce a functional macrophage population within the tumor mass, which has the ability to selectively kill neoplastic cells, would be of significant clinical importance. These macrophages would not only tend to function to eliminate neoplastic cells as such, but their *in vivo* events associated with macrophage antigen processing and initiation of both T and B cell responsiveness would contribute to a decrease in tumor cell dissemination. This concept is well supported by the findings of Vorbrodt *et al.* (38). Vorbrodt *et al.* (38) have reported that during x-ray therapy of human skin cancers, macrophages were found to be actively engaged in tumor cell destruction. Intimate contact between "invading macrophages" and cancer cells with concomitant formation of cytoplasmic bridges and fusion zones were frequently observed following radiation therapy. In subsequent investigations to pursue this finding, Vorbrodt *et al.* (39) demonstrated that radiation of macrophage and tumor cells in culture was associated with macrophage activation, increase in lysosomes and phagolysosomes, as well as associated macrophage adherence to cancer cells and the presence of phagocytized cancer cells. Vorbrodt *et al.* (40) suggested that x-irradiation of the tumor cells results in alterations in the tumor cell membrane which promotes adhesion and contact between the macrophage and the tumor cell and, in an as yet unknown fashion, leads to degeneration of the tumor cell and phagocytosis of the cell by the macrophages.

The anti-tumor effect of yeast glucan is clearly evident by the present experimental studies as well as our previous clinical endeavors. Glucans obtained from a variety of other sources have also been demonstrated to have anti-tumor activity in various experimental systems. Sakai *et al.* (41) have compared the anti-tumor action of certain glucans against the Sarcoma 18-in ascites form and attempted to relate antitumor action to chemical structure. Those glucans possessing a linear β 1→3 linked D glucose structure were most effective. Glucans composed of alpha-configurations were ineffective. With the exception of a tendency for a slight loss in body weight, no other ill effects were observed in the glucan-treated groups.

Singh *et al.* (42) reported that anti-tumor action of a scleroglucan derived from *Sclerotium glucanicum*. This glucan possesses a main chain of (1→3) β-D-glucopyranosyl units with every third or fourth unit carrying a (1→6) β-D-glucopyranosyl group. Singh *et al.* indicated that scleroglucan did not show toxic effects in the test animals. The absence of overt toxicity of various glucans may be of future significance in their consideration as immunostimulants.

Chihara *et al.* (43) have reported that the glucans which are very effective in modifying tumor growth in experimental animals were ineffective in modifying growth of tumor cell cultures, denoting that the action is host mediated and not directly cytocidal. When our yeast glucan preparation was incubated with tumor cells *in vitro*, no direct cytotoxicity was manifested, confirming the observation of Chihara *et al.* (43) that the antitumor effect of glucan is host mediated.

Dennert and Tucker (44) have reported that lentinan, a linear β 1,3 glucan, obtained from the mushroom lentiusedodes possesses pronounced antitumor activity. Antitumor effect was found in normal, but not in neonatally thymectomized mice denoting that an intact T cell system was a prerequisite for the demonstrated antitumor effect of lentinan. It remains to be established whether yeast glucan is also a T cell adjuvant and whether its antitumor activity is mediated through the proliferation and activation of macrophages or an enhancement in T cell populations and function. Lentinan apparently does not exert its antitumor activity by macrophage stimulation, or by an enhancement in cell or humoral immunity (45), but may exert its effect by stimulation of histamine or serotonin (45).

An area which as yet remains essentially unexplored is the influence of specific macrophage stimulants on not only the effectiveness of chemotherapeutic agents but also on the alteration of responsiveness of tumor-bearing animals to bacterial and viral challenges. The previous studies of Sokoloff *et al.* (46) may well be significant in denoting effectiveness of combined macrophage activation and chemotherapy. Sokoloff *et al.* reported that zymosan administered to mice bearing Sarcoma 180 and Ehrlich carcinoma transplants. considerably increased the tumor oncolytic effect of mitomycin C, while reducing its toxicity. Further studies will be required to denote whether effectiveness of glucan in controlling tumor growth can be enhanced by antineoplastic agents and likewise, whether it will be possible to reduce the required dose of chemotherapeutic agents by glucan or other such macrophage stimulants and thus reduce problems of drug toxicity.

There is little question, in view of the diverse reports of various investigators, that glucans derived from various sources, but possessing a $1 \rightarrow 3$ β-configuration, have significant antitumor activity against a variety of tumors in diverse animal species, including man. It is obvious that glucan is a unique agent not only relative to its ability to activate host defense mechanisms, including those directed against malignant and non-malignant allogenic and xenogenic cells (47), but also as a chemically defined agent employable in evaluation of the concept of immunotherapy and immunoprophylaxis.

It is generally presently considered that immunotherapy, as exemplified by the employment of BCG, is only effective against a small number of tumor cells which approximate 10^5 cells. In the present study involving two animal species and three different tumors, initial numbers of tumor cells injected were on the order of 10^6. In the acute myelogenous leukemia model we have also found it possible to completely reverse the tumor state when glucan is injected on days 5-7 post-tumor cell transplantation. At this time the primary tumor is 2-3% of body weight, normally 4-6 g, and considerable metastasis has already occurred to liver, lung and spleen. The effectiveness of glucan in this regard may be due to its non-viable state since the use of viable organisms and the induction of septicemia presents to the organism the choice of diverting macrophages from tumor target cells to control the infectious episode induced in the host. Indeed, in view of the apparent significant role macrophages play in controlling tumor growth and dissemination, facilitation of tumor growth under instances of BCG therapy may well reflect the diversion of the macrophage population from what should be their primary dedication, namely the destruction of tumor cells within the internal environment, to an attempt to control the infectious episode. While further studies will be essential to evaluate these possibilities, the potential danger of employing living, still partially pathogenic bacteria has also been stressed by Weiss (48).

Our composite studies clearly establish the importance of macrophages as host defense cells against the growth of various tumor cells, as well as the importance of macrophages in determining dissemination of malignant leukemic cell populations. It can well be anticipated that through a further delineation of the role of macrophages in tumor cell destruction, as well as the importance of macrophage populations of tumors to tumor growth and dissemination, an appreciation of host defense mechanisms against neoplastic states will be forthcoming.

ACKNOWLEDGEMENT

This study was supported in part by USPHS grant CA 13746.

REFERENCES

1. Pillemer, L. and E. E. Ecker (1941). Anticomplementary factor in fresh yeast. *J. Biol. Chem. 137*:139-142.

2. Benacerraf, B. and M. M. Sebestyen (1957). Effect of bacterial endotoxins on the reticuloendothelial system. *Res. Proc. 16*:860-866.

3. Northcote, D. H. and R. W. Horne (1952). The chemical composition and structure of the yeast cell wall. *Biochem. J. 51*:232-236.

4. Di Carlo, F. J. and J. V. Fiore (1958). On the composition of zymosan. *Science 127*:756-757.

5. Mundkur, B. (1960). Electron microscopical studies of frozen-dried yeast. *Exp. Cell Res. 20*:28-42.

6. Cutler, J. L. (1960). The enhancement of hemolysin production in the rat by zymosan. *J. Immunol. 84*:416-419.

7. Diller, I. C. and Z. T. Mankowski (1960). Response of sarcoma 37 and normal cells of the mouse host to zymosan and hydroglucan. *Ext. de Acta Internatl Contre le Cancer 16*:584-587.

8. Mankowski, Z. T., I. C. Diller and W. J. Nickerson (1958). The action of hydroglucan on experimental mouse tumors. *Proc. Am. Assoc. Cancer Res. 2*:324.

9. Old, L. J., D. A. Clarke, B. Benacerraf and M. Goldsmith (1960). The reticuloendothelial system and the neoplastic process. *Ann. N.Y. Acad. Sci. 88*:265-280.

10. Thiele, E. H. (1974). Induction of host resistance in different mouse strains. *Proc. Soc. Exp. Biol. Med. 146*:1067-1070.

11. Riggi, S. J. and N. R. Di Luzio (1961). Identification of a reticuloendothelial stimulating agent in zymosan. *Am. J. Physiol. 200*:297-300.

12. Hassid, W. Z., M. A. Joslyn and R. M. McCready (1941). The molecular constitution of an insoluble polysaccharide from yeast, Saccharomyces cerevisiae. *J. Am. Chem. Soc. 63*:294-298.

13. Bacon, J. S. D., V. C. Farmer, D. Jones and I. F. Taylor (1969). The glucan components of the cell wall of Baker's yeast (Saccharomyces cerevisiae) considered in relation to its ultrastructure. *Biochem. J. 114*:557-567.

14. Sears, W., J. Strickland, and N. R. Di Luzio, unpublished observations.

15. Di Luzio, N. R. (1975). Macrophage recognition factors and neoplasia. *The Reticuloendothelial System.* International Academy of Pathology Monograph. Williams and Wilkins Co.

16. Mansell, P. W. A., H. Ichinose, R. J. Reed, E. T. Krementz, R. McNamee and N. R. Di Luzio (1975). Macrophage-mediated destruction of human malignant cells *in vivo. J. Natl. Cancer Inst. 54*:571-580.

17. Di Luzio, N. R. (1975). The role of plasma recognition factors in neoplasia. *Trace Components of Plasma: Isolation and Clinical Significance.* Am. Natl. Red. Cross, in press.

18. Di Luzio, N. R., R. McNamee, E. Jones, S. Lassoff, W. Sear and E. O. Hoffmann. Inhibition of growth and dissemination of Shay myelogenous leukemic tumor in rats by glucan and glucan activated macrophages. *Proceedings of the VII International Congress of the Reticuloendothelial Soc.* Plenum Press, New York, in press.

19. Palm, J. and D. B. Wilson (1974). The ag-B locus of rats: A major histocompatibility complex. *Immunobiology of Transplantation.* F. H. Bach, Ed. Grune and Stratton, New York.

20. Shay, H., M. Gruenstein, H. E. Marx and L. Glazer (1951). Development of lymphatic and myelogenous leukemia in Wistar rats following gastric instillation of methylcholanthrene. *Cancer Res. 11*:29-34.

21. Lapis, K. and I. Benedeczky (1967). Electron microscopic study of the Shay chloroleukemia. *Cancer Res. 27*:1544-1564.

22. Handler, E. E. and E. S. Handler (1970). Experimental leukemias: Model systems for the study of hematopoiesis. *Regulation of Hematopoiesis.* A. S. Gordon, Ed. Appleton-Century Crofts, New York.

23. Hassid, W. Z., M. A. Joslyn, and R. M. McCready (1941). The molecular constitution of an insoluble polysaccharide from yeast Saccharomyces cerevisiae. *J. Am. Chem. Soc. 63*:295-298.

24. Di Luzio, N. R., E. R. Miller, R. McNamee and J. C. Pisano (1972). Alterations in plasma recognition factor activity in experimental leukemia. *J. Reticuloendothel. Soc. 11*:186-197.

25. Di Luzio, N. R., R. McNamee, E. F. Miller and J. C. Pisano (1972). Macrophage recognition factor depletion after administration of particulate agents and leukemic cells. *J. Reticuloendothel. Soc. 12*:314-323.

26. Di Luzio, N. R., R. McNamee, I. Olcay, A. Kitahama and R. H. Miller (1974). Inhibition of tumor growth by recognition factors. *Proc. Soc. Exp. Biol. Med.* *145*:311-315.

27. Amos, D. B. (1960). Possible relationships between the cytotoxic effects of isoantibody and host cell function. *Ann. N.Y. Acad. Sci.* *87*:273-292.

28. Bennett, B., L. J. Old and E. A. Boyse (1964). The phagocytosis of tumor cells *in vitro. Transplantation* *2*:183-202.

29. Krahenbuhl, J. L. and L. H. Lambert, Jr. (1975). Cytokinetic studies of the effects of activated macrophages on tumor target cells. *J. Natl. Cancer Inst.* *54*:1433-1437.

30. Clark, R. A., S. J. Klebanoff, A. B. Einstein and A. Fefer (1975). Peroxidase H_2O_2 halide system: Cytotoxic effect on mammalian tumor cells. *Blood* *45*:161-170.

31. Haskill, J. S., J. W. Proctor and Y. Yamamura (1975). Host responses within solid tumors. I. Monocytic effector cells within rat sarcomas. *J. Natl. Cancer Inst.* *54*:387-393.

32. Birbeck, M. S. C. and R. L. Carter (1972). Observations on the ultrastructure of two hamster lymphomas in hamsters with particular reference to infiltrating macrophages. *Int. J. Cancer* *9*:249-257.

33. Gershon, R. K., R. L. Carter and N. J. Lane (1967). Studies on homotransplantable lymphomas in hamsters. IV. Observations on macrophages in the expression of tumor immunity. *Am. J. Pathol.* *51*:1111-1133.

34. Baum, M., D. Sumner, M. H. Edwards and P. Smythe (1973). Macrophage phagocytic activity in patients with breast cancer. *Br. J. Surg.* *60*:899-900.

35. Keller, R. (1973). Evidence for compromise of tumour immunity in rats by a non-specific blocking serum factor that inactivates macrophages. *Br. J. Exp. Pathol.* *54*:298-305.

36. Eccles, S. A. and P. Alexander (1974). Macrophage content of tumours in relation to metastatic spread and host immune reaction. *Nature* *250*:667-669.

37. Eccles, S. A. and P. Alexander (1974). Sequestration of macrophages in growing tumours and its effect on the immunological capacity of the host. *Br. J. Cancer* *30*:42-49.

38. Vorbrodt, A., A. Hliniak, S. Krzyzowska-Gruca and S. Gruca (1972). Ultrastructural studies on the behaviour of macrophages in the course of x-ray therapy of human skin cancer. *Acta Histochem.* *43*:270-280.

39. Vorbrodt, A., A. Grabska, S. Krzyzowska-Gruca and S. Gruca (1973). Cytochemical and ultrastructural studies on the contact formation between macrophages and irradiated cancer cells *in vitro. Folia Histochem. Cytochem.* *11*:357-358.

40. Vorbrodt, A., A. Grabska, S. Krzyzowska-Gruca and S. Gruca (1973). The formation of contacts between macrophages and neoplastic cells. *Folia Histochem. Cytochem.* *11*:185-190.

41. Sakai, S., S. Takada, T. Kamasuka, Y. Momoki and J. Sugayama (1968). Antitumor action of some glucans: Especially on its correlation to their chemical structure. *Gann.* *57*:507-512.

42. Singh, P. P., R. L. Whistler, R. Tokuzen and W. Nakahara (1974). Scleroglucan, an antitumor polysaccharide from Sclerotium glucanicum. *Carbohydrate Res.* *37*:245-247.

43. Chihara, G., J. Hamuro, Y. Y. Maeda, Y. Arai and F. Fukuoka (1970). Fractionation and purification of the polysaccharides with marked antitumor activity, especially lentinan from Lentinus edodes (Berk.) Sing. (an edible mushroom). *Cancer Res.* *30*:2776-2781.

44. Dennert, G. and D. Tucker (1973). Antitumor polysaccharide lentinan – a T cell adjuvant. *J. Natl. Cancer Inst.* *51*:1727-1729.

45. Maeda, Y. Y., J. Hamuro, Y. O. Yamada, K. Ishimura and G. Chihara (1973). The nature of immunopotention by the anti-tumour polysaccharide lentinan and the significance of biogenic amines in its action. *Immunopotentiation.* Elsevier, New York.

46. Sokoloff, B., Y. Toda, M. Fujisawa, K. Enomoto, C. Saelhof, L. Bird and C. Miller (1961). Experimental studies in mitomycin C. 4. Zymosan and the RES. *Growth 25*:249-263.

47. Wooles, W. R. and N. R. Di Luzio (1964). Inhibition of homograft acceptance and homo- and hetero-graft rejection in chimeras by reticuloendothelial system stimulation. *Proc. Soc. Exp. Biol. Med. 115*:756-759.

48. Weiss, D. W. (1975). *Immunobiology of Tumor-Host Relationship.* R. T. Smith and M. Landy, Eds. Academic Press, New York, 327-330.

MACROPHAGES IN REGRESSING AND PROGRESSING MOLONEY SARCOMAS*

Stephen W. Russell, William F. Doe
and Charles G. Cochrane

INTRODUCTION

Macrophages can mediate injury *in vitro* to neoplastic cells, either specifically or nonspecifically, through a number of different pathways (1). These observations, coupled with the finding that various kinds of tumors in several species contain substantial numbers of this inflammatory cell type (2,3), have contributed to the growing awareness that macrophages may play a significant role in host defense against neoplasia.

To understand better the role of tumor macrophages *in vivo*, we have recently been analyzing cells of this type recovered from progressing and regressing Moloney sarcomas. The following is a summary of studies performed to date.

TUMOR MODEL

The neoplasm used in these studies is the Moloney sarcoma induced by intramuscular injection of cultured MSC cells (4). Among experimental tumor systems it offers the advantage that either regressing or progressing sarcomas can be induced in adult mice, predictably and consistently, by varying the size of the tumor cell inoculum (4). Regressing tumors result from injection of 10^4 MSC cells, while progressing neoplasms are produced by inoculation of 10^6 cells.

Following an initial acute inflammatory response, developing tumors are infiltrated by mononuclear inflammatory cells (4). This response is similar to that described earlier by Fefer and his colleagues (5) in virus-induced Moloney sarcomas. Regressing tumors are uniformly infiltrated by inflammatory cells, while the host inflammatory response is restricted to the peripheries of

*This is manuscript number 996 from the Department of Immunopathology, Scripps Clinic and Research Foundation, 476 Prospect Street, La Jolla, California 92037. The work was supported by USPHS contract N01-CB-44001; USPHS grants AI 07007 and CA 17720; California Division-American Cancer Society Junior Fellowship J-235; and the Lilly International Fellowship Foundation. The authors thank Mr. Ronald Hoskins and Ms. Ann Tozier for their excellent technical assistance.

progressing sarcomas (4,6). Pulmonary metastases develop in mice bearing progressing tumors, attesting to the truly malignant nature of the neoplasm. Karyotypic analyses and identification of abnormal, marker chromosomes characteristic of MSC cells have confirmed that pulmonary lesions are true metastases and not new primary tumors induced by the systemic spread of murine sarcoma virus (7).

DISAGGREGATION OF TUMORS

In terms of total cell yield and cell recovery (6,8), enzymatic methods have proved 15-20 times more efficient in our hands than mechanical means (homogenizing, screening, mincing, etc.) of disaggregating tumors. Proteases with pH optima in the physiologic range were tested to determine their efficacy in disaggregation systems. Of those evaluated (carboxypeptidase A, chymopapain, chymotrypsin, papain, pronase and trypsin), papain gave the highest cell yields and percent recoveries and had the least deleterious effect on the inflammatory cell surface markers examined. All of the proteolytic enzymes tested were markedly increased in their disaggregation efficiency if employed in conjuction with collagenase. DNAse was needed to prevent the formation of nucleic acid gels. The papain/collagenase/DNAse mixture used to disaggregate tumors has yielded up to 6.5×10^8 viable cells/g tumor and DNA recoveries as high as 50-60%.

MACROPHAGE CONTENT OF TUMORS

Sarcomas begin to regress or to progress inexorably 11-13 days post-inoculation. Table 1 summarizes the results of a detailed analysis of the macrophage content of tumors made during this critical period (6).

TABLE 1.
*Numbers of Macrophages in Progressing and Regressing Moloney Sarcomas**

	Progressing Tumors (Mean ± 1 SEM)	Regressing Tumors (Mean ± 1 SEM)
Tumor Weight (mg)	763 ± 126	146 ± 17
DNA (mg/g tumor)	8.0 ± 0.3	8.9 ± 0.4
% (DNA) Recovery	55.2 ± 2.5	32.5 ± 3.5
% Macrophages**	18.5 ± 2.6	45.4 ± 5.1
Macrophages per Tumor	$1.3 \times 10^8 \pm 0.4$	$1.3 \times 10^8 \pm 0.4$
Macrophages/g Tumor	1.7×10^8	8.9×10^8

*5 progressing and 10 regressing sarcomas analyzed 11–13 days postinoculation. Reprinted by permission of the Journal of Immunology (6).

**Of total cells recovered.

As was the case 8 days postinoculation (6), the percentage of macrophages in regressing tumors after 11-13 days was 2-3 times that found in progressing sarcomas. However, the total number of macrophages per tumor was the same (1.3×10^8) for each type. These absolute values may be misleading if the difference in size between the two types of tumor is not considered, since the number of macrophages per gram is approximately 5 times greater in smaller, regressing sarcomas than in progressing neoplasms.

As mentioned earlier, inflammatory cells were distributed throughout regressing tumors, but were confined to the peripheries of progressing neoplasms. The actual difference between macrophage concentrations in the central portions of the two types of tumors therefore was far greater than was suggested by the overall 5-fold difference reported above.

ASSOCIATION OF TUMOR MACROPHAGES WITH CYTOSTASIS *IN VIVO* AND *IN VITRO*

Coincident with the appearance of inflammatory infiltrates, mitotic activity in regressing tumors all but ceases (4). Further analysis of both regressing and progressing tumors (6) has confirmed the intimate association of cytostasis with the presence of mononuclear inflammatory cells: mitotic activity was suppressed throughout regressing neoplasms, but was diminished only at the edges of progressing sarcomas. By contrast, the centers of progressing sarcomas, which were devoid of inflammatory elements, exhibited many mitotic figures.

Macrophages appear to be the most abundant inflammatory cell in Moloney sarcomas (9). To determine if the cytostatic effect observed *in vivo* can be associated with macrophages, studies of how tumor macrophages affect the replication of tumor cells *in vitro* have begun. The results of initial experiments, comparing the effects of adherent cells from either the peritoneal cavity of normal mice or disaggregated, regressing Moloney sarcomas, are summarized in Table 2.

Before seeding, peritoneal cells were stirred for 30 min. with the enzymes used to disaggregate tumors. Percent macrophages in starting suspensions was determined and the same number of normal and tumor macrophages (10^6) were seeded/well in Linbro plates. After washing and overnight incubation, monolayers of adherent cells were seeded with 5×10^4 target cells/well. Forty hours later cells were pulsed (3 hr.) with ^{3}H-thymidine (1μCi/ml, sp.ac. 5 Ci/mmol) and harvested using trypsin. DNA was precipitated with 5% cold TCA and analyzed for radioactivity in a liquid scintillation counter.

When compared to target cells cultured with normal peritoneal cells (>95% macrophages), washed monolayers of adherent cells from disaggregated tumors suppressed the uptake of thymidine by both MSC and SV40 (55 and 30% suppression, respectively). Adherent cells from tumors and normal

TABLE 2.
*Suppression of ^{3}H-Thymidine Incorporation**

Target Tumor Cell	Tumor Cells Alone	Source of Adherent Effector Cells		Percent Suppression**
		Normal Peritoneum	Disaggregated Tumor	
None	–	1,180 ± 21	4,239 ± 628	–
MSC	44,208 ± 1,789	26,705 ± 1,337	15,649 ± 2,051	55
SV40 3T3 Cell	22,308 ± 2,872	12,089 ± 993	11,335 ± 965	30

*Mean (triplicate) CPM ± 1 S.D.

$$\text{**Percent suppression} = 100 - \left(\frac{\text{Tumor Macs + Target Cells} - \text{Tumor Macs Alone}}{\text{Normal Macs + Target Cells} - \text{Normal Macs Alone}} \times 100 \right)$$

peritonea both suppressed incorporation if target cells cultured alone were considered as the control. In this instance, the cells recovered from tumors were the most efficient effector population. The elevated background count for cells from the disaggregated tumor was due to the presence of wells in neoplastic elements explanted from tumors along with macrophages.

Preliminary results indicate that treatment of effector cell monolayers with antimacrophage serum and complement substantially reduces the suppressive effect, suggesting that tumor macrophages are at least partly responsible for the inhibition of thymidine uptake obtained in this system.

DISCUSSION

The quantitative and functional studies summarized here strengthen the hypothesis that macrophages help to mediate the regression of Moloney sarcomas. First, mononuclear inflammatory cells are intimately associated with the regression of this tumor (4,5), and are absent from all but the edges of neoplasms which run a progressive course (4,6). Macrophages appear to be the most common inflammatory cell type in these infiltrates (9).

Secondly, there is a marked quantitative difference between the macrophage content of progressing and regressing Moloney sarcomas. The concentration of macrophages in smaller, regressing tumors is as much as 5 times that found in progressing sarcomas. This observation is in basic agreement with the work of Stutman (10), which showed that progressing, virus-induced Moloney sarcomas in nude-athymic (nu/nu) mice contained fewer macrophages than similar, regressing neoplasms in normal heterzygotes. Stutman's finding of a reduced macrophage content in progressing tumors of T lymphocyte-deficient mice may indicate, among other things, a need for this cell type in the recruitment of macrophages in tumors.

A third consideration is the histologic evidence of cytostasis that is related in sarcomas to the presence of infiltrating mononuclear inflammatory cells. This effect, at least in part, may be mediated by macrophages. There is ample evidence to support this assertion from studies conducted *in vitro* using macrophages from the peritoneum and various lymphoid organs (11-15). In addition, we and Holden and his colleagues (16) have shown independently that macrophages recovered directly from disaggregated Moloney sarcomas interfere with the incorporation of ^{3}H-thymidine into tumor cells – a result which suggests interference with tumor cell replication (13-15). Suppression appears to be nonspecific, in that a neoplastic cell type (SV40) other than the one used to induce tumors (MSC) was affected.

These studies implicate the macrophage as being important in host defense against neoplasia. Proof of this point, however, awaits additional investigations conducted *in vitro* with purified cell populations prepared from tumors, as well as depletion and adoptive transfer studies performed *in vivo*. Our current efforts are directed to these ends.

SUMMARY

Regressing and progressing Moloney sarcomas were examined histologically and after disaggregation with enzymes. Regression was associated with mononuclear cell infiltration. The concentration of macrophages in regressing sarcomas was 5 times that found in progressing tumors. Macrophages obtained from disaggregated tumors suppressed the uptake of ^{3}H-thymidine into two unrelated types of neoplastic cells *in vitro*, and appeared intimately associated with suppression of mitotic activity in tumors. The implication of these data is that macrophages help to mediate the regression of Moloney sarcomas.

REFERENCES

1. Cerottini, J.-C. and K. T. Brunner (1974). Cell-mediated cytotoxicity, allograft rejection, and tumor immunity. *Advances in Immunol. 18*:67-132.

2. Evans, R. (1972). Macrophages in syngeneic animal tumor. *Transplantation 14*:468-473.

3. Wood, G. W., G. Y. Gillespie and R. F. Barth (1975). Receptor sites for antigen-antibody complexes on cells derived from solid tumors: Detection by means of antibody sensitized sheep erythrocytes labeled with technetium-99m. *J. Immunol. 114*:950-957.

4. Russell, S. W. and C. G. Cochrane (1974). The cellular events associated with regression and progression of murine (Moloney) sarcomas. *Int. J. Cancer 13*:54-63.

5. Fefer, A., J. L. McCoy, K. Perk and J. P. Glynn (1968). Immunologic, virologic and pathologic studies of regression of autochthonous Moloney sarcoma virus-induced tumors in mice. *Cancer Res. 28*:1577-1585.

6. Russell, S. W., W. F. Doe, and C. G. Cochrane (1976). Number of macrophages and distribution of mitotic activity in regressing and progressing Moloney sarcomas. *J. Immunol. 116*: In press.

7. Russell, S. W., U. Francke, L. Buettner and C. G. Cochrane (1974). Modes of growth and spread of a transplantable, virus-producing murine (Moloney) sarcoma: Karyotypic analysis. *J. Natl. Cancer Inst.* *53*:801-806.

8. Meinke, W., D. A. Goldstein and M. R. Hall (1974). Rapid isolation of mouse DNA from cells in tissue culture. *Analyt. Biochem.* *58*:82-88.

9. Russell, S. W., W. F. Doe and A. Tozier (1975). The relative occurrence of macrophages in regressing and progressing Moloney sarcomas. *Fed. Proc.* *34*:268.

10. Stutman, O. (1975). Delayed tumour appearance and absence of regression in nude mice infected with murine sarcoma virus. *Nature* *253*:142-144.

11. Owen, J. J. T. and R. C. Seeger (1973). Immunity to tumours of the murine leukaemia-sarcoma virus complex. *Br. J. Cancer 28, Suppl. I*:26-34.

12. Seeger, R. C. and J. J. T. Owen (1974). Anti-tumour cytotoxic effects mediated by minor and major cell populations of lymph nodes. *Nature* *252*:420-421.

13. Senik, A., L. de Giorgi, E. Gomard and J. P. Levy (1974). Cytostasis of lymphoma cells in suspension: Probable non-thymic origin of the cytostatic lymphoid cells in mice bearing MSV-induced tumors. *Int. J. Cancer* *14*:396-400.

14. Keller, R. (1975). Cytostatic elimination of syngeneic rat tumor cells *in vitro* by nonspecifically activated macrophages. *J. Exptl. Med.* *138*:625-644.

15. Krahenbuhl, J. L. and J. S. Remington (1974). The role of activated macrophages in specific and nonspecific cytostasis of tumor cells. *J. Immunol.* *113*:507-516.

16. Holden, H. T., J. S. Haskill, H. Kirchner and R. B. Herberman. Two functionally distinct antitumor effector cells isolated from primary murine sarcoma virus-induced tumors. Submitted for publication.

DISCUSSION

Osias Stutman, Chairman

Although active questioning of the speakers during their presentation cleared many or all the small queries concerning techniques or methodological approaches, several conceptual problems were developed during the discussion.

Dr. Golde's presentation generated three main questions: 1) What is the origin of the alveolar macrophage? It was accepted especially from animal studies, that there was evidence for two populations, one locally derived (or "fixed") and one of immigrant (blood monocytes, bone marrow derived?) origin. Dr. Golde's data from a human bone marrow transplantation chimera indicated that the main component recovered after bronchial lavage is of immigrant (bone marrow) origin. 2) What are the control mechanisms that regulate alveolar macrophage turnover? It became apparent that since macrophages can generate colony stimulating factors, they may regulate their own turnover, although this is still hypothetical. (The role of chronic irritation, as in smokers, deserves study). 3) A possible protective role in surveillance for alveolar macrophages from smokers was considered. These macrophages showed signs of activation, i.e., adhered to and killed targets more efficiently. The "immigrant" origin of these cells was considered to perhaps relate to chronic irritation.

Dr. DiLuzio's presentation generated questions concerning the actual efficiency of the treatment of established tumors with glucan. Although a substantial reduction of tumor mass was achieved, it was not clear if there was actual prolongation of life. This brought up the concept of a possible local macrophage insufficiency in relation to tumor mass, as well as the problem of macrophage production and mobilization to the tumor site.

Dr. Russell's presentation generated a series of methodological as well as conceptual questions. What are the appropriate controls for the study of activated macrophages? Several participants indicated the possible activation by endemic chronic infections, thus increasing activity of "normal" macrophages. In the Moloney sarcoma virus (MSV) system, it is apparent that there is a correlation between macrophage content within the tumor and progressive growth (i.e. progressively growing tumors have less macrophages than tumors that will regress). Are there any differences between "progressor" versus "regressor" macrophages in this system? What are the effects of the virus proper on macrophage function and activation? How do these factors influence macrophage localization within the tumor? Due to tumor mass, the actual absolute numbers of macrophages per tumor are comparable in progressive and regressive tumors; however, clear differences appear when the results are expressed as macrophages per gram of tumor, the regressive tumors containing almost 10 times more macrophages. Another problem concerning functional study of macrophages obtained from tumors relates to "selection" by the fractionation procedures. Although no definitive answers to these questions were produced during the discussion, it became apparent that the awareness of the researchers of such problems represents a major force to clarify these issues.

SESSION V
Stimulation of Macrophage Function and Applied Therapy

Chairman: Ole A. Holtermann

INTRODUCTION

Ole A. Holtermann, Chairman

The speakers of this session will address themselves to the general theme of stimulation of the reticuloendothelial system (RES) and the possible application of such stimulation in the management of neoplastic disease. As the RES is being recognized to occupy a central position in host defense against neoplastic or potentially neoplastic cells, efforts to delineate the optimal conditions for stimulation and augmentation of the function of this system to the advantage of the host is becoming increasingly urgent. Several of the workshop participants have already touched upon this subject and in the opening session, Dr. DiLuzio presented a comprehensive list of agents that may act as stimulants of the RES. A number of these agents may have a direct activating effect on the RES, whereas others may act via the immune system or other mechanisms.

A representative of the agents that may act as a direct RES stimulant is the microbial polysaccharide glucan. This polysaccharide has the remarkable property of inducing an inflammatory infiltrate which is composed almost exclusively of histiocytes at the site of injection. A clinical investigation of the potential antitumor effect of local administration of this substance will be presented by Dr. Mansell.

One of the agents that has been most extensively investigated with regard to RES stimulation is BCG. The mode of action of this microorganism is undoubtedly complex and may comprise both direct and indirect effects on the RES as well as stimulation of specific antitumor immunity. Certain aspects of the mechanism by which macrophages are activated by BCG and the interaction of such activated macrophages with neoplastic cells will be discussed by Dr. Meltzer.

As compared to lymphocytes from tumor immune animals, macrophages exhibit a very high efficiency in their cytocidal effect on neoplastic cells. In isolated lymphocyte populations, macrophages may be present as a minor contaminant. The contribution of these contaminating macrophages to the cytotoxicity of such lymphocyte populations will be discussed by Dr. Fidler. Transfer of activated macrophages to tumor bearing hosts may increase their tumor resistance and Dr. Fidler will present experience with macrophage transfer in an animal tumor model system.

PERITONEAL MACROPHAGES FROM BCG-INFECTED MICE: TUMOR CYTOTOXICITY AND CHEMOTACTIC RESPONSES *IN VITRO*

Monte S. Meltzer[1], Mary M. Stevenson[2], Robert W. Tucker[3] and Edward J. Leonard[1]

The anti-tumor effects of infection with *Mycobacterium bovis*, strain BCG (BCG) have been well documented (1). BCG infection and host response to this infection can be exploited for successful immunoprophylaxis and immunotherapy of tumors. This has been demonstrated in many animal model systems and has been extended into clinical trials with human neoplasms. The optimal conditions and mechanisms of these anti-tumor effects are only partially known and have been targets of continued and intensive investigation in our laboratory (2) and by others. Sequelae of BCG infection are complex; the major locus of action for BCG in both immunoprophylaxis and immunotherapy of tumors, however reside in the mononuclear phagocyte system. BCG immunotherapy by intratumor injection of living organisms induces a sequence of immunologically specific and nonspecific events, each of which in turn amplifies multiple tumoricidal mechanisms. A simplified representation of this tumoricidal amplification system is shown in Figure 1. The cell type which dominates this reaction both histologically (3) and functionally is the BCG activated macrophage. Changes in macrophage function which can occur during BCG immunotherapy include: (a) increased adherence to culture substrates (4,5), (b) increased particle phagocytosis (5), (c) alterations of intracellular metabolism and metabolic events at the cell surface (5,6), (d) changes in gross cellular and ultrastructural morphology (4,5,7), (e) increased resistance to a variety of faculative or obligate intracellular pathogens (8), (f) increased responsiveness to chemotactic stimuli (9), and (g) ability to induce cytostatic (growth inhibition) and/or cytotoxic changes for tumor cells

[1] *Tumor Antigen Section, Biology Branch, National Cancer Institute.*
[2] *Guest Worker, Biology Branch, National Cancer Institute*
[3] *Cell Physiology and Oncogenesis Section, Laboratory of Biochemistry, National Cancer Institute.*

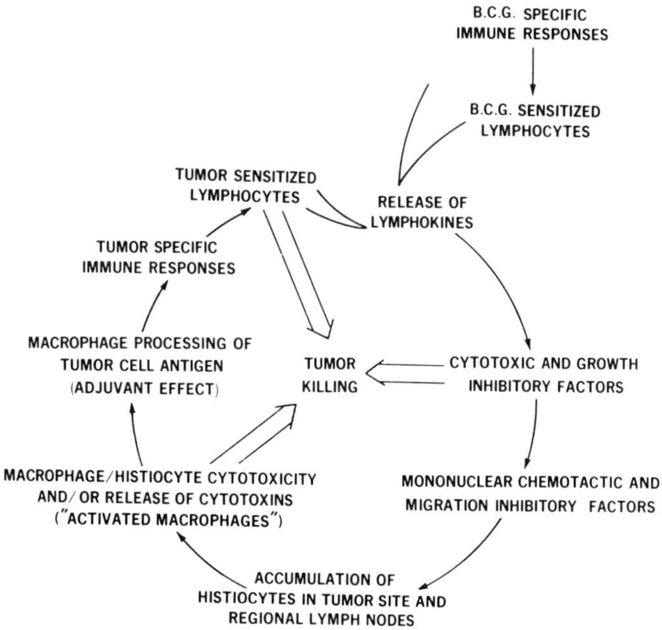

Fig. 1. *Tumoricidal mechanisms in BCG immunotherapy by intralesional injection.*

(10,11). Whether all of these changes occur simultaneously with macrophage "activation" or can occur independently is not known. There have been a number of reports which suggest a dissociation of macrophage induced tumor cytotoxicity with other criteria of macrophage activation (10-12). We have directed our efforts in defining two areas of macrophage function which are modified with BCG infection – macrophage mediated tumor cytotoxicity and macrophage response to chemotactic stimuli. Both of these macrophage functions play important roles in the anti-tumor effects of BCG and have thus far been closely correlated.

Intrapertoneal (ip) injection of BCG induces a chronic murine infection. Viable BCG organisms can be isolated from peritoneal macrophages 6 months after ip injection. Macrophages [phagocytic, substrate adherent mononuclear peritoneal cells (PC)] from BCG infected mice were cytotoxic to tumor cells *in vitro* (11,13). This cytotoxicity was simply and dramatically illustrated by macrophage induced plaques on tumor monolayers (Figure 2). Nonadherent PC from BCG infected mice, PC from uninfected (normal) mice, viable BCG organisms (10-fold the number of organisms recovered from BCG activated macrophages) or mixtures of normal PC and BCG organisms *in vitro* did not induce tumor monolayer plaques (11). While the mechanisms of this *in vitro* macrophage-tumor cell reaction remain to be defined, some features of this reaction are known: (a) Intimate macrophage-tumor cell contact was required, although actual phagocytosis of whole tumor cells was not observed

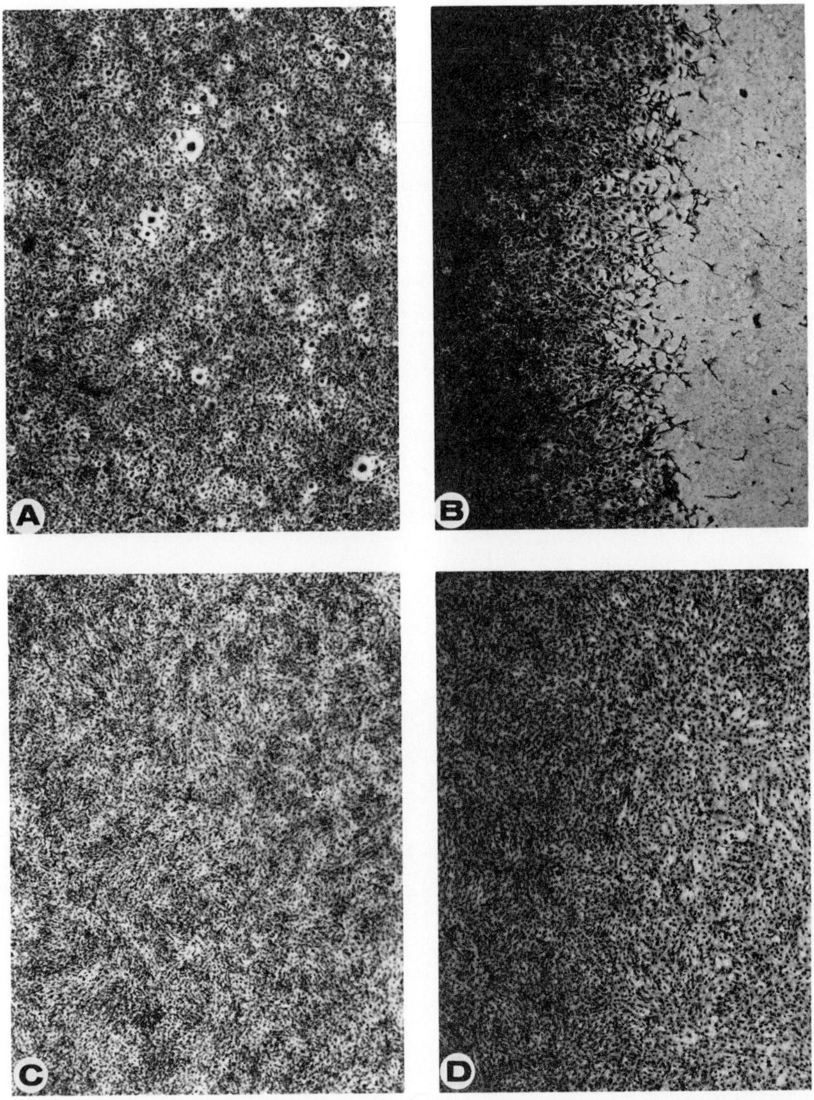

Fig. 2. *Normal and BCG activated macrophages on neoplastic and nonneoplastic cell monolayers.*

Neoplastic (tumor 7943) and the paired nonneoplastic (cell line 8407) cell monolayers were cultured with adherent PC from BCG infected or uninfected syngeneic mice for 60 hours. Cell cultures were washed and stained. These photographs represent the boundary between central macrophage-containing areas (right of photo) and peripheral macrophage-free areas (left of photo). (A) Normal macrophages on tumor 7943. (B) BCG activated macrophages on tumor 7943. Note complete absence of tumor cells in center of culture and sharp center/periphery boundary. (C) Normal macrophages on cell line 8407. (D) BCG activated macrophages on cell line 8407. Note that target cell density in center is less than that of periphery. Magnification 23 ×.

(10,11,14). Soluble cytotoxic factors released by macrophages or by macrophage-tumor cell interactions have not been described (10-12,15,16). (b) Tumor monolayer destruction occurred at relatively low macrophage/tumor cell ratios (1-5 macrophages/tumor cell) and was the net result of both cytostatic and cytotoxic effects (12,16,17). BCG activated macrophages were also affected, at least morphologically, by this intense reaction to become rounded and to detach from the culture substrate (11,18). (c) While this reaction was antigenically nonspecific, there was a spectrum of target cell susceptibility. With the same pool of BCG activated macrophages, tumor cells (viral- or chemical carcinogen-induced or spontaneous syngeneic and non-syngeneic tumors) were quantitatively more susceptible to macrophage cytopathic effects than were nonneoplastic cells (11,19). This lowered susceptibility of nonneoplastic cells to BCG activated macrophages occurred across xenogeneic histocompatibility barriers (11,20). Nonneoplastic cells were also more resistent to immunologically nonspecific lymphocyte and/or soluble mediator induced cytopathic mechanisms initiated by BCG infection (21).

While the macrophage induced plaque assay defined the basic system, quantitative analysis was difficult. This difficulty was bypassed as we developed a cytotoxic assay system using: (a) defined target cells: neoplastic and nonneoplastic cell line pairs. Each member of the cell line pair had common growth characteristics and was derived from a single cloned syngeneic embryo cell line (the cell pairs were kindly provided by Dr. K. K. Sanford, Cell Physiology and Oncogenesis Section, Laboratory of Biochemistry, National Cancer Institute, NIH) and (b) defined end point: release of ^{3}H-thymidine (^{3}H-TdR) from prelabeled target cells into supernatant culture fluids (16). BCG activated macrophages were cytotoxic to the neoplastic cell pair member (Figure 3). Significant release of ^{3}H-TdR could be detected by 24 hours and with macrophage/tumor cell ratios of 1:1 and less. Macrophages from uninfected mice released much less target cell label throughout the 3 day assay. The differential susceptibility of neoplastic and nonneoplastic target cells was documented and quantified in this cytotoxic system with two different syngeneic cell pairs (Figure 4). Furthermore, with a mixture of neoplastic and noneoplastic target cells among BCG activated macrophages, significant release of radiolabel was detected only from tumor cells. No "innocent bystander" killing of nonneoplastic cells during the BCG activated macrophage-tumor cell reaction was evident (Table 1.)

Using these defined neoplastic/nonneoplastic cell line pairs we examined macrophage-target cell interactions by time-lapse cinemicrographic analysis (18). BCG activated macrophage-tumor cell interaction was characterized by the following target cell changes: (a) Complete and permanent cytostasis was observed from the outset of filming (3-4 hours of culture) and continued throughout the 3 day assay. (b) Tumor cell movement progressively slowed

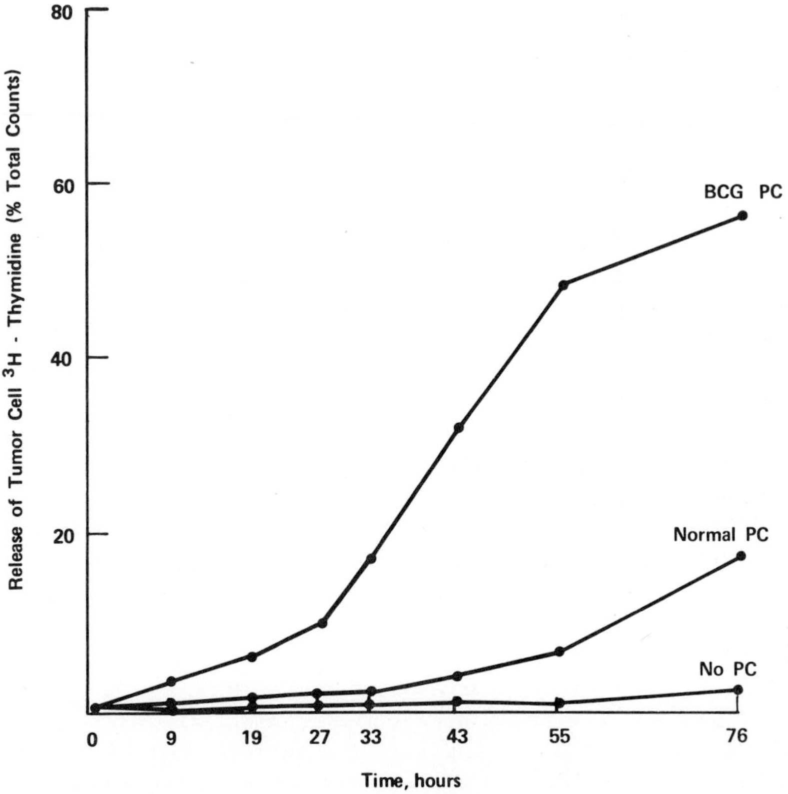

Fig. 3. *Tumor cytotoxicity of BCG activated macrophages.*

PC (2 × 10^5 macrophages) from BCG infected or control mice were added to prelabeled tumor 7943 monolayers (0.4 × 10^5 cells). After 3-4 hours of incubation, nonadherent PC were removed by washing. Culture supernatant fluids were assayed for release of ^{3}H-TdR at various times. Cytotoxicity was expressed as percent total counts. Each time point represents mean of triplicate cultures.

and by 24-32 hours degenerative morphological changes were evident (slowing of nuclear rotation, increased granularity of cytoplasm with vacuolization, decreased attachment to culture substrate, elongated and irregular cytoplasmic processes). (c) By 48 hours, no viable tumor cells were present in the microscopic field. (d) In areas of the culture without macrophages (periphery) tumor cells divided and grew to a confluent multilayer. Tumor cell cultures with normal macrophages showed continued cell division throughout the 3 day assay and cell morphology was identical to tumor cells in cultures without macrophages. The division of nonneoplastic target cells was also decreased among BCG activated macrophages, however, changes in cell morphology or cell death were not observed. The cytostatic effect of BCG activated

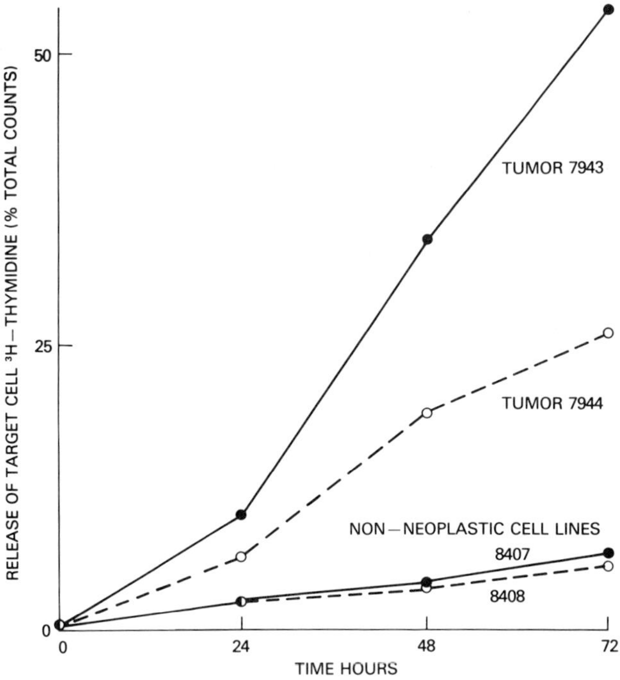

Fig. 4. *Cytotoxicity of BCG activated macrophages: neoplastic and nonneoplastic paired cell lines.*

Tumor 7943 and the paired nonneoplastic cell line 8407 as well as tumor 7944 and the paired nonneoplastic cell line 8408 were all derived from a single cloned cyngeneic embryo cell line. PC (2 × 10^5 macrophages) from BCG infected mice were added to cultures of prelabeled neoplastic and nonneoplastic cell monolayers (0.4 × 10^5 cells). After 3-4 hours of incubation, nonadherent PC were removed by washing. Culture supernatant fluids were assayed for release of ^{3}H-TdR at 24, 48, and 72 hours. Cytotoxicity was expressed as percent total counts. Each point represents mean of triplicate cultures.

macrophages on nonneoplastic cells was transient. By 42 hours of culture, target cell division was again observed and by 72 hours, the monolayer of nonneoplastic target cells was confluent, although at a lower density than the monolayer in the macrophage-free periphery (Figure 2.) This macrophage induced cytostasis was not observed in cultures of nonneoplastic cells with normal macrophages.

The responses of effector macrophages to neoplastic and nonneoplastic cell lines were as dramatic as the changes observed in the target cells. Movement of BCG activated macrophages around, over, and under tumor cells was an early and conspicuous feature. Macrophage-tumor cell interactions were characterized by repeated and relatively short (about 2 hours) periods of

TABLE 1.
BCG activated macrophage cytotoxicity: mixed neoplastic and nonneoplastic target cells

	Adherent PC From: No PC	Control PC 1.2×10^6	BCG PC 0.3×10^6
Target Cells	Percent Release Target Cell ^{3}H-TdR (72 hr)		
^{3}H-Neoplastic cells with:			
Neoplastic cells	9	15	71
Nonneoplastic cells	9	21	66
^{3}H-Nonneoplastic cells with:			
Neoplastic cells	7	13	25
Nonneoplastic cells	11	23	25

PC from BCG infected mice and from control mice were added to culture wells. After 3-4 hours of incubation, nonadherent PC were removed by washing. Mixtures of neoplastic (tumor 7943) and nonneoplastic (cell line 8407) cells were added to macrophage monolayers (2×10^4 ^{3}H-TdR labeled cells plus an equal number of unlabeled cells). Culture supernatant fluids were assayed for release of ^{3}H-TdR at 72 hours. Cytotoxicity was expressed as percent total counts. Each point represents mean of triplicate cultures.

contact. A single macrophage would help from a cluster around a tumor cell, remain attached for a short time, then move to another tumor cell. The departing macrophage was quickly replaced by other macrophages so that while continuous macrophage-tumor cell contact was maintained, there was constant turnover of the individual macrophages involved. The interaction of BCG activated macrophages with the nonneoplastic cell line or normal macrophages with either cell line was qualitatively similar at this level of analysis. The important difference in the BCG activated macrophage-tumor cell interaction was frequency. The translational movement of BCG activated macrophages among tumor cells was 4-5 fold greater than their movement among nonneoplastic cells or the movement of normal macrophages among tumor cells (Figure 5). This increased BCG activated macrophage movement combined with complete cytostasis of tumor cells (not seen with normal macrophages) could markedly increase the potential number of macrophage-tumor cell contacts. BCG activated macrophage movement among tumor cells was maximal at 28-32 hours and then decreased. The decrease in macrophage movement paralleled the decreased number of tumor cells, so that by 46 hours, when no viable tumor cells were present, macrophage movement was identical to that observed in BCG activated macrophage cultures without target cells.

Cinemicrographic observations of BCG activated macrophages among tumor cells suggested that activated macrophages were more responsive (at least *in vitro*) to the presence of neoplastic cells than were normal macro-

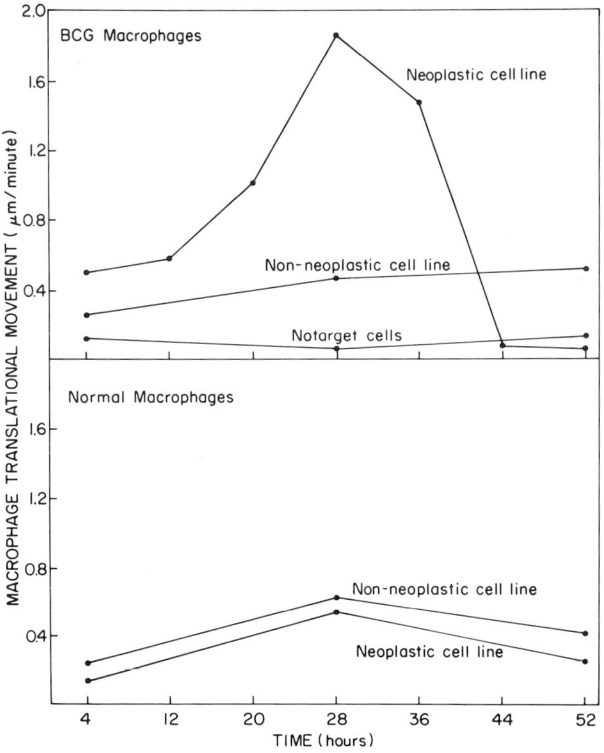

Fig. 5. *Macrophage translational movement among neoplastic and nonneoplastic cell monolayers.*

Cultures of peritoneal macrophages from BCG infected and normal mice with neoplastic and nonneoplastic cell monolayers were filmed by time-lapse cinemicroscopy. Translational cell movement was determined by mapping locations of macrophages and measuring the distance traveled by each macrophage over a 10 minute interval (10 frames). At least 15-20 macrophages were followed for 6 consecutive 10 minute intervals to obtain average translational movement/hour. Standard errors of mean translational movement/hour (90-120 measurements) were less than 5% of the mean. Measurements were converted to microns/minute by comparison with a stage micrometer filmed at the same magnification.

phages. This increased responsiveness was reflected in the markedly increased macrophage movement in tumor cultures. We analyzed and quantitated macrophage movement by measuring the chemotactic responses of peritoneal macrophages (4×10^5 macrophages/chemotactic chamber) to lymphocyte-derived (72 hour supernatant fluids from mitogen-stimulated spleen cell cultures, LDCF) and complement-derived (mouse serum incubated with bacterial endotoxins, EAMS) stimuli (22). The *in vitro* chemotactic response of tumoricidal BCG activated macrophages was greater than the response of macrophages from uninfected mice in terms of rate, magnitude and sensitivity (Figure 6). Macrophage cytotoxicity and chemotactic response were closely correlated when measured at varying times after BCG ip infection (Figure 7). Both of these macrophage functions were increased by 10 days after BCG infection and remained increased through 6 weeks. Mice injected with other agents which induced tumoricidal macrophages were also more responsive to chemotactic stimuli than were macrophages from untreated mice (9). Peritoneal macrophages from exudates induced by irritants (mineral oil or fluid thioglycollate) were not cytotoxic to tumor cells and were not more responsive to chemotactic stimuli (Table 2). Thus among the agents tested, those which induced tumoricidal capacity also increased chemotactic responsiveness.

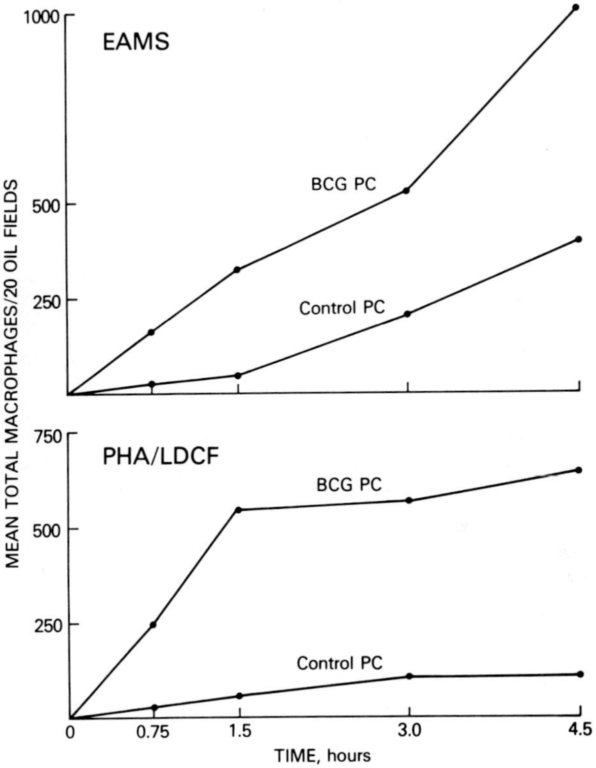

Fig. 6. *Chemotactic responses of macrophages from BCG infected and uninfected mice.*

PC from BCG ip infected and normal mice were collected 7 days after ip injection. Chemotactic responses of peritoneal macrophages were assayed to dilutions of LDCF or EAMS. Each point represents mean of triplicate filters.

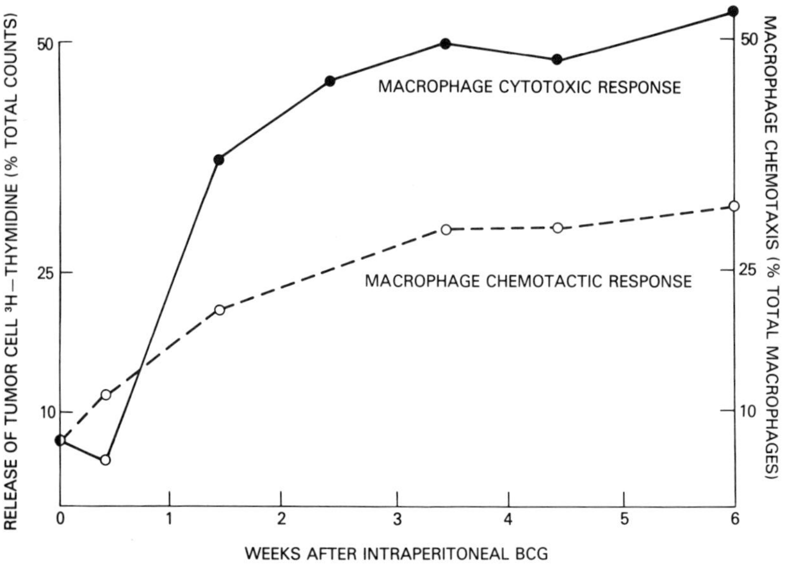

Fig. 7. *Chemotactic and cytotoxic responses of BCG activated macrophages at various times after BCG ip injection.*

Mice were injected ip with BCG. PC from BCG infected mice were collected at various times after ip injection. Chemotactic responses of peritoneal macrophages were assayed to dilutions of LDCF after 3 hours of incubation. Chemotactic response was expressed as percent migration (mean migrated macrophages per 20 oil fields extrapolated to total filter area/total macrophages added to chamber for triplicate filters). Cytotoxic response (percent total counts) was assayed by measuring the ^{3}H-TdR released from prelabeled tumor 7943 cells into culture fluids by adherent PC from BCG infected mice. Each point represents mean of triplicate cultures.

The chemotactic response of macrophages from normal mice was 5-10% of the total macrophages added to the chemotactic chamber over the 3 hour assay. This percentage was remarkably consistent from experiment to experiment and was independent of the total number of macrophages added (in the range of 1-10 $\times$ 10^5 macrophages/chamber). With BCG infection, the percentage of responsive macrophages was 20-50% dependent upon the time of PC harvest after infection. One explanation for these percentages would be that chemotactic responsiveness is an index for measuring a subpopulation of activated macrophages. Normal mice thus have a small activated macrophage subpopulation which could increase with infection, such as BCG, and/or specific and nonspecific immune stimulation. These activated macrophages may account for the increased tumor resistance in animals treated with macrophage activation agents; a deficiency in this macrophage subpopulation could contribute to or be associated with overt neoplastic disease. Recently reported defects of mononuclear cell chemotaxis in cancer patients would be

TABLE 2.
Macrophages from mice treated with macrophage activation agents or peritoneal irritants: chemotaxis and tumor cytotoxicity.

PC from mice injected with:	Chemotactic response (macrophages/ 20 oil fields ± SEM in response to:)		Cytotoxic Response (72 hour release of tumor cell ^{3}H-TdR: percent total counts)
	Diluent	LDCF	
No treatment	2 ± 2	83 ± 4	14
BCG ip	64 ± 4	486 ± 12	47
LPS ip	43 ± 1	411 ± 15	36
Mineral oil ip	3 ± 1	65 ± 1	8
Thioglycollate ip	0 ± 0	23 ± 3	13

Mice were injected with BCG, E coli lipopolysaccharide (LPS), mineral oil or fluid thioglycollate medium ip. PC were collected 7 days after ip injection. Chemotactic responses of peritoneal macrophages were assayed after 3 hours of incubation. Cytotoxic responses were assayed by measuring the ^{3}H-TdR released from prelabeled tumor 7943 cells into culture supernatant fluids by adherent PC from treated mice.

consistent with this model (23). We have extended this clinical observation into the mouse model system. Peritoneal macrophages from mice with subcutaneous syngeneic fibrosarcomas have depressed responsiveness to both lymphocyte and complement-derived chemotactic stimuli (Figure 8.) Mice treated with tissue culture medium, fetal calf serum, syngeneic spleen cells or incomplete Freund's adjuvant did not have depressed macrophage chemotactic responsiveness *in vitro* (24). The tumor-induced defect in macrophage chemotaxis occurred before the tumor became palpable and persisted until the death of the animal. The depression of chemotactic responsiveness to both stimuli remained fairly constant (about 50% of the normal response) after the first week despite increasing tumor size, increasing duration of tumor and decreasing recovery of peritoneal macrophages. This constant depression again suggests that the defect may be associated with changes in a reactive subpopulation of macrophages.

Stimulation of mononuclear phagocyte function by infection with BCG in normal mice was also evident in tumor bearing mice. Peritoneal macrophages from BCG infected normal and tumor bearing mice were cytotoxic to tumor cells *in vitro* and were more responsive to chemotactic stimuli than were macrophages from uninfected mice. Furthermore, BCG activated macrophages from normal and tumor bearing mice had comparable tumoricidal and chemotactic responses even though the chemotactic responses of uninfected tumor bearing mice were markedly depressed both *in vivo* (PC/mouse in response to BCG ip) and *in vitro*. (Table 3) BCG infection would thus appear to restore and/or bypass the depression of mononuclear phagocyte function associated with neoplastic disease.

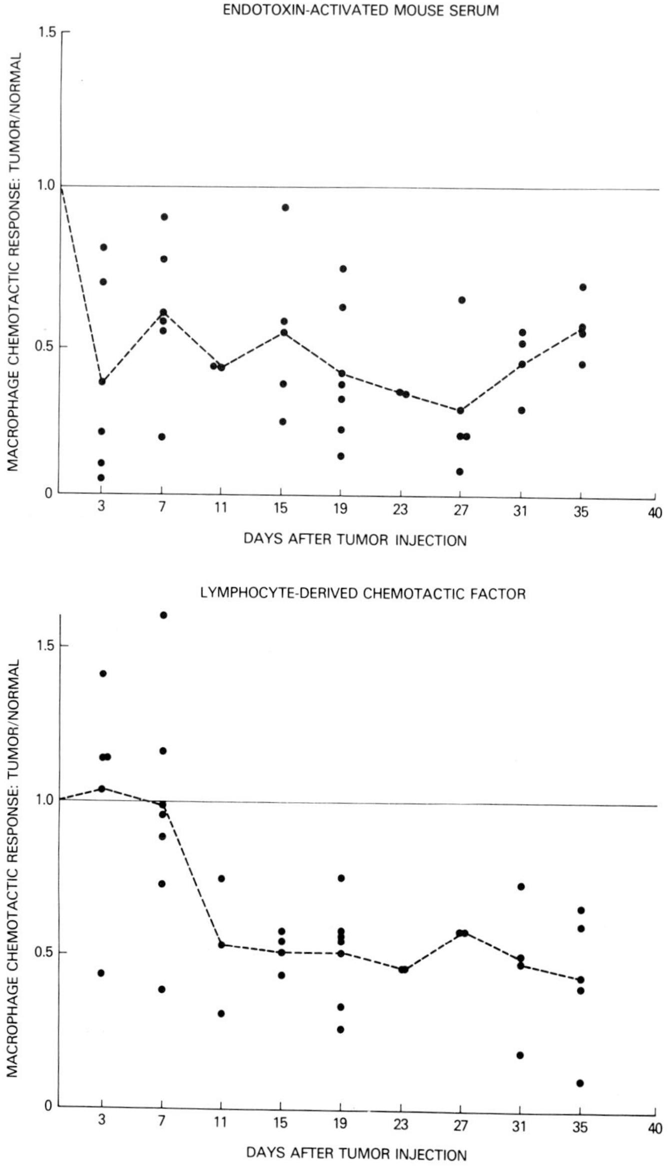

Fig. 8. *Chemotactic response of peritoneal macrophages from tumor bearing and normal mice.*

Mice were innoculated with 1.0 × 10^6 tumor 1038 cells into the right rear footpad. At various times after tumor injection, PC were collected from groups of 6-10 mice. Chemotactic responses of pooled peritoneal macrophages to dilutions of LDCF or to dilutions of EAMS were assayed after 3 hours of incubation. Macrophage chemotaxis was expressed as percent of normal response. Normal response was defined as 1.0 for each experiment. Each point represents mean of triplicate filters. Mean chemotactic responses at each time after tumor injection are connected by the dotted line.

TABLE 3.
Chemotactic and cytotoxic responses of macrophages from BCG infected normal and tumor bearing mice.

PC from mice with:	Footpad size(mm)	PC/mouse × 10^{-6}		Macrophage chemotaxis	Tumor cytotoxicity	
		total	macrophage		tumor 1038	tumor 1023
					percent total counts	
NO TUMOR						
No treatment	2.1	4.6	2.3	650 ± 60 (16)	24	12
BCG ip	2.1	18.6	6.9	910 ± 60 (23)	48	22
2 WEEK TUMOR						
No treatment	4.6	3.9	1.7	200 ± 60 (5)	26	12
BCG ip	3.3	17.3	9.0	1220 ± 60 (30)	49	23
4 WEEK TUMOR						
No treatment	9.0	4.0	1.6	170 ± 10 (4)	20	11
BCG ip	9.4	6.6	3.5	1660 ± 140 (41)	55	26
6 WEEK TUMOR						
No treatment	12.5	5.5	3.0	140 ± 10 (4)	18	10
BCG ip	13.0	5.4	2.7	960 ± 130 (24)	40	20

Normal mice and mice innoculated with 1.0×10^6 tumor 1038 cells into the footpad were injected ip with BCG. PC were collected 10 days after ip injection. Chemotactic responses to dilutions of LDCF were measured after 3.5 hours of incubation. Chemotactic responses were expressed as mean total macrophages/ 20 oil fields ± SEM for triplicate filters and as percent of total macrophages given in parenthesis (migrated macrophages/total macrophages added). Cytotoxic responses were assayed by measuring the ^{3}H-TdR released from prelabeled tumor 1038 cells and antigenically different tumor 1023 cells into the culture supernatant fluids by adherent PC at 48 hours of incubation. Each point represents mean of triplicate cultures.

REFERENCES

1. Bast, R. C., B. Zbar, T. Borsos and H. J. Rapp (1974). BCG and cancer. *N. Engl. J. Med. 290*:1413-1420, 1458-1469.

2. Rapp, H. J. (1973). A guinea pig model for tumor immunology: A summary. *Israel J. Med. Sci. 9*:366-374.

3. Hanna, M. G., Jr., M. J. Snodgrass, B. Zbar and H. J. Rapp (1973). Histologic and ultrastructural studies of tumor regression in inbred guinea pigs after intralesional injection of *Mycobacterium bovis* (BCG). *Natl. Cancer Inst. Monogr. 39*:71-84.

4. Mooney, J. J. and B. J. Waksman (1970). Activation of normal rabbit macrophage monolayers by supernatants of antigen-stimulated lymphocytes. *J. Immunol. 105*:1138-1145.

5. Nathan, C. F., M. L. Karnovsky and J. R. David (1971). Alterations of macrophage functions by mediators from lymphocytes. *J. Exp. Med. 133*:1356-1376.

6. Remold-O'Donnell, E. and H. G. Remold (1974). The enhancement of macrophage adenylate cyclase by products of activated lymphocytes. *J. Biol. Chem. 249*:3622-3627.

7. Dvorak, A. M., M. E. Hammond, H. F. Dvorak and M. J. Karnovsky (1972). Loss of cell surface material from peritoneal exudate cells associated with lymphocyte-mediated inhibition of macrophage migration from capillary tubes. *Lab. Invest. 27*:561-574.

8. Krahenbuhl, J. L. and J. S. Remington (1971). *In vitro* induction of nonspecific resistance in macrophages by specifically sensitized lymphocytes. *Infect. Immun. 4*:337-343.

9. Meltzer, M. S., E. E. Jones and D. A. Boetcher (1975). Increased chemotactic responses of macrophages from BCG-infected mice. *Cell. Immunol. 17*:268-276.

10. Hibbs, J. B., Jr., L. H. Lambert, Jr. and J. S. Remington (1972). Possible role of macrophage mediated non-specific cytotoxicity in tumour resistance. *Nature New Biol. 235*:48-50.

11. Cleveland, R. P., M. S. Meltzer and B. Zbar (1974). Tumor cytotoxicity *in vitro* by macrophages from mice infected with *Mycobacterium bovis* strain BCG. *J. Natl. Cancer Inst. 52*:1887-1895.

12. Keller, R. (1973). Cytostatic elimination of syngeneic rat tumor cells *in vitro* by non-specifically activated macrophages. *J. Exp. Med. 138*:625-644.

13. Hibbs, J. B., Jr. (1973). Macrophage nonimmunologic recognition: target cell factors related to contact inhibition. *Science 180*:868-870.

14. Evans, R. and P. Alexander (1970). Cooperation of immune lymphoid cells with macrophages in tumor immunity. *Nature (Lond.) 228*:620-622.

15. Hibbs, J. B., Jr. (1974). Heterocytolysis by macrophages activated by bacillus Calmette-Guérin:lysome exocytosis into tumor cells. *Science 184*:468-471.

16. Meltzer, M. S., R. W. Tucker, K. K. Sanford and E. J. Leonard (1975). Interaction of BCG-activated macrophages with neoplastic and nonneoplastic cell lines *in vitro*: quantitation of the cytotoxic reaction by release of tritiated thymidine from prelabeled target cells. *J. Natl. Cancer Inst. 54*:1177-1184.

17. Grant, C. K., G. D. Currier and P. Alexander (1972). Thymocytes from mice immunized against an allograft render bone marrow cells specifically cytotoxic. *J. Exp. Med. 135*:150-164.

18. Meltzer, M. S., R. W. Tucker and A. C. Breuer (1975). Interaction of BCG-activated macrophages with neoplastic and nonneoplastic cell lines *in vitro*: cinemicrographic analysis. *Cell. Immunol. 17*:30-42.

19. Hibbs, J. B., Jr., L. H. Lambert, Jr. and J. S. Remington (1972). *In vitro* nonimmunologic destruction of cells with abnormal growth characteristics by adjuvant activated macrophages. *Proc. Soc. Exp. Biol. Med. 139*:1049-1052.

20. Holtermann, O. A., E. Klein and G. P. Casale (1973). Selective cytotoxicity of peritoneal leukocytes for neoplastic cells. *Cell. Immunol. 9*:339-352.

21. Meltzer, M. S. and G. L. Bartlett (1972). Cytotoxicity *in vitro* by products of specifically stimulated spleen cells: susceptibility of tumor cells and normal cells. *J. Natl. Cancer Inst. 49*:1439-1443.

22. Boetcher, D. A. and M. S. Meltzer (1975). Mouse mononuclear cell chemotaxis: description of system. *J. Natl. Cancer Inst. 54*:795-799.

23. Boetcher, D. A. and E. J. Leonard (1974). Abnormal monocyte chemotactic response in cancer patients. *J. Natl. Cancer Inst. 52*:1091-1099.

24. Stevenson, M. M. and M. S. Meltzer. Depressed macrophage chemotaxis in tumor bearing mice. *J. Natl. Cancer Inst.*, submitted.

THE *IN VIVO* DESTRUCTION OF HUMAN TUMOR BY GLUCAN ACTIVATED MACROPHAGES

Peter W. A. Mansell, M. D., F.R.C.S.

Division of Oncology
Royal Victoria Hospital and
McGill University Cancer Research
Unit, Montreal

Nicholas R. Di Luzio, Ph.D.

Department of Physiology
Tulane University Medical School
New Orleans, La. 70112

INTRODUCTION

Until recently the role of the macrophage in the host's reaction to tumor was not well recognized, partly because of the undue emphasis put upon the lymphocyte as the effector cell and partly because of the difficulty of studying the macrophage as an isolated cell. Morphologically the macrophage was described almost a hundred years ago (1) but it is not until the last few years that the cell has received recognition as an antigen processing, phagocytic and tumoricidal cell in its own right (2-10). It has also been shown that defective macrophage function occurs in immunological deficiency induced by malnutrition (11), infections (12), and malignant conditions (13).

Macrophages as part of the reticuloendothelial system (RES) can only function effectively in the presence of a factor occurring in normal human plasma which has been called humoral recognition factor (HRF) (14,15,16). This factor, an α 2-macroglobulin (15,16), is markedly decreased in the plasma in a number of conditions – following major surgery (17) and burns (18) and in malignant disease (19,20,21). Recent studies using the sequential measurement of HRF levels in patients with cancer have shown that there is a relationship between the stage of the disease and the level of HRF in the plasma (22). More strikingly it has been shown that treatment of the patient with curative measures such as radical surgery or radiation is followed by a restoration of the HRF levels towards normal (19) and recently the use of the RES stimulant BCG was shown to be followed by a similar rise (22,23).

Extensive animal studies have shown agreement with the situation in man (24) but have also clarified the action of HRF to some extent. The factor has been shown not only to promote phagocytosis but to be chemotactic (25). Using the Shay chloroleukaemia rat tumor as a model it has been shown possible to inhibit tumor growth and the production of metastases by treatment with HRF (24,25).

One of the most potent RES stimulators is the substance Glucan, a β 1-3 glycosidic polysaccharide prepared from the inner part of the outer membrane of the yeast *Saccharomyces cerevisiae,* the molecular structure of which is graphically presented below (26-34): When this substance is given to

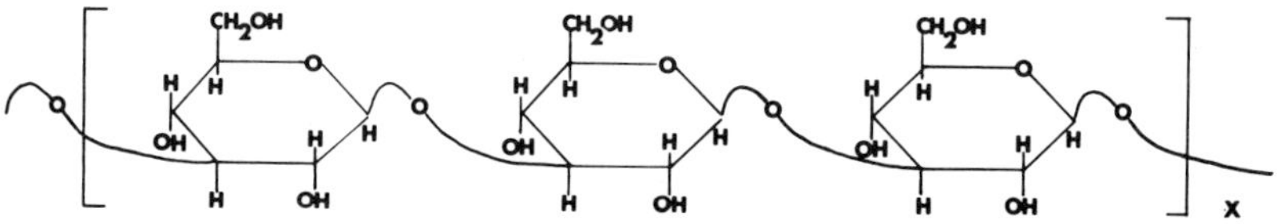

GLUCAN

experimental animals it is possible to prevent the growth of a primary tumor by pretreatment, simultaneous treatment at the time of tumor implant and post treatment. It is also possible to prevent the occurrence of and to cure metastases. It can be shown that the animal initially given tumor and Glucan simultaneously is protected against subsequent challenge with tumor (24). These findings were originally made in the rat Shay chloroleukaemia model but have recently been confirmed in two other models, the mouse B16 melanoma and an adenocarcinoma model (24,35).

As a result of these findings a small clinical pilot study was undertaken to test the efficacy of administering HRF alone, HRF plus Glucan and Glucan alone in a controlled situation to patients with a variety of malignant diseases in order to enhance the activation of macrophages and their recognition of tumor cells. These initial attempts were markedly successful in that they showed that Glucan was a potent agent capable of activating and mobilizing macrophages within a tumor and that a tumor thus treated showed necrosis within a short length of time which appeared to be mediated by macrophages (23,35). Marked rises in the patient's plasma level of HRF were recorded during this event.

This report expands the previous clinical experience while the experimental data are presented elsewhere (24).

MATERIALS AND METHODS

Patients

The patients in this present study were those being treated at the Division of Oncology, Royal Victoria Hospital, Montreal. They all had advanced malignant disease with easily accessible subcutaneous nodules. They consisted of seven patients, three with malignant melanoma and four with carcinoma of the breast.

Evaluation

All patients had biopsy proven malignant disease and were followed at weekly intervals in the out-patient clinic. In four of the patients biopsy of the injected lesions was possible; in one post-mortem; in the other cases this was not possible. Lesions were injected directly with Glucan in amounts adjusted to the size of the lesion, it having been previously shown that the effect is to some extent dose dependent. Control injections of dextrose saline were used in other lesions.

Minimal reactions were observed at the site of injection. Mild discomfort occurred lasting up to 96 hours. No systemic side effects were observed. In one case a very large breast lesion which had been injected six months earlier developed a tense fluid filled cyst which was aspirated on several occasions with the production of blood stained fluid containing large numbers of macrophages.

Preparation of Glucan

Glucan was prepared as described (26,30) originally in a lipid emulsion base (23,37) but recently it has been possible to produce a more highly soluble form for injection at a concentration of up to 100mgm. / ml in dextrose saline (38). This enables the Glucan to be injected at a higher concentration and since the particle size is much smaller, less than 1μ, it is much easier to inject. No untoward reactions have been noticed using this preparation. It has not been possible as yet to make a preparation that is injectable intravenously in man.

RESULTS

Clinical

The clinical results remain essentially the same as those reported earlier (22,23,39). In all cases, except one, a striking clinical regression of the tumor was seen. This one case was that of a 58 year old patient with widely recurrent skin nodules from cancer of the breast. The nodules covered the whole chest wall and invaded the skin of the neck. Many different types of treatment had been tried in this case, all without success. The nodules were very slow growing and fibrotic in character. It was never possible to inject these lesions successfully and the attempt was painful; injections were made under the lesions, however, and in 48 hours a typical inflammatory type of reaction was seen which subsided after about five days. This patient would not permit a biopsy and there was no clinical evidence of tumor regression.

In all other cases the usual course of events was as follows: Injections were made into, and around, the tumor nodules, varying the amount of injectate to suit the amount of tumor present since it has been shown that the response is dose dependent (23). On no occasion, with the exception of the slight pain associated with any percutaneous injection, did the patients complain of any discomfort at the time of injection. In no case were any constitutional symptoms seen. Within 48 hours in all cases an easily recognized erethematous reaction occurred with some edema which gradually subsided by the fifth day. In all cases a fluctuant swelling became apparent during this time with a greater or lesser amount of residual nodule adjacent to it. In the series already reported it was noted that the very small lesions simply disappeared in a small pocket of exudate containing large numbers of macrophages (23). This was not seen on this occasion, probably because the lesions treated were on the whole larger. However, the results of this series are in agreement with those of the former.

One case, a man of 31 with widespread malignant melanoma, had several subcutaneous nodules injected and, although he died of widespread disease shortly after the injections, it was possible to observe the clinical course of the treatment and to obtain biopsy material. Another patient with stage four melanoma had two subcutaneous nodules, one of which was injected with Glucan and the other with dextrose saline as a control. The injected lesion underwent the changes described and was biopsied. No change was seen in the control lesion.

A third patient, a 47 year old woman with cancer of the breast, had had a variety of treatments before coming to us with a large 6 cm. diameter residual tumor in the lower inner quadrant of the right breast. At the time of that initial examination there was no evidence of distant disease. An injection of 400 mgm. of Glucan in lipid emulsion was made and ten days later what appeared to be a breast abcess burst in the patient's home. This was treated by her own doctor symptomatically and found to be sterile. Six months later she returned with a tense, sore swelling in the breast at the site of injection. This was aspirated and 120 ml. of blood stained fluid were removed. A smear performed on this fluid showed that it contained large numbers of dead tumor cells and, apart from many red blood cells, a large number of macrophages. During the ensuing two months repeated aspirations were performed with much the same result. Finally a simple mastectomy was done, there still being no evidence of distant disease. At operation a large blood filled cyst was found surrounded by necrotic and viable tumor tissue. The patient continues to do well.

Histological

All the biopsies reviewed have shown to a greater or lesser extent evidence of tumor necrosis and infiltration by macrophages. The macrophages have a distinctive character enabling them to be easily distinguished (Figures

1-3) since their cytoplasm is vacuolated and has a foamy appearance. These macrophages appear not only within the tumor itself but, most strikingly, along the "battlefront" between viable and non-viable tumor (Figures 1-3).

Electron micrographs of the breast tumor showed large macrophages containing several particles of Glucan (Figures 5,7). Some of these particles contain the characteristic electron dense centre (Figures 8,9) which may represent a minute amount of protein or other nitrogen containing substance left within the Glucan particle at the time of preparation.

The amount of frank necrosis varies from specimen to specimen. In some cases there is coagulative necrosis (Figures 1,5), while in other areas there is the appearance of apoptosis (40) (Figures 4,7). Particularly in the breast case the necrotic tissue contains macrophages as well as dead tumor cells in close apposition to apparently healthy tumor (Figures 5,7). The appearance of macrophages in the two melanoma specimens is more obvious (Figures 1-4,6) since in many cases they contain melanin and the biopsies were taken early, 48 hours (Figure 6) and 96 hours (Figures 1-4); whereas the breast biopsy was

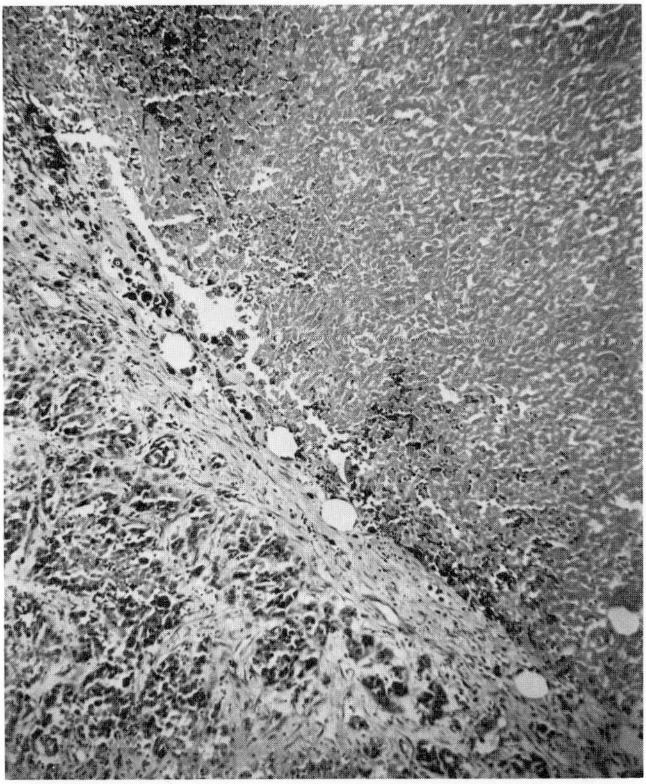

Fig. 1. *Melanoma showing the border between the viable tumor, lower left, and the necrotic area with an interface of macrophages and dead cells. H and E ×80.*

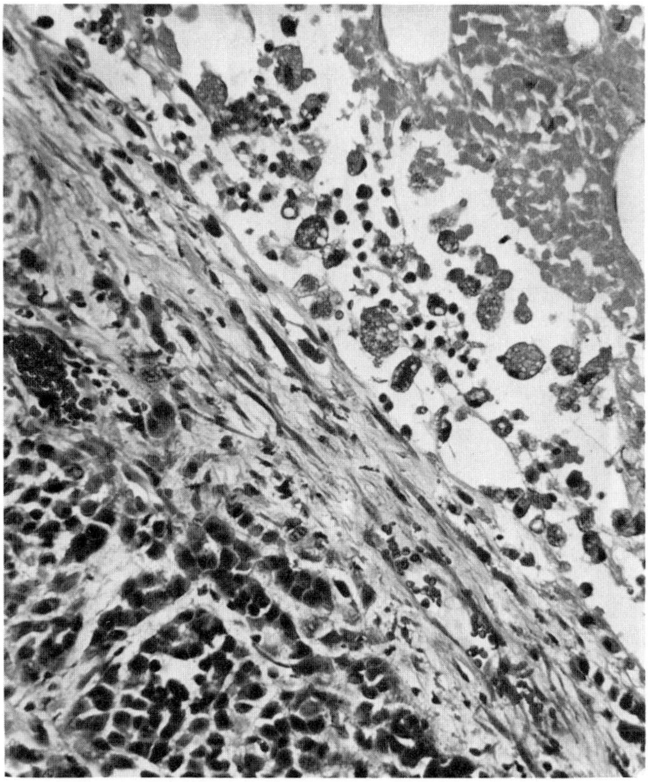

Fig. 2. *Higher power view of Figure 1. H and E ×200.*

obtained eight months after the first Glucan injection and the only remaining evidence of its action is the strikingly large areas of necrosis within the tumor. No free Glucan particles were seen in this specimen whereas they are clearly visible in the melanoma cases (Figure 6).

In summary, the histological appearance of a Glucan injected nodule depends to some extent upon the amount of Glucan injected and the length of time between the injection and the biopsy. In general, however, the appearance is one of mobilization and activation of macrophages. The macrophages assume a characteristic appearance as a result of the ingestion of Glucan particles and appear at the leading edge of the area of necrosis as well as actually invading the tumor tissue. Other cells, such as polymorphonuclear leucocytes and plasma cells, are often seen as well (Figure 7) and in many instances actual cell to cell contact can be seen between macrophages and tumor cells (Figure 6). The precise mechanism of macrophage mediated tumor

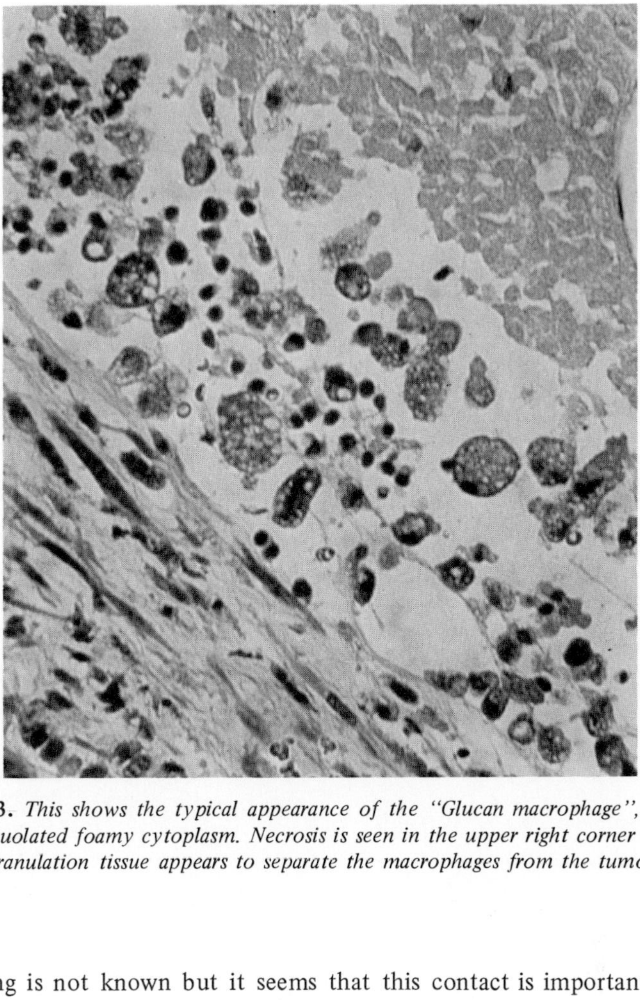

Fig. 3. *This shows the typical appearance of the "Glucan macrophage", a large cell with a vacuolated foamy cytoplasm. Necrosis is seen in the upper right corner and a band of early granulation tissue appears to separate the macrophages from the tumor. H and E ×320.*

cell killing is not known but it seems that this contact is important (41) and that it can be achieved by very small numbers of macrophages relative to the numbers of tumor cells (42), thus showing a distinct advantage for the macrophage over the lymphocyte in this respect.

DISCUSSION

The results of this small series, taken in conjunction with those previously reported (23) and another series still being performed (43), clearly show that Glucan is a potent macrophage activator *in vivo* in man and that when used intralesionally can induce the destruction of the injected tumor, with little, if any, side effects. The striking feature of the tumor destruction is that it

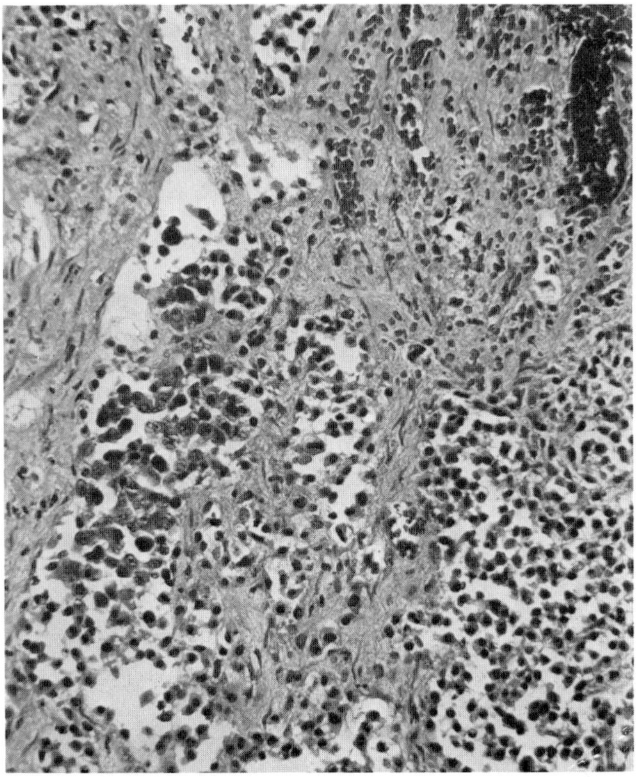

Fig. 4. *A small pocket of melanoma tissue is seen surrounded and infiltrated by macrophages. The cells in the lower right area present the typical appearance of apoptosis. H and E ×200.*

appears to be carried out by means of an enormously increased population of activated macrophages of distinctive histological appearance.

It is well known that the metastatic potential of a tumor is governed, to some extent, by the number of resident macrophages (44). It is of great interest that recent studies in this laboratory have shown that the antitumor response, in terms of circulating antibody directed against specific membrane antigen, can be predicted by assessing the number of macrophages seen within a tumor, particularly in the case of melanoma (45). Thus, a tumor having a high resident population is likely to occur in a patient with well developed immunity whereas the reverse is true. The question as to whether the macrophage response seen in the Glucan treated tumor represents recruitment and activation of an already resident macrophage population or the induction

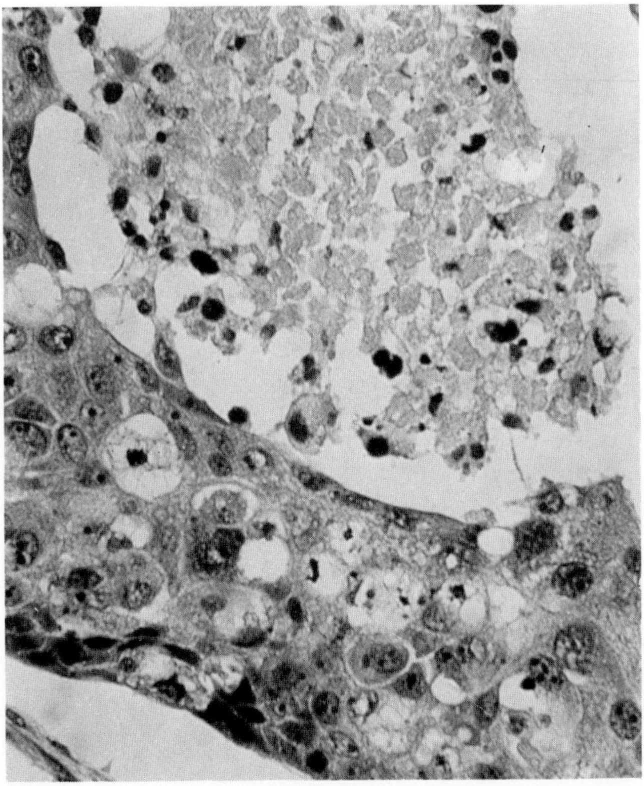

Fig. 5. *Breast cancer showing the tumor and a pocket of necrotic tissue with macrophages with typically foamy cytoplasm. H and E ×320.*

of an entirely new population remains to be solved. It is known that HRF is an efficient chemotactic agent and since the use of Glucan is followed by a rise in the plasma level of HRF it seems likely that both these possibilities are true to a varying extent within each individual.

The problem at the present time is that this effect is simply because the route of administration is a purely local one; although there is very preliminary evidence to suggest that a systemic effect can be seen when large "depot" injections are made in individuals whose tumor is not easily accessible (23). There is no doubt that the most potent effects of Glucan in the experimental animal (24) are seen, as BCG and *C parvum*, both RES stimulants, when the agent is given intravenously (47).

With the increasing interest in the macrophage content of tumors as an index of host resistance (41,45,47,48) and the alterations in monocyte

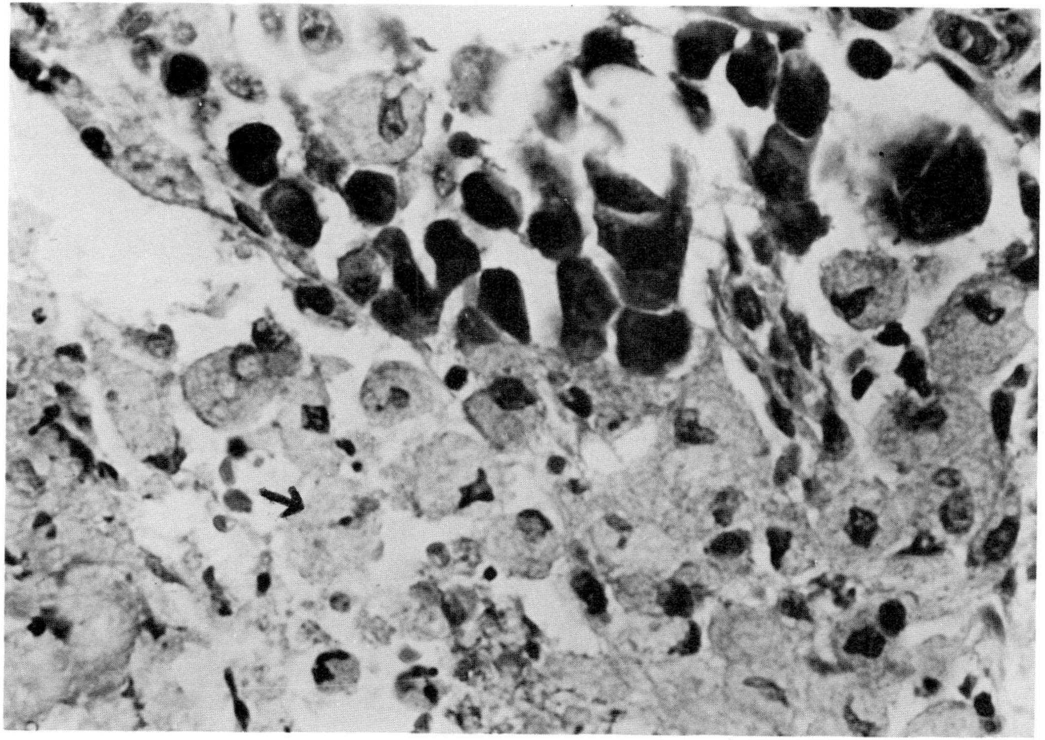

Fig. 6. *Melanoma. The macrophages can be seen in close apposition with the tumor cells. A fragment of Glucan is arrowed. H and E* $\times 1000$.

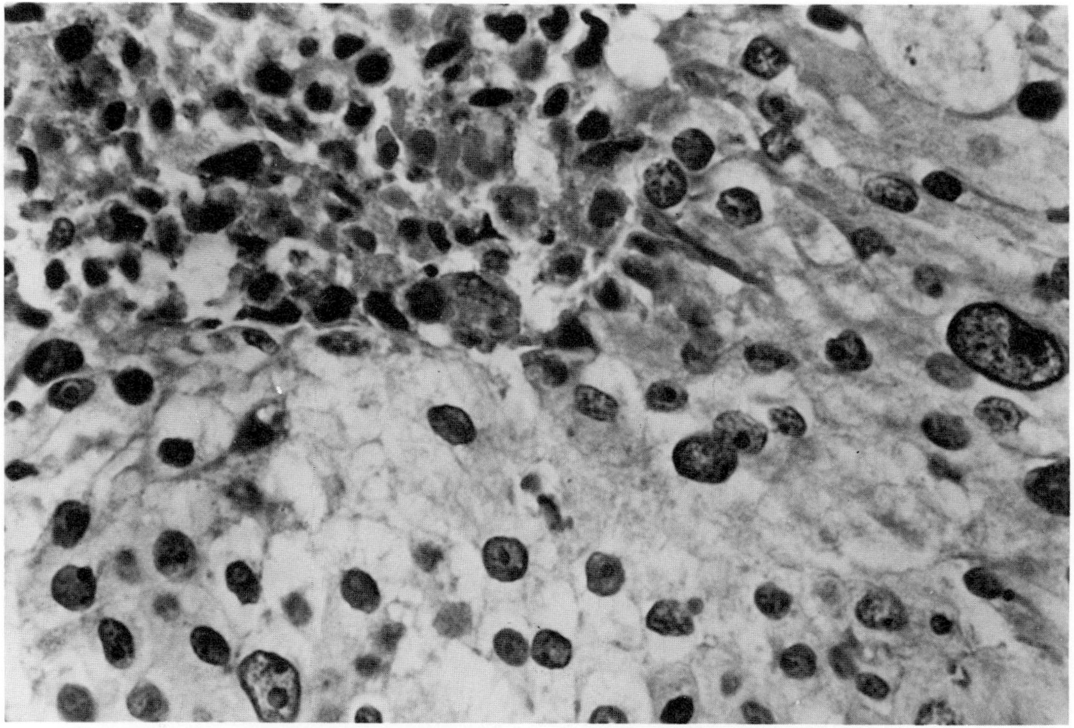

Fig. 7. *Breast cancer. A higher power view showing the close contact between the tumor cells and the area of necrosis containing macrophages and apoptotic cells. H and E ×800.*

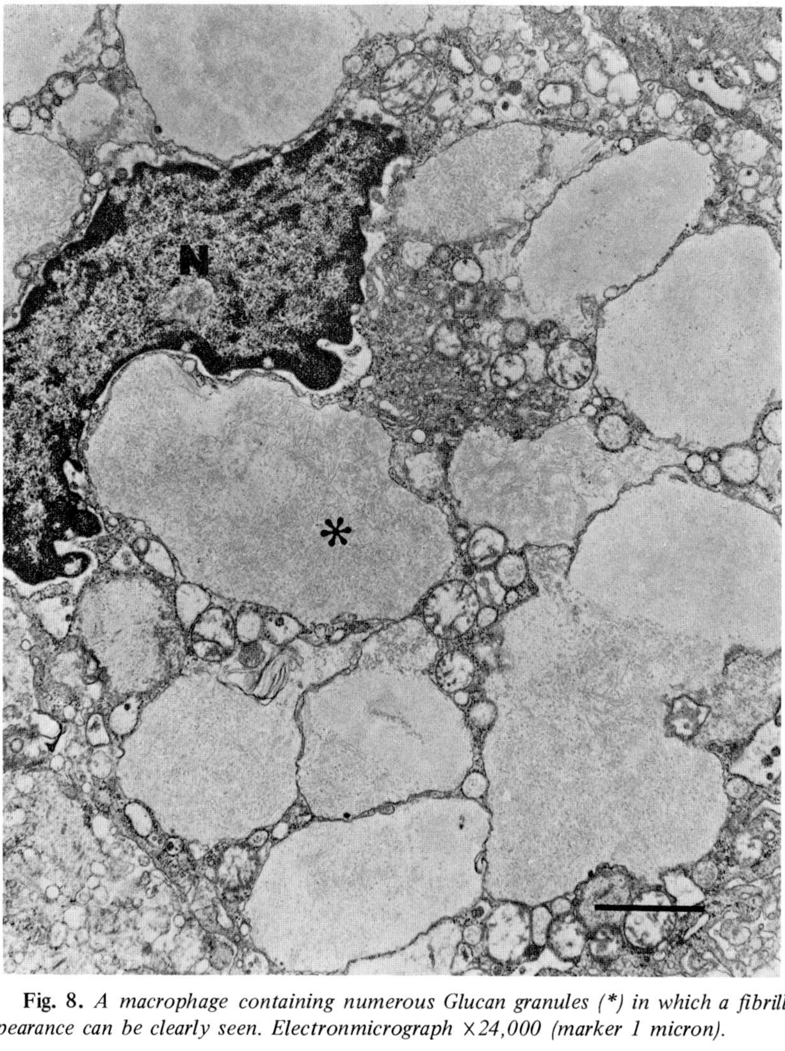

Fig. 8. *A macrophage containing numerous Glucan granules (*) in which a fibrillary appearance can be clearly seen. Electronmicrograph ×24,000 (marker 1 micron).*

chemotaxis in advanced disease states (13,49), it is to be hoped that in the very near future it will be possible to dissect out the role that these cells play in the control of malignant disease. One of the newer tools in this search is the development, in this laboratory, and others (48,50), of reliable anti-macrophage antisera with which the dissection of macrophage function will be made easier. One of the questions that remains to be answered is whether defects in the various migration tests that are in vogue at present (51)

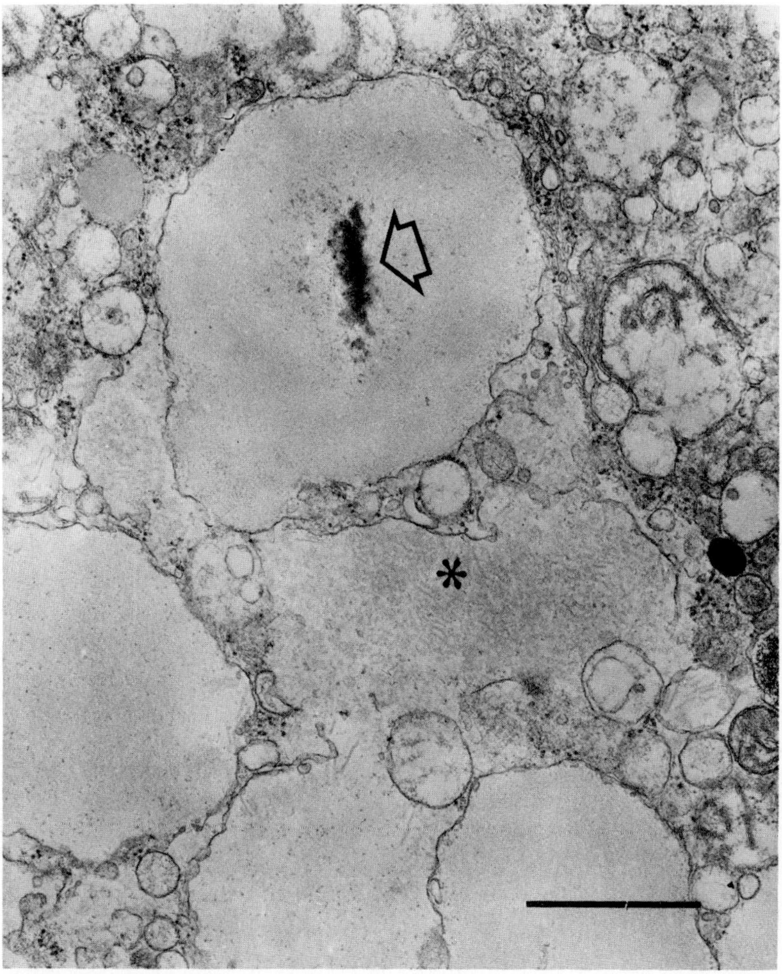

Fig. 9. *Glucan particles enclosed within a macrophage. The membrane surrounding the particles is clearly seen, as is the fibrillary structure (*). One of the particles, arrowed, shows the central electron dense core which is sometimes seen. Electron-micrograph ×38,000. (marker 1 micron).*

represent a defect in the production of lymphokine on the part of the antigen stimulated lymphocyte or a defect primarily resident in the migratory cell, which, either because of the absence of a factor or some inherent defect, is unable to respond to the stimulus even when correctly delivered.

More and more emphasis is now being put on the use of immunotherapy as adjunctive therapy in cancer (52) and the results are at last beginning to show that nonspecific stimulation of the RES using either BCG, C.parvum, Levamisole or Glucan is an intelligent way to initiate or maintain an antitumor reaction in the host. Recently it has been shown that adoptive immunotherapy can actually be achieved using immune macrophages themselves (53).

So far as the nonspecific immune stimulants go, Glucan has certain very definite advantages over others in current use. It is a chemically defined product whose end point of metabolism is glucose. It is not a viable or killed organism. It contains no protein, it is totally nontoxic and it is known to be effective. If this agent could be used in man intravenously, as it is in animals (23,25), there is no reason to suppose that it might not provoke a generalized stimulation of the RES which might lead to the control, or cure, of the malignant process; particularly if used in conjunction with other immunotherapeutic and chemotherapeutic modalities. Of particular interest is the possibility, as yet supported only by very preliminary evidence in men and animals, that Glucan may, as well as being a macrophage activator, be a B cell mitogen (54). This aspect of its function is also in urgent need of investigation.

ACKNOWLEDGEMENTS

I am indebted to Dr. M. G. Lewis for his opinion on the histopathology, Dr. G. Rowden for the electronmicroscopy, and Dr. J. W. Proctor for the animal experiments, all of the McGill University Cancer Research Unit, Montreal.

SUMMARY

Macrophages are an essential, and relatively little studied, part of the host's immune defenses against tumor. Macrophages will only function efficiently in the presence of a plasma factor, humoral recognition factor (HRF), which is present in lesser amounts than normal in the cancer bearing patient. The lowered level of HRF corresponds in general with the clinical stage of the tumor. HRF and the polysaccharide Glucan, which is a potent reticuloendothelial system (RES) stimulant, have been found capable of inducing tumor regression, both of the primary and metastases, in animal models. In man, HRF and Glucan have been shown to induce macrophage mediated regression of injected tumor nodules in every case of a small series studied. Glucan has many advantages as a nonspecific immune stimulant and none of the disadvantages which are seen with such agents as BCG or *C. parvum*, currently in vogue. It is suggested, on the basis of these findings, that Glucan is worthy of further study, both in animals and man.

REFERENCES

1. Jacoby. F. (1959). *Macrophages in Cells and Tissues in Culture.* Academic Press, London and New York.

2. Halpern, B. N. (1959). The role and function of the reticuloendothelial system in immunological process. J. Pharm. Pharmacol. 11:321-338.

3. Kauffman, H. M., L. J. Humphrey, L. D. Hanback, F. Davis, G. E. Madge and M. S. Rittenbury (1967). Inhibition of the afferent arc of the rental homograft response with a reticuloendothelial depressant. *Transplantation 5*:1217-1222.

4. Wooles, W. R., N. R. DiLuzio (1963). Reticuloendothelial function and the immune response. *Science 142*:1078-1080.

5. Zembala, M., W. Ptak, M. Hanczowska (1973). Macrophage and lymphocyte co-operation in target cell destruction *in vitro. Clin. Exp. Immunol. 15*:461-466.

6. Ariyan, S., R. K. Cerson (1973). Augmentation of the adoptive transfer of specific tumor immunity by nonspecifically immunized macrophages. *J. Natl. Cancer Inst. 51*:1145-1148.

7. Amos, D. B. (1962). The use of simplified systems as an aid to the interpretation of mechanisms of graft rejection. *Prog. Allergy 6*:468-538.

8. Baker, P., R. S. Weiser, J. Gutila, C. A. Evans and R. J. Blandau (1962). Mechanisms of homograft rejection: The behavior of the Sarcoma I ascites tumor in the A/Jax in the C57BL/6K mouse. *Ann N.Y. Acad. Sci. 101*:46-63.

9. Bennet, B., L. J. Old and E. A. Boyse (1964). The phagocytosis of tumour cells *in vitro. Transplantation 2*:183-202.

10. Chambers, V. C. and R. S. Weiser (1972). The ultrastructure of Sarcoma I cells and immune macrophages during their interaction in the peritoneal cavities of immune C57BL/6 mice. *Cancer Res. 32*:413-419.

11. Passwell, J. H., M. W. Steward and J. F. Soothill (1974): The effects of protein malnutrition on macrophage function and the amount and affinity of antibody response. *Clin. Exp. Immunol. 17*:491-495.

12. Watson, S. R., V. S. Sljvic and I. N. Brown (1975). Defect in macrophage function in the antibody response to sheep erythrocytes in systemic mycobacterium lepraemurium infection. *Nature (Lond.) 256*:206-207.

13. Cline, M. J. (1973). Defective mononuclear phagocyte function in patients with myelomonocytic leukaemia and in some patients with lymphoma. *J. Clin. Invest. 52*:2185-2190.

14. Pisano, J. C., J. P. Filkins and N. R. DiLuzio (1968). Phagocytic and metabolic activities of isolated rat Kupffer cells. *Proc. Soc. Exp. Biol. Med. 128*:912-922.

15. Pisano, J. C. and N. R. DiLuzio (1970). Purification of an opsonic protein fraction from rat serum. *J. Reticuloendothel. Soc. 7*:386-396.

16. Allen, C., T. M. Saba and J. Molvar (1973). Isolation, purification and characterisation of opsonic protein. *J. Reticuloendothel. Soc. 13*:410-423.

17. Saba, T. M. and N. R. DiLuzio (1969). Reticuloendothelial blockade and recovery as a function of opsonic activity. *Am. J. Physiol. 216*:197-206.

18. Mansell, P. W. A., N. R. DiLuzio, R. McNamee and R. Dietrich. In preparation.

19. Pisano, J. C., N. R. DiLuzio and N. K. Salky (1970). Absence of macrophage humoral recognition factor(s) in patients with neoplasia. *J. Lab. Clin. Med. 76*:141-150.

20. DiLuzio, N. R., J. C. Pisano and N. K. Salky (1971). Humoral recognition factor activity and neoplasia: Clinical and experimental considerations. *Laryngoscope 81*:737-749.

21. Pisano, J. C., J. P. Jackson, N. R. DiLuzio and H. Ichinose (1972). Dimensions of humoral recognition factor depletion in carcinomatous patients. *Cancer Res. 32*:11-15.

22. Mansell, P. W. A., E. T. Krementz, N. R. DiLuzio, I. Olcay, R. McNamee and E. Hoffmann (1974). Role of macrophages and recognition factors in tumour cell recognition and inhibition: An experimental and clinical study. *Proc. XI Internat. Cancer Congr. 4*:696-697.

23. Mansell, P. W. A., H. Ichinose, R. J. Reed, E. T. Krementz, R. McNamee and N. R. DiLuzio (1975). Macrophage-mediated destruction of human malignant cells *in vivo. J. Nat. Cancer Inst. 54*:571-580.

24. DiLuzio, N. R., R. McNamee, E. Jones, J. A. Cook and E. Hoffmann (1976). The employment of Glucan and Glucan activated macrophages in the enhancement of host resistance to malignancies in experimental animals. *The Macrophage in Neoplasia.* Mary A. Fink, Ed. Academic Press, New York.

25. DiLuzio, N. R., R. McNamee, I. Olcay, A. Kitahama and R. H. Miller (1974). Inhibition of tumour growth by recognition factors. *Proc. Soc. Exp. Biol. Med. 145*:311-315.

26. Riggi, S. G. and N. R. DiLuzio (1961). Identification of a reticuloendothelial stimulating agent in zymosan. *Am. J. Physiol. 200*:297-300.

27. Ashworth, C. T., N. R. DiLuzio and S. A. Riggi (1963). A morphologic study of the effect of reticuloendothelial stimulation upon hepatic removal of minute particles from the blood of rats. *J. Exp. Mol. Pathol. (suppl). 1*:83-103.

28. Wooles, W. R. and N. R. DiLuzio (1963). Reticuloendothelial function and the immune response. *Science 142*:1078-1080.

29. DiLuzio, N. R., W. R. Wooles and S. H. Morrow (1964). The effect of splenectomy and x-irradiation on antibody formation in reticuloendothelial hyperfunctional mice. *J. Reticuloendothel. Soc. 1*:429-441.

30. DeLuzio, N. R. and S. J. Riggi (1970). The effects of laminarian, sulfated glucan and oligosaccharide of glucan on reticuloendothelial activity. *J. Reticuloendothel. Soc. 8*:465-473.

31. Wooles, W. R. and N. R. DiLuzio (1962). Influence of reticuloendothelial hyperfunction on bone marrow transplantation. *Am. J. Physiol. 203*:404-408.

32. DiLuzio, N. R. and C. G. Crafton (1970). A consideration of the role of the reticuloendothelial system (RES) in endotoxin shock. *Adv. Exp. Med. Biol. 9*:27-57.

33. Trejo, R. A. and N. R. DiLuzio (1972). Influence of reticuloendothelial (RES) functional modification on endotoxin detoxification by liver and spleen. *J. Reticuloendothel. Soc. 10*:515-525.

34. DiLuzio, N. R. Macrophages, recognition factors and neoplasia. *The Reticuloendothelial System.* Int. Acad. Pathol. Monogr. Williams & Wilkins, Baltimore. In press.

35. Proctor, J. W. Personal communication.

36. DiLuzio, N. R., E. F. Miller, R. McNamee and J. C. Pisano (1972). Alterations in plasma recognition factor activity in experimental leukaemia. *J. Reticuloendothel. Soc. 11*:186-197.

37. DiLuzio, N. R., R. McNamee, E. F. Miller and J. C. Pisano (1972). Macrophage recognition factor depletion after administration of particulate agents and leukaemic cells. *J. Reticuloendothel. Soc. 12*:314-323.

38. McNamee, R. Personal communication.

39. Mansell, P. W. A., E. T. Krementz, N. R. DiLuzio (1975). Clinical experiences with immunotherapy of melanoma. *Behring Inst. Mitt. 56*:256-262.

40. Wyllie, A. H. (1973). Death in normal and neoplastic cells. *J. Clin. Path. 27 (Suppl. 7)* 35-42.

41. Evans, R. (1973). Macrophages and the tumour bearing host. *Br. J. Cancer. 28* (*Suppl. 1*) 19-25.

42. Keller, R. (1973). Cytostatic elimination of syngeneic rat tumour cells *in vitro* by nonspecifically activated macrophages. *J. Exp. Med. 138*:625-644.

43. Carter, R. D. and N. R. DiLuzio. Unpublished results.

44. Birbeck, M. S. and R. L. Carter (1972). Observations of the ultrastructure of two hamster lymphomas with particular reference to infiltrating macrophages. *Int. J. Cancer. 9*:249-257.

45. Lewis, M. G. and P. W. A. Mansell. Unpublished results.

46. Whittaker, J. A., J. S. Lilleyman, A. Jacobs and I. Balfour (1973). Immunotherapy with intravenous BCG. *Lancet. ii:* 1454.

47. Roubin, R., J-P Cesarini, W. H. Fridman, J. Pavie-Fischer and H. H. Peter (1975). Characteristics of the mononuclear cell infiltrate in human malignant melanoma. *Int. J. Cancer 16*:61-73.

48. Gauci, C. L. (1975). The macrophage content of human malignant melanoma. *Behring Inst. Mitt. 56*:73-78.

49. Brosman, S. A. (1975). Alterations of monocyte chemotaxis in patients with genitourinary carcinoma. *Proc. Symp. Neoplasm Immunity: Mechanisms,* Chicago.

50. Greaves, M. F., J. A. Falk and R. E. Falk. Antisera to human macrophages. In press.

51. Cochran, A. J., C. E. Ross, R. M. Mackie, R. M. Grant and D. E. Hoyle (1975). The immune status of patients with malignant melanoma. *Behring Inst. Mitt. 56*:125-130.

52. Morton, D. L. (1974). Cancer immunotherapy: An overview. *Sem. Oncol. 1*:297-310.

53. Dullens, H. F. J. and W. Den Otter (1974). Therapy with allogeneic immune peritoneal cells. *Cancer Res. 34*:1726-1730.

54. Proctor, J. W., P. W. A. Mansell, L. M. Jerry and M. G. Lewis. Unpublished results.

MACROPHAGE DEFICIENCY IN TUMOR BEARING ANIMALS: CONTROL OF EXPERIMENTAL METASTASIS WITH MACROPHAGES ACTIVATED *IN VITRO*[1]

I. J. Fidler, D.V.M., Ph.D.

Frederick Cancer Research Center
Basic Research Program
Frederick, Maryland 21701

INTRODUCTION

We have recently reported the results of the interaction of normal, sensitized or concanavalin A-stimulated syngeneic, or xenogeneic lymphocytes with the B16 melanoma, C57BL/6, or A mouse embryo cells in an *in vitro* colony inhibition-stimulation system. Sensitized lymphocytes at ratios up to 1000:1 repeatedly and significantly enhanced the growth of the target cells. At higher lymphocyte ratios, target cell inhibition occurred (1). In studies with spontaneous canine tumors, low doses of lymphocytes in the absence of autologous serum brought about stimulation of target cells *in vitro*. Serum from tumor bearing dogs, while blocking lymphocyte-mediated cytotoxicity, actually potentiated the tumor growth seen with low numbers (100:1) of sensitized lymphocytes. Again, high doses of lymphocytes brought about a significant inhibition of target cells *in vitro* (2).

Prehn has advanced the theory that antigenic tumors or a weak incipient immune response may bring about a cellular immune reactivity that initially is stimulatory to the tumor cell growth. When the immune response is active, inhibition to tumor growth could occur (3-4). Subsequently, Prehn (3) demonstrated that low ratios of specifically sensitized spleen cells mixed with a constant number of tumor cells and then injected s.c. into immunosuppressed mice actually aided the growth of the tumor, while high ratios inhibited growth. Our investigations with an experimental metastasis system in mice demonstrated that a low number of normal or sensitized syngeneic

[1] Research sponsored by the National Cancer Institute under Contract No. N01-C0-25423 with Litton Bionetics, Incorporated.

lymphocytes mixed *in vitro* with the B16 melanoma increased the number of pulmonary metastases in C57BL/6 mice given i.v. injections of the tumor-lymphocyte mixture. However, once a critical ratio of immune cells to tumor cells was exceeded, inhibition of tumor metastases was clearly demonstrated (5).

These and other (6-8) studies have demonstrated the dual role that immune cells have in their interaction with syngeneic tumors. However, the mechanism responsible for the phenomenon has remained unclear. Several explanations are possible: (a) We are dealing with one population of immune cells (lymphocytes) that produce lymphotoxins (lymphokines), which at low concentrations stimulate but at high concentrations inhibit tumor growth (9); (b) there are two (or more) subclasses of lymphocytes which produce stimulatory or inhibitory growth effects; and (c) there are two distinct populations of immune cells, one principally responsible for stimulation of tumor growth (lymphocyte) and the other responsible for tumor inhibition (macrophages).

Studies were performed to determine if a small number of syngeneic macrophages, hidden within a "purified" lymphocyte preparation, may have been responsible for the inhibition observed with high doses of lymphocytes. Effects on tumor growth by syngeneic lymphocytes, macrophages, or both were tested *in vitro*. Various numbers of lymphocytes alone, macrophages alone, or both were added to B16 cells and cultured for several days. The data demonstrate that high numbers (10,000:1) of lymphocytes from immunized, but not from normal mice, inhibited tumor growth *in vitro*. Macrophages from normal mice had no effect on the tumor, while small numbers of macrophages (100:1) from immunized mice significantly inhibited tumor growth. This suggested that, even at a 1% contamination, macrophages within lymphocyte populations could have contributed to the observed *in vitro* cytotoxicity.

The ability of interacting lymphocytes and macrophages to effect syngeneic tumor cytotoxicity, both *in vivo* and *in vitro*, has been recognized (11-17). Normal macrophages, although not demonstrably cytotoxic to tumor cells, can be activated (made cytotoxic) by supernatants derived from cultures of syngeneic spleen cells sensitized *in vivo* and grown with tumor cells *in vitro* or by incubation with sensitized thymocytes (12,14,15,18). Once activated, the macrophages show increased adherence to glass, as well as increased mobility, phagocytic capability, and enzymatic activity (19). Such activated macrophages are also cytotoxic *in vitro* to tumor cells (12,14,15,18).

The cooperation of lymphocytes and macrophages in the mediation of cellular reactivity to syngeneic tumors raises several questions. In an animal bearing a progressively growing tumor, is the failure of tumor rejection due to lack of cellular cooperation? Is the activation of macrophages by lymphocyte mediators strain- or species-specific? Do lymphocytes from tumor bearing animals suppress macrophage-mediated cytotoxicity? What is the role of the normal or activated macrophage in the phenomenon of immune stimulation-inhibition to tumor cell arrest and growth *in vivo*? Moreover, can normal or activated syngeneic macrophages abrogate the stimulation to tumor growth mediated by low numbers of syngeneic lymphocytes? The present report concerns these and other related questions.

MATERIALS AND METHODS

Animals. – Inbred mouse strain A (H-2^a) was obtained from the Jackson Laboratories (Bar Harbor, Maine). Fischer 344 rats and C57BL/6 (H-2^b) mice were supplied by Frederick Cancer Research Center, Experimental Animal Breeding Facility (Frederick, Maryland).

Tumors and tumor cultures. – The transplantable B16 melanoma, originating in C57BL/6 mice, and the Walker 256 carcinosarcoma, transplanted in Fischer 344 rats, were used. The tumors were grown *in vitro* in enriched media as described previously (1,5,20).

Sensitization of animals. – C57BL/6 mice were immunized to the syngeneic B16 melanoma by s.c. injections of 1×10^6 melanoma cells that had been exposed to 15,000 rads of X-radiation and mixed with complete Freund's adjuvant (CFA). Mice received injections three times at 2-week intervals (CFA was used only with the initial injection) and then were challenged with 1×10^5 viable unirradiated B16 cells injected s.c. Only mice that completely rejected the normally lethal dose of viable tumor cells were classified as immunized animals; their spleens, lymph nodes, and peritoneal exudate cells were collected aseptically. Ten-twelve week old A mice and Fischer rats (150 g) were given 2 s.c. injections, one week apart, of 5×10^6 X-irradiated B16 melanoma cells. Animals were killed 7-10 days after the second injection, and their peritoneal exudate cells (PEC), spleens, and lymph nodes were collected aseptically.

Macrophage cultures. – Three ml of thioglycollate was injected i.p. into normal or sensitized mice, and 4-5 days later the animals were killed and their peritoneal exudate cells (PEC) were harvested by washing with Hank's Balanced Salt Solution (HBSS) containing heparin, 2 units/ml. The PEC were centrifuged and resuspended in complete minimal essential medium (CMEM) (1,5,20) and 1×10^7 cells were plated into 100 20-mm plastic petri dishes which were placed into a humidified 37°C incubator containing 5% CO_2 atmosphere. The cultures were washed and refed with CMEM 1 hour after plating in order to remove all non-plastic-adherent cells (primarily lymphocytes). PEC cultures were then refed once a day for three days to remove all granulocytes (5). On day 3 all the remaining adherent cells phagocytized carbon particles, had the typical macrophage morphology, and were utilized in the subsequent *in vitro* cytotoxicity studies.

Preparation of lymphocyte supernatants and in vitro activation of macrophages. – Spleens and lymph nodes from normal mice, from mice sensitized to tumor *in vivo*, and from rats were collected aseptically, placed into HBSS, and pressed through a wire mesh sieve (E-C Apparatus, St. Petersburg, Florida). The cell suspensions were filtered through a glass-wool column and centrifuged; and the cellular pellets were resuspended in CMEM. Viability, as determined by the trypan blue exclusion test, was about 95%, and most cells appeared to be lymphocytes. The various nonadherent lymphocytes were added to nonconfluent monolayers of B16 melanoma cells at a ratio of 1000:1 (lymphocyte to tumor). After 24 h the culture media were collected, as well as media from B16 tumor cells grown alone, centrifuged at 6000 rpm for 10 minutes, and filtered through a 0.2-μm Millipore filter. The cell-free supernatants were then either stored at 80°C or added immediately to 3-4 day old cultures of macrophages. After 48 h, these cultures were washed twice with HBSS and harvested with the aid of a soft, wide-tipped rubber policeman. Cell counts and viability were determined, and the macrophages were placed into cold HBSS to prevent clumping prior to *in vitro* or *in vivo* assays.

Macrophage-mediated cytotoxicity in vitro. – The procedure was described in detail previously (21,22). B16 melanoma cells, growing *in vitro* in exponential growth phase, were labeled for 24 h with 0.25 μCi of [^{125}I]iododeoxyuridine (^{125}IUDR). The activity of ^{125}IUDR was 100 mCi/μmole per ml of medium (New England Nuclear Corporation, Boston, Mass.). After the labeling period and before the assays, the cultures were washed with HBSS to remove all unbound radioisotopes. The labeled B16 cells were then harvested by a short trypsinization (0.25% trypsin, 1 minute), centrifuged and suspended in CMEM. Single cell suspensions of labeled target cells were mixed with macrophages at various ratios and rotated for 1 h on a platform at room temperature. The mixtures were then plated into culture dishes and incubated for a total of 5 days, after which cytotoxicity was evaluated by monitoring remaining radioactivity in adherent, presumably viable, target cells. Each sample was counted 3 times for 5 min each. As mentioned above, appropriate controls were included to demonstrate that macrophages did not reincorporate ^{125}IUDR released from dead tumor cells. Percentage cytotoxicity was computed by comparing cpms of adherent target cells alone to cpms of target cells plus normal or activated macrophages. The results were analyzed for statistical significance by Student's *t*-test (2-tailed).

Effects of activated macrophages on artificial pulmonary tumor metastases. – B16 melanoma cells grown *in vitro* were harvested during their exponential growth phase by a short trypsinization (0.25% trypsin:EDTA solution for 1 min), washed twice, and resuspended in HBSS. The number of single viable tumor cells was determined and adjusted to 50,000 cells/ml

HBSS. Tumor cells were injected i.v. into the tail vein of normal C57BL/6 mice. Inoculum volume per mouse for all experiments was 0.2 ml (10,000 cells). After 48 h the mice were divided randomly into several treatment groups and injected i.v. with either 0.9% NaCl solution or macrophages from one of the several supernatant treatments. The experimental groups were coded, and 2 or 3 weeks later all mice were killed. The number of pulmonary metastases was determined, with the aid of a dissecting microscope, by two independent observers.

RESULTS

Macrophage-mediated Cytotoxicity *In Vitro*

A. *Activation by syngeneic mediators.* Macrophages harvested from normal C57BL/6 mice, C57BL/6 mice with subcutaneous B16 melanoma, and C57BL/6 mice immunized against B16 melanoma were treated *in vitro* with lymphocyte supernatants. After 48 h, all treated and control macrophages were harvested, mixed with viable ^{125}IUDR labeled B16 cells, and plated *in vitro*; tumor cytotoxicity was then assayed. The *in vitro* cytotoxic effects of the syngeneic macrophages are summarized in Table 1. The data demonstrated that macrophages from normal mice were not cytotoxic to B16 melanoma

TABLE 1.
Activation of C57BL/6 Mouse Macrophages by Syngeneic Lymphocytes Supernatants

Macrophages	Lymphocyte mediator	Average cpm in live target cells on day 5 (mean cpm ± SD)[1]	Percentage significant cytotoxicity
None (tumor cells alone)	None	1010 ± 30	
Normal C57BL/6	None (B16 culture)	1020 ± 80	
	Normal C57BL/6	1000 ± 60	
	Tumor bearing C57BL/6	890 ± 50	
	Immunized C57BL/6	700 ± 30	31(p<0.01)
Tumor bearing C57BL/6	None	950 ± 50	
	Normal C57BL/6	950 ± 50	
	Tumor bearing C57BL/6	870 ± 37	
	Immunized C57BL/6	400 ± 20	60(p<0.005)
Immunized C57BL/6	None	570 ± 100	44(p<0.005)
	Normal C57BL/6	530 ± 40	48(p<0.005)
	Tumor bearing C57BL/6	510 ± 25	50(p<0.005)
	Immunized C57BL/6	430 ± 40	57(p<0.005)

[1] 10,000 ^{125}IUDR labeled B16 melanoma cells plated with macrophages. Macrophage tumor cell ratio 100:1. Values are means of triplicate five-day cultures.

even at a 100:1 ratio (macrophage to tumor cells). However, these macrophages could be rendered cytotoxic to the tumor by incubation with mediators released from lymphocytes of syngeneic mice immunized to the tumor. Supernatants from cultures containing either normal lymphocytes or lymphocytes from tumor bearing mice had no effect on macrophages from normal mice. Macrophages from tumor bearing mice were not cytotoxic to the B16 cells *in vitro*, although again, such macrophages were rendered highly cytotoxic by incubation with mediators released from syngeneic lymphocytes of immunized mice. Incubation with supernatants from cultures containing lymphocytes from normal mice or tumor bearing mice had no such effect. On the other hand, untreated macrophages harvested from mice immunized to the B16 melanoma were highly cytotoxic to the tumor. Their cytotoxicity was not abrogated or inhibited by supernatants from cultures containing lymphocytes from either normal or tumor bearing mice. This study suggested that macrophages of tumor bearing (syngeneic) mice were potentially cytotoxic to the tumor target. Apparently the failure of these macrophages to destroy the syngeneic B16 melanoma cells was not due to their inhibition by lymphocyte products.

B. *Activation by allogeneic mediators.* When the B16 melanoma cells are injected into A mice, the allogeneic tumor is rejected. This led us to ask the questions: was there a cooperation between lymphocytes and macrophages and if so, can it be demonstrated *in vitro*? In this experiment, untreated macrophages from normal A mice, from A mice sensitized to B16 melanoma *in vivo*, and from C57BL/6 mice bearing subcutaneous B16 melanoma were assayed for their *in vitro* cytotoxicity to the B16 melanoma. Macrophages from tumor bearing C57BL/6 mice were incubated with supernatants from cultures containing either lymphocytes from normal A mice or lymphocytes from A mice sensitized *in vivo* to the B16 melanoma. The cytotoxicity of the treated and untreated macrophages to B16 cells was then assayed *in vitro*.

The data summarized in Table 2 demonstrated that while macrophages from normal A mice were not cytotoxic to the B16 melanoma, macrophages from the A mice sensitized to the B16 *in vivo* had significant cytotoxic properties. Macrophages from C57BL/6 mice bearing B16 melanoma were not cytotoxic to B16 cells *in vitro*. However, such macrophages were rendered cytotoxic following their incubation with supernatants of cultures containing lymphocytes from A mice sensitized *in vivo* to the B16 melanoma but not after incubation with supernatants from normal, nonsensitized A lymphocytes.

C. *Activation by xenogeneic mediators.* Macrophages from normal C57BL/6 mice were incubated with supernatants of B16 cells cultured with either normal rat lymphocytes or those from rats sensitized *in vivo* to the B16 melanoma. The results (Table 3) demonstrated that incubation of macrophages from normal C57BL/6 mice (non cytotoxic) with supernatants from cultures

TABLE 2.
Activation of C57BL/6 Mouse Macrophages by Allogeneic Lymphocytes Supernatants

Macrophages	Lymphocyte mediator	Average cpm in live target cells on day 5 (mean cpm ± SD)[1]	Percentage significant cytotoxicity
None (tumor cells alone)	None	2770 ± 450	
Normal A	None	2200 ± 400	
Sensitized A	None	1200 ± 170	57(p<0.005)
Tumor bearing C57BL/6	None	2600 ± 500	
	Normal A	2650 ± 300	
	Sensitized A	1380 ± 300	50(p<0.005)

[1] 20,000 ^{125}IUDR labeled B16 melanoma cells plated with macrophages. Macrophage to tumor cell ratio 50:1. Values are means of triplicate 5 day cultures.

of normal (nonsensitized) rat lymphocytes and B16 melanoma cells had no effect on the cytoxicity of the mouse macrophages. However, C57BL/6 mouse macrophages could be made highly cytotoxic to the B16 cells by their incubation with supernatants from cultures of xenogeneic lymphocytes from rats sensitized *in vivo* to the mouse tumor.

Effects of C57BL/6 macrophages activated with xenogeneic lymphocyte mediators on tumor cells in vivo. – Macrophages were harvested from C57BL/6 mice bearing a progressively growing B16 melanoma s.c. These macrophages were cultured *in vitro* with various supernatants obtained from xenogeneic rat lymphocytes after their interaction with the tumor *in vitro* or with supernatants from tumor cultures alone. Following this incubation (activation), the macrophages were injected i.v. into C57BL/6 mice that 48 h previously, had been injected i.v. with 10,000 viable B16 cells. The *in vivo* effects of these syngeneic macrophages are shown in Tables 4 and 5.

TABLE 3.
Activation of C57BL/6 Mouse Macrophages by Xenogeneic Lymphocytes Supernatants

Macrophages	Lymphocyte mediator	Average cpm in live target cells on day 5 (mean cpm ± SD)[1]	Percentage significant cytotoxicity
None (tumor cells alone)	None	1100 ± 30	
Normal C57BL/6	None	1020 ± 80	
	Normal Rat	1000 ± 70	
	Rat sensitized to B16	520 ± 20	53(p<0.005)

[1] 10,000 ^{125}IUDR labeled B16 melanoma cells. Macrophage to tumor cell ratio 100:1. Values are means of triplicate 5 day cultures.

TABLE 4.
Effects of Syngeneic C57BL/6 Mouse Macrophages Activated by Xenogeneic Lymphocyte Supernatants on Experimental Metastasis

Macrophage treatment *in vitro*	Number of pulmonary metastases[1]
Tumor cells alone[2]	205 ± 45
Supernatants of B16 melanoma cultures alone	227 ± 36
Supernatants of B16 melanoma cultures and normal rat lymphocytes	185 ± 30
Supernatants of B16 melanoma cultures and rat lymphocytes sensitized to B16 melanoma	74 ± 30[3]

[1] Six mice/group. Pulmonary metastases were counted 14 days post i.v. injection of 200,000 viable macrophages.

[2] 10,000 viable B16 melanoma line F-11 injected i.v.

[3] $p<0.01$

In these experiments, we used different B16 melanoma tumor lines. Line F-3 is a low metastasis producer, while line F-11 produces a relatively high number of pulmonary metastases following i.v. injection (21). Although the number of pulmonary metastases varied from one experiment to the other, the results were very similar.

The data demonstrated that the i.v. injection of untreated macrophages from tumor bearing mice did not affect the outcome of the experimental pulmonary metastasis. Similarly, macrophages, that were cultured *in vitro* with supernatants of either B16 melanoma cells alone or normal nonsensitized rat lymphocytes and B16 melanoma cells and then injected i.v., had no inhibitory effects on established pulmonary metastases. The i.v. injection of macrophages treated with supernatants obtained from *in vitro* cultures of B16 melanoma cells and rat lymphocytes sensitized *in vivo* to an A mouse tumor (adenocarcinoma 15091) led to some inhibitory effects on artificial metastasis ($p<0.01$) (Table 4).

Macrophages treated with supernatants obtained from *in vitro* cultures of B16 melanoma cells and lymphocytes from rats sensitized *in vivo* to C57BL/6 normal lymphocytes demonstrated significant inhibitory activity to pulmonary metastases ($p<0.01$). By far, the most significant inhibition of pulmonary metastases formation was observed following the i.v. injection of macrophages treated *in vitro* with supernatants of B16 melanoma cell cultures incubated with rat lymphocytes sensitized to the B16 melanoma *in vivo*. The difference between the number of pulmonary metastases in control animals and those injected with activated macrophages was highly significant ($p<001$).

The decrease in pulmonary metastases effected by injection of syngeneic macrophages was related to macrophage treatment *in vitro*, the number of

TABLE 5.
Effects of Syngeneic C57BL/6 Mouse Macrophages Activated by Xenogeneic Lymphocyte Supernatants on Experimental Metastasis

	Experiment #1 No. of pulmonary metastases[1]		Experiment #2 No. of pulmonary metastases[1]
	Day 14	Day 21	Day 14
No macrophages, Tumor cells alone[2]	14 ± 6	28 ± 5	30 ± 3
Supernatants of B16 melanoma cultures	12 ± 5	29 ± 8	31 ± 2
Supernatants of B16 melanoma cultures and rat lymphocytes sensitized to a.c. 15091	9 ± 2	16 ± 3[3]	30 ± 2
Supernatants of B16 melanoma cultures and rat lymphocytes sensitized to C57BL/6	10 ± 2	12 ± 4[3]	18 ± 3
Supernatants of B16 melanoma cultures and rat lymphocytes sensitized to B16 melanoma	6 ± 3	4 ± 2[4]	4 ± 1[4]

[1] Six mice/group. Pulmonary metastases were counted on Days 14 or 21 post i.v. injection of 500,000 macrophages.

[2] Ten mice/group. Pulmonary metastases were counted 14 days post i.v. injection of 1,000,000 macrophages.

[3] $p<0.01$

[4] $p<0.001$

injected macrophages, and the duration of their activity *in vivo*. This is noted in Table 5. In this experiment mice were killed either 14 or 21 days following the i.v. injection of the *in vitro*-activated macrophages. It appeared that day 21 post-macrophage injection, the number of pulmonary metastases had actually increased in all mice except those given injections of macrophages activated by supernatants of rat lymphocytes sensitized *in vivo* to B16 melanoma. In contrast, mice injected with activated macrophages had fewer lung metastases on day 21 post-treatment than on day 14 post-treatment.

DISCUSSION

Lymphocytes incubated *in vitro* with an antigen to which they have been previously sensitized release a variety of substances into the culture medium. The substances are chemotactic to macrophages, inhibit the migration of macrophages, can be cytotoxic *in vitro* to target cells, can cause skin reactions similar to delayed hypersensitivity, can bring about blastogenesis of nonsensitized lymphocytes, and in some cases may render macrophages cytotoxic (23). In another biological system, it has been suggested that a product of sensitized lymphocytes can enhance the antibacterial properties of macrophages (24).

Many studies support the hypothesis that successful *in vivo* rejection of a syngeneic tumor may require the cooperation of lymphocytes and macrophages. In animals with a primary spontaneous neoplasm or transplantable syngeneic tumor, such cooperation may be absent, either due to a defect in synthesis and/or release of lymphocyte mediators or because the macrophages fail to respond to mediators. In addition, it is possible that lymphocytes in tumor bearing animals may interact with circulating tumor antigen and release mediators at a distant site, thus preventing local accumulation and activation of macrophages. Finally, the functional defect in tumor rejection may reside in both lymphocytes and macrophages of the tumor host.

The present experiment confirmed our past observations and those of other investigators (12,14,15,18,19,25) that macrophages from mice bearing a tumor can be rendered cytotoxic to the tumor by several related methods. In a syngeneic system, supernatants collected from cultures of sensitized spleen cells and tumor cells as well as macrophages, can render normal macrophages cytotoxic (25). Specifically, thymocytes from sensitized mice released a macrophage-activating factor when cultured with the target cells. The factor that renders normal macrophages cytotoxic has been reported to be a product of thymus-dependent lymphocytes; once released, it could render allogeneic or syngeneic macrophages cytotoxic. Another possibility is that a cytophilic antibody released by lymphocytes could enhance macrophage-mediated cytotoxicity (27).

Our studies confirm the results of others and demonstrate that macrophages from tumor bearing mice, while not innately cytotoxic to their syngeneic tumor, can be made cytotoxic by xenogeneic lymphocyte activation. The *in vivo* experiments dealt with activation of macrophages by a factor released by non-plastic-adhering xenogeneic lymphocytes obtained from normal and/or sensitized rats. It appeared that only the lymphocytes from rats that were sensitized *in vivo* to the B16 melanoma and to a lesser degree to the C57BL/6 lymphocytes, and then cultured with the tumor target *in vitro* released a factor capable of activating the mouse macrophages from tumor bearing mice. This finding agrees with earlier published reports dealing with syngeneic or allogeneic activation of macrophages and confirms the observation that the mechanism responsible for the release of lymphocytic mediators is antigen specific. Our studies also utilized an *in vivo* experimental metastasis assay to determine the effects of i.v. injected activated syngeneic macrophages on tumor cells disseminated *in vivo*.

In our earlier studies of the quantitative analysis of cancer metastasis (28), we demonstrated that the majority of circulating tumor cells rapidly die; but tumor cells which by 1-2 days post-i.v. injection are established in the lung parenchyma will continue to grow progressively and kill the recipient animals (20,28). In the present experiment we studied in the *in vivo* inhibitory effects of the *in vitro*-activated syngeneic macrophages on established pulmonary metastases. The macrophages obtained from the mice bearing the B16 melanoma s.c. were either not cytotoxic *in vivo* or not sufficiently effective, as seen by the constant and rapid progression of tumor growth leading to death of the host. It is, therefore, most significant that these macrophages could be rendered cytotoxic by the xenogeneic lymphocyte supernatants. Indeed, this approach to macrophage activation could be a method of overcoming or even bypassing the possible defect in the autochthonous response to neoplasm.

SUMMARY

Macrophages from normal C57BL/6 mice, mice with a subcutaneous B16 melanoma, and mice immunized against the B16 tumor were examined for *in vitro* cytotoxicity to B16 tumor cells. Macrophages were treated by incubation with supernatants from B16 cells grown alone or in cultures containing syngeneic, allogeneic or xenogeneic lymphocytes from B16 sensitized animals. The various treated and untreated macrophages were then cultured for 5 days with viable B16 cells prelabeled with ^{125}IUDR. Of the untreated macrophages, only those from immunized mice were cytotoxic to the tumor cells; macrophages from normal and tumor bearing mice became cytotoxic following incubation with supernatants from cultures containing lymphocytes from immunized syngeneic mice, sensitized allogeneic mice, or sensitized rats.

In addition, the ability of *in vitro* treated macrophages from C57BL/6 mice to inhibit established pulmonary metastases *in vivo* was studied. The data demonstrated that specifically *in vitro*-treated macrophages injected i.v. into mice significantly reduced their number of established pulmonary metastases. Moreover, it appeared that the *in vivo* inhibition of tumor nodules was continuing at the time of sacrifice.

These results support the experimental data that cytotoxic macrophages may play an important role in the defense against neoplasia. Furthermore, the application of xenogeneic activation of macrophages from tumor bearing animals that renders them cytotoxic may provide a possible approach to therapy.

REFERENCES

1. Fidler, I. J. (1973). *In vitro* studies of cellular mediated immunostimulation of tumor growth. *J. Nat. Cancer Inst. 50*:1307-1312.

2. Fidler, I. J., R. S. Broday and S. Bech-Nielson (1974). *In vitro* immune stimulation-inhibition to spontaneous canine tumors of various histologic types. *J. Immunol. 112*:1051-1060.

3. Prehn, R. T. (1972). The immune reaction as a stimulator of tumor growth. *Science 176*:170-171.

4. Prehn, R. T. (1971). Immunostimulation theory of tumor development. *Transplant. Rev.* 7:26-54.

5. Fidler, I. J. (1974). Immune stimulation-inhibition of experimental cancer metastases. *Cancer Res. 34*:491-498.

6. Medina, D. and G. Heppner (1973). Cell-mediated "immunostimulation" induced by mammary tumor virus-free BALB/c mammary tumors. *Nature 242*:329-330.

7. Jeejeebhoy, H. F. (1974). Stimulation of tumor growth by the immune response. *Int. J. Cancer 13*:665.

8. Shearer, W. T., Philpott and C. W. Parker (1975). Humoral immunostimulation. II. Increased nucleoside incorporation, DNA synthesis, and cell growth in L cells treated with anti-L cell antibody. *Cellular Immunology* 17:447-459.

9. Kolb, W. P. and G. A. Granger (1970). Lymphocyte *in vitro* cytotoxicity: Characterization of mouse lymphotoxin. *Cellular Immunology 1*:122-130.

10. Fidler, I. J. and D. E. Peterson (1975). *In vitro* tumor growth inhibition by syngeneic lymphocytes and/or macrophages. *7th International Congress of the Reticuloendothelial Society,* in press.

11. Lipsky, P. E. and A. S. Rosenthal (1975). Macrophage-lymphocyte interaction. II. Antigen-mediated physical interactions between Guinea pig lymph node lymphocytes and syngeneic macrophages. *J. Exp. Med. 141*:138-150.

12. Alexander, P., R. Evans and C. K. Grant (1972). The interplay of lymphoid cells and macrophages in tumor immunity. *Ann. Inst. Pasteur 122*:645-658.

13. Gottlieb, A. A. and S. R. Waldman (1972). The multiple functions of macrophages in immunity. *Macrophages and Cellular Immunity,* A. Laskin and H. Lechevalier, Eds., p. 13. CRC Press, Cleveland.

14. Evans, R. and P. Alexander (1971). Rendering macrophages specifically cytotoxic by a factor released from immune lymphoid cells. *Transplantation 12*:227-229.

15. Lohmann-Matthes, M. L., F. G. Ziegler and H. Fischer (1973). Macrophage cytotoxicity factor. A produce *in vitro* sensitized thymus-dependent cells. *Eur. J. Immunology 3*:56-58.

16. North, R. J. (1974). T-cell dependence of macrophage activation of mobilization during infection with *Mycobacterium* tuberculosis. *Infection and Immunity 10*:66-71.

17. Feldman, M. (1974). Cell to cell interactions in the immune response. *Ser. Haemat.* 7:593-609.

18. Grant, C. K., G. A. Currie and P. Alexander (1972). Thymocytes from mice immunized against an allograft render bone marrow cells specifically cytotoxic. *J. Exp. Med. 135*:150-164.

19. Alexander, P. and R. Evans (1971). Endotoxins and double stranded RNA render macrophages cytotoxic. *Nature New Biol. 232*:76-78.

20. Fidler, I. J. (1975). Biological behavior of malignant melanoma cells correlate to their survival *in vivo. Cancer Res. 34*:218-224.

21. Norbury, K. C. and I. J. Fidler (1975). *In vitro* tumor cell destruction by syngeneic mouse macrophages: Methods for assaying cytotoxicity. *J. Immunol. Methods* 7:109-122.

22. Fidler, I. J. Activation *in vitro* of mouse macrophages by syngeneic, allogeneic or xenogeneic lymphocyte supernatants. *J. Nat. Cancer Inst.*, in press.

23. David, J. R. (1975). A brief review of macrophage activation by lymphocyte mediators. *The Phagocytic Cell In Host Resistance.* J. A. Bellanti, and H. Dayton, Eds. Raven Press, New York.

24. Mackanness, G. B. (1971). Cell-mediated immunity. *Cellular Interactions in the Immune Response.* S. Cohen, G. Cudkowicz and R. T. McCluskey, Eds. Karger AG, Basel.

25. Piessens, W. F., W. H. Churchill and J. R. David (1975). Macrophages activated *in vitro* with lymphocyte mediators kill neoplastic but not normal cells. *J. Immunol. 114*:293-299.

26. Fidler, I. J. (1974). Inhibition of pulmonary metastasis by intravenous injection of specifically activated macrophages. *Cancer Res. 34*:1074-1078.

27. Pels, E. and W. Den (1974). The role of cytophilic factor from challenged immune peritoneal lymphocytes in specific macrophage cytotoxicity. *Cancer Res. 34*:3089-3094.

28. Fidler, I. J. (1970). Metastasis: Quantitative analysis of distribution and fate of tumor emboli labeled with ^{125}I-5-iodo-2′ deoxyuridine. *J. Nat. Cancer Inst. 45*:773-782.

DISCUSSION

Ole A. Holtermann, Chairman

STUDIES ON LOCAL ADMINISTRATION OF MATERIAL WITH LYMPHOKINE ACTIVITY TO NEOPLASMS INVOLVING THE SKIN

Ole A. Holtermann, Benjamin W. Papermaster,
Dutzu Rosner and Edmund Klein

Regression of neoplasms involving the skin has been observed after repeated local inductions of delayed hypersensitivity reactions to chemical haptens or microbial antigens (1,2,3). It has been proposed that the mechanism for the tumor regressions is a selective destruction of tumor cells by the leukocytes of the inflammatory infiltrate of the delayed hypersensitivity reactions. Since lymphokines are mediators of delayed hypersensitivity reactions, it was considered to be of interest to explore the potential antitumor effect of local administration of material with lymphokine activity.

Supernatant fluids from primary cultures of human lymphocytes stimulated with the mitogens concanavalin A or phytohemagglutinin were used in initial studies (3). Intracutaneous injections of 0.1 ml. volumes of such fluids induced +++ reactions of induration and erythema measuring up to 40 mm. in diameter reaching peak intensity at 6-8 hours after injection. Microscopic examination of the sites of reaction 24 hours after injection revealed a mixed inflammatory infiltrate consisting predominantly of large and small mononuclear cells with smaller numbers of polymorphonucleated granulocytes. Intracutaneous injections of control fluid from cultures of lymphocytes incubated in the absence of mitogens or culture medium containing the mitogens incubated without lymphocytes both induced reactions of slight (+) induration and faint erythema measuring up to 5 mm. in diameter. Thus, the major reactive components of the fluids of the stimulated lymphocyte culture were products of mitogen-lymphocyte interaction, rather than residual mitogen.

Material from mitogen-stimulated lymphocyte cultures was used for local treatment in two patients with multiple superficial basal cell carcinomas and in two patients in the plaque stage of mycosis fungoides (M.F.). The treated lesions were all relatively small, measuring no more than 10-20 mm. in

TABLE 1.
Effect of Local Administration of Material with Lymphokine Activity to Neoplasms Involving the Skin

	Number of Patients	Number of Lesions Showing Regression	
		Grossly	Microscopically
A. Material from Primary Lymphoid Cell Cultures			
Diagnoses			
Basal Cell Carcinoma	2	3/3	1/3
Mycosis Fungoides	2	2/4	0/4
B. Material from Established Lymphoid Cell Cultures			
Diagnoses			
Mammary Carcinoma	3	8/18	2/18
Reticulum Cell Sarcoma	2	6/7	1/7
Mycosis Fungoides	1	1/2	0/2

diameter. By repeated local injections of active material, reactions were maintained almost continuously at the tumor sites for periods ranging from 3-5 weeks. This regimen resulted in measurable regression of all of the three treated basal cell carcinomas and in two of the four treated plaques of M.F. (Table I). Microscopic examination of tissue obtained from the treated lesions at the time of termination of the study did not reveal malignant cells at the site of one of the basal cell carcinomas. Biopsies of the remaining treated lesions revealed the presence of residual tumor cells.

These studies have recently been extended to the use of material with lymphokine activity obtained from the 1788 line of human lymphoid cells (4). This line of cells was established from peripheral blood leukocytes of a normal donor. Culture fluids were passed through an "Amicon XM100" membrane with a nominal pore size corresponding to particles of a molecular weight of 100,000 Daltons. The filtrate was concentrated 20 fold over an "Amicon PM10" membrane with a nominal pore size corresponding to 10,000 Daltons. Intracutaneous injections of the concentrated material resulted in reactions that both grossly and microscopically were similar to the reactions induced by the material obtained from mitogen stimulated lymphocytes. The results of repeated local injections of this material at the sites of cutaneous lesions of mammary carcinoma, reticulum cell sarcoma and M.F. are summarized in Table I.

The immediate accessibility of tumors involving the skin offers possibilities of direct observation and manipulation. In the exploration of immunological approaches to the treatment of neoplasms, skin tumors have proven to be a most valuable model system. It has been established that induction of regression of a wide spectrum of human tumors by immunological means is feasible (1-4). Destruction of neoplastic cells by activated mononuclear phagocytes recruited to the tumor sites could be the mechanism of tumor regression after local induction of delayed hypersensitivity challenge reactions to haptens or microbial antigens. An alternative approach to the activation and recruitment of these mononuclear effector cells is passive administration of lymphokines. The results of these preliminary studies on administration of lymphokines to tumors involving the skin indicate that an extension of this approach to inaccessible tumors warrants exploration.

Supported by grants No. 1 RO1 CA17205-01 and 9 RO1 CA13599-03 and contracts No. NIH-NCI-71-2137 and NO1-CP-33373 from the National Cancer Institute, National Institutes of Health, Bethesda, Maryland; the Cancer Research Institute, New York, New York; and the Albert and Mary Lasker Foundation, New York.

REFERENCES

1. Klein, E. (1969). Hypersensitivity reactions at tumor sites. *Cancer Research* *29*:2351-2362.

2. Levis, W. R., K. H. Kraemer, W. G. Klinger, G. L. Peck and W. D. Terry (1973). Topical immunotherapy of basal cell carcinomas with dinitrochlorobenzene. *Cancer Research 33*:3036-3042.

3. Holtermann, O. A., B. Papermaster, D. Rosner, H. Milgrom and E. Klein (1975). Regression of cutaneous neoplasm following delayed-type hypersensitivity challenge reactions to microbial antigens or lymphokines. *J. Med. Exp. Clin. 6*:157-168.

4. Papermaster, B. W., O. A. Holtermann, E. Klein, I. Djerassi, D. Rosner, T. Dao and J. J. Costanzi. Preliminary observations on tumor regressions induced by local administration of a lymphoid cell culture supernatant fraction in patients with cutaneous metastatic lesions. *Clin. Immunol. Immunopath.*, in press.

ANTAGONISM OF IMMUNOSUPPRESSION BY BCG

Richard I. Murahata and Malcolm S. Mitchell

Yale University School of Medicine

Bacillus Calmette-Guérin (BCG) is of considerable value as a nonspecific adjuvant in the immunotherapy of neoplasia. Mice infected with BCG show an overall increase in function of the reticuloendothelial system (RES) and demonstrate an increased clearance rate of *E. coli* endotoxin and carbon particles. Treatment with BCG or some of its cell-free derivatives such as methanol-extraction residue (MER) increase antibody synthesis, and this effect is presumed to be due to an increased number of immunologically reactive cells. BCG has been shown to reverse the immunodepressant effect of methylcholanthrene, and MER can protect against the immunosuppressive effects of antilymphocyte serum both *in vivo* and *in vitro*. BCG pretreatment is protective against tumor development after irradiation, injection of an oncogenic virus or transplantation of live tumor cells. BCG can produce activated macrophages which are nonspecifically cytotoxic to transformed cells *in vitro*. We have reported that BCG increases the production of Lymphocyte-Activating Factor (LAF) by macrophages, and that it elicits nonspecifically cytotoxic nonadherent spleen cells (1). It was of interest to see if BCG could also prevent immunosuppression caused by a cancer chemotherapeutic agent, cytosine arabinoside (Ara-C), thereby increasing the therapeutic efficacy of combined chemotherapy and immunotherapy.

BCG derived from the Tice strain was obtained from the National Institutes of Health, Bethesda, Maryland. The lyophilized material was reconstituted with Minimal Essential Medium to a concentration of 2.5 mg per ml, and groups of mice (C57BL/6J, 8-10 weeks old) were injected in the lateral tail vein with 0.5 mg. (approximately 1.5×10^7 viable units). Ten days later the mice received 20X10 x-irradiated (2800 r) L-1210 leukemia cells intraperitoneally. This dose of allogeneic tumor cells leads to suboptimal immunization. On days 3-7 following immunization, one group of animals received 20 mg/kg Ara-C i.p. Other groups included mice injected with BCG alone, mice injected with L-1210 alone, mice pretreated with BCG and immunized with L-1210, and mice immunized with L-1210 and treated with Ara-C. Mice were sacrificed 14-17 days after immunization with tumor. The original 48-hour *in vitro* cytotoxicity assay of Brunner *et al.* (2) was used to quantitate spleen cell-mediated immunity (CMI) to H-2d alloantigens utilizing the DBA mastocytoma P-815Y as the target cell. Results are expressed as "per cent lysis," or

$$100 \times \left(1 - \frac{\text{No. of tumor cells in experimental tube}}{\text{No. of tumor cells in control tube}}\right)$$

As shown in the Table, BCG significantly augmented CMI above levels in mice given 20×10^6 L-1210 alone.

TABLE

BCG Pretreatment	Ara-C	CMI ± S.E.
–	–	47.7 ± 4.5
+	–	75.5 ± 2.8
–	+	12.8 ± 6.0
+	+	49.1 ± 3.5

All groups received antigen (L-1210 cells.)

Ara-C had a pronounced immunosuppressive effect. Pretreatment with BCG protected against immunosuppression by Ara-C. The mice showed neither the augmented immunity seen with BCG and antigen (L-1210), nor the suppression found with Ara-C, but instead had a stabilization of their immune response, which was similar to controls given only antigen. The BCG potentiation of CMI here appeared to be specific, in that no killing of a C3H hepatoma (H-129) was observed in any group. Removal of glass- or plastic-adherent cells had no effect on the CMI nor did treatment with antitheta serum (rabbit antithymocyte serum twice absorbed with normal mouse liver cells) and complement. Further evidence for the lack of participation of the classical "killer T-lymphocyte" was the lack of activity of these spleen cells in a 6-hour chromium release assay (3). Treatment of the spleen cells with rabbit anti-mouse gamma globulin and complement resulted in a significant decrease in the cytotoxic effect as did treatment with carbonyl iron particles and removal with a magnet. Sequential treatment of the spleen cells with both of these techniques is in progress to determine if one type of cell has both characteristics, or if two distinct subpopulations are involved. Our current presumption is that a phagocytic nonadherent effector cell is induced by BCG and L-1210 cells and is a member of the monocytic series, armed with specific cytophilic antibody.

REFERENCES

1. Mitchell, M. S., D. Kirkpatrick, M. B. Mokyr and I. Gery (1973). On the mode of action of BCG. *Nature New Biology 243*:216-218.

2. Brunner, K. T., J. Mauel and R. Schindler (1966). *In vitro* studies of cell bound immunity: Cloning assay of the cytotoxic action of sensitized lymphoid cells on allogeneic target cells. *Immunology 11*:499-506.

3. Brunner, K. T., J. Mauel, J. C. Cerottini and B. Chapuis (1968). Quantitative assay of the lytic action of immune lymphoid cells on ^{51}Cr-labeled allogeneic target cells *in vitro*: Inhibition by isoantibody and by drugs. *Immunology 14*:181-196.

Dr. Luka Milas: We have investigated whether peritoneal macrophages from C_3Hf/Bu mice treated with anaerobic corynebacteria (*C. parvum* or *C. granulosum*) are capable of destroying *in vitro* cultures of a syngeneic fibrosarcoma, tumorgeneic mouse L-P59 cells (allogeneic cells) and human malignant melanoma cells. (Basic *et al., J. Natl. Cancer Inst. 52*:1839, 1974; *Ibid., J. Natl. Cancer Inst. 55*:589, 1975). All of these malignant cell cultures were destroyed by *C. granulosum* activated macrophages. In contrast the growth of allogeneic fibroblasts and kidney epithelial cells was not affected by the presence of activated macrophages. The aggregation and adherence of macrophages to neoplastic cells preceded the lysis of these cells, which suggests that cell-to-cell contact was a necessary prerequisite for target cell destruction.

The following observations from my laboratory may suggest that *in vivo* antitumor resistance caused by treatment of mice with *C. parvum* or *C. granulosum* is also partly mediated by activation of macrophages:

a) The peritoneal cavity, the spleen and the liver of mice treated with these bacteria contain numerous macrophages (Milas *et al., J. Natl. Cancer Inst. 52*:1875, 1974; *Ibid, Cancer Res. 35*:2365, 1975).

b) Macrophages heavily infiltrate fibrosarcomas which undergo regression in mice injected with *C. granulosum.* Many of these macrophages are found to contain cellular debris (Milas *et al., Cancer Res. 34*:2470, 1974).

c) Immunosuppression of mice by whole body irradiation causes a remarkable increase in the number of pulmonary metastases generated by intravenously injected fibrosarcoma cells. Treatment of animals with *C. granulosum* before irradiation not only abolished this effect or irradiation, but also produced an antitumor response equal to that in mice treated with the bacteria alone. This radioresistant antitumor response might be ascribed to activated macrophages (Milas *et al., J. Natl. Cancer Inst. 52*:1875, 1974).

d) Peritoneal cells from mice treated with *C. parvum* prevented the appearance of tumors in mice when admixed to fibrosarcoma cells prior to the inoculation of this admixture into the peritoneal cavity of normal mice.

A 6
B 7
C 8
D 9
E 0
F 1
G 2
H 3
I 4
J 5